THIRD EDITION

INFORMATICS
AND NURSING:
Competencies
& Applications

Linda Q. Thede, PhD, RN-BC
Editor, CIN Plus

Jeanne P. Sewell, RN, MSN
Assistant Professor
Georgia College and State University
Milledgeville, Georgia

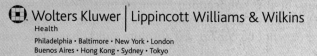
Wolters Kluwer | Lippincott Williams & Wilkins
Health
Philadelphia • Baltimore • New York • London
Buenos Aires • Hong Kong • Sydney • Tokyo

Acquisitions Editor: Hilarie Surrena
Development Editor: Michelle Clarke
Director of Nursing Production: Helen Ewan
Managing Editor/Production: Erika Kors
Designer: Holly Reid McLaughlin

Cover Designer: Lou Fuiano
Art Director, Illustration: Brett MacNaughton
Manufacturing Coordinator: Karin Duffield
Production Services/Compositor:
  Macmillan Publishing Solutions

3rd Edition

9 8 7 6 5 4 3 2

Printed in China

Library of Congress Cataloging-in-Publication Data

Thede, Linda Q.
  Informatics and nursing : competencies & applications / Linda Q. Thede, Jeanne P. Sewell.—3rd ed.
    p. cm.
  ISBN-13: 978-0-7817-9597-5
  ISBN-10: 0-7817-9597-4
  1. Nursing informatics. I. Sewell, Jeanne P. II. Title.
  RT50.5.T483 2010
  610.73--dc22

2009000986

Care has been taken to confirm the accuracy of the information presented and to describe generally accepted practices. However, the authors, editors, and publisher are not responsible for errors or omissions or for any consequences from application of the information in this book and make no warranty, expressed or implied, with respect to the currency, completeness, or accuracy of the contents of the publication. Application of this information in a particular situation remains the professional responsibility of the practitioner; the clinical treatments described and recommended may not be considered absolute and universal recommendations.

LWW.com

CCS1009

Contributors

Deborah Ariosto, MSN, RN
Assistant Director of Clinical Informatics
Deborah Heart and Lung Center
Browns Mills, New Jersey

Pam Correll, RN, BSN
Nursing Informatics Consultant
Maine Center for Disease Control
    and Prevention
Public Health Nursing Program
Bangor, Maine

Karen H. Frith, PhD, RN, CNAA
Associate Professor
University of Alabama in Huntsville
College of Nursing
Huntsville, Alabama

Judy Hornbeck, MHSA, BSN, RN
Highland, Illinois

Reviewers

Mary T. Bouchard, MSN, CNS, RN, CRRN
Nursing Faculty
Thomas Jefferson University
School of Nursing
Philadelphia, Pennsylvania

Fran Cornelius, PhD, MSN, RN, CNE
Coordinator of Informatics Projects
Assistant Clinical Professor
Drexel University
School of Nursing
Philadelphia, Pennsylvania

Betsy Frank, RN, PhD
Professor
Indiana State University
College of Nursing, Health,
    and Human Services
Terre Haute, Indiana

Judith Holland, PhD, MSN
Assistant Professor
Hawaii Pacific University
School of Nursing
Kaneohe, Hawaii

Pamela D. Korte, RN, MS
Associate Professor
Monroe Community College
School of Nursing
Rochester, New York

Kay Lake, RN, MS
Faculty
Indiana Wesleyan University
Swayzee, Indiana

Rebecca B. Shaheen, RN, MSN
Department Chairperson, Professor, Adjunct
    Faculty
Computer Department
School of Nursing
Community College of Allegheny County
Monroeville, Pennsylvania

Debra P. Shelton, EdD, APRN-CS,
CAN, OCN, CNE
Associate Professor, Assistant to the Director
    of Undergraduate Studies
Northwestern State University
Shreveport, Louisiana

Kellie Smith, RN, MSN
Instructor
School of Nursing
Jefferson University
Philadelphia, Pennsylvania

Cindy Versteeg, RN, MScN
Professor
Nursing Studies
Algonquin College
Ottawa, Canada

iv

Preface

Writing a text in a field like informatics, in which today's news is easily outdated within months, is a challenge. In this third edition, we have tried to keep the best of the second edition, add topics that have entered the field since the last edition, and make it all interesting – and yes, thought provoking – to you, the reader. Information technology is being used more and more, leaving it vulnerable to problems that inevitably arise with new methods. We have tried to present a fair picture of both the benefits and drawbacks of some of these technologies. The most important factor that we hope you will take away from this text is the realization that the intelligent use of information technology rests with humans: humans who understand both the promise of technology and its limitations, as well as how it can be integrated into the workflow.

Besides providing information for anyone who is just beginning to learn about nursing informatics, the book has been designed to be used either as a text for a course in nursing informatics or with a curriculum in which informatics is a vertical strand. The first two units, Informatics Basics and Computers and Your Professional Career, provide background information that would be useful in first-year courses, or as an introduction to computers. The third unit, Information Competency, would be useful at any point in a curriculum. Units four and five, The New Healthcare Paradigm and Healthcare Informatics, provide information that would be useful at more senior levels, whereas the last unit, Computer Uses in Healthcare Beyond Clinical Informatics, can either be used as a whole or its individual chapters matched with a course.

This book comes with a set of instructor resources that can be accessed on thePoint, LWW's very popular Web-based content portal. With the materials you find on thePoint, you will be able to enhance your lectures with PowerPoint presentations, which provide an easy way for you to integrate the textbook with your students' classroom experience through either slide shows or handouts. In addition to the PowerPoint slides, the Test Generator lets you put together exclusive new tests from a bank containing over 250 questions, to help you in assessing your students' understanding of the material. These questions are formatted to match the NCLEX (National Council Licensure Examination), so that your students can have practice in preparing for this important examination. Additionally, the authors have provided a Web site that includes all Web addresses in the book, more information to supplement the text, and Web sites that are pertinent to each chapter. The Web page can be found at http://dlthede.net/Informatics/ Informatics.htmhttp://dlthede.net/Informatics/ Informatics.htm

Linda Q. Thede, PhD, RN-BC
Jeanne P. Sewell, RN, MSN

Acknowledgments

Few writers, if any, know enough about a topic to write entirely from their own knowledge bank and what they can learn from the literature and the Web, even with two authors, as is the case with this edition of the text. We wish to thank Andy Salner, MD, for his help regarding the CHESS (Comprehensive Health Enhancement Support System) program. We also appreciate the help of both Kathy Lesh, RN, EdM, MS, technical manager of clinical informatics for the KEVRIC Company, and Susan Matney, MSN, RN, for help with Chapter 16, and Karen Martin, RN, MSN, FAAN. Thanks also to Barry Lung, MSN, RN, BC, informatics clinical consultant; Jill Williams, MSN, RN, CPHQ, MCSM, system analyst/program administrator; and Karen Childers, MSN, RN, system analyst, for adding their expertise to Chapters 19, 20, and 21. In addition, we thank Karen Frith, PhD, RN, for writing Chapters 24 and 25.

In an effort to add a personal touch, there are three displays, whose authors freely gave of their time to write: Deborah Ariosto, MS, RN, tells of her experiences with an online support program, CHESS, in Chapter 15. In Chapter 17, Pam Correll, RN, BSN, writes about why she finds standardized terminologies helpful, and Judi Hornback, MHSA, BSN, RN, again contributes her typical day as an informatics nurse in Chapter 18. We hope you find these entertaining as well as informative. There were numerous others who assisted us in editing and rewriting; we are truly indebted to you for all of your guidance and assistance.

Contents

UNIT I   Informatics Basics   1

1 Introduction to Nursing Informatics: Managing Healthcare Information   3

2 Meet the Computer   21

3 Software: Information Management   44

4 Understanding Computer Concepts: Common Features   58

5 Computers and Networking   77

UNIT II   Computers and Your Professional Career   99

6 Professional Networking   101

7 Word Processing   120

8 Presentation Software: Looking Professional in the Spotlight   133

9 Spreadsheets: Making Numbers Talk   144

10 Databases: Creating Information From Data   160

UNIT III   Information Competency   183

11 The Internet: One Road to Health and Evidence-Based Practice Information   185

12 Finding Knowledge in the Digital Library Haystack   199

13 Mobile Computing: Finding Knowledge in the Palm of Your Hand   215

UNIT IV   The New Healthcare Paradigm   229

14 The Consumer and the Electronic Health Record   231

15 The Empowered Consumer   248

16 Interoperability at the International and National Level   266

17 Nursing Documentation: Is It Valuable?   286

UNIT V   Healthcare Informatics   307

18 The Informatics Discipline   309

19 Basic Electronic Healthcare Information Systems   329

20 Specialized Electronic Healthcare Information Systems   347

21 Electronic Healthcare System Issues   359

22 Carrying Healthcare to the Client   376

UNIT VI   **Computer Uses in Healthcare Beyond Clinical Informatics**   **389**

23 Educational Informatics: e-Learning   391

24 Administration Tools for Efficiency   409

25 Informatics and Research   423

26 Legal and Ethical Issues   436

Index   447

UNIT I

000 10100 01010

Informatics Basics

CHAPTER 1 Introduction to Nursing Informatics: Managing Healthcare Information

CHAPTER 2 Meet the Computer

CHAPTER 3 Software: Information Management

CHAPTER 4 Understanding Computer Concepts: Common Features

CHAPTER 5 Computers and Networking

INFORMATICS is too often viewed solely as one of its components instead of as a whole. Its primary goal is information management, but knowledge of each of these divisions is a necessary part of informatics. This unit, which opens the book, provides an introduction to these components and then focuses on the tool of informatics, the computer. The following units will examine the others.

Chapter 1 presents a brief overview of informatics, what it is, the factors that are making it more important in healthcare, and a look at its components: information management, computer competency, and information literacy. Chapter 2 investigates the computer: its characteristics, types, parts, how it works, and the storage of data. Also included is a section on batteries, a subject that becomes more important with the advent of mobile computers, and a section about peripherals. Software, the brains of computers, is addressed in Chapter 3, where operating systems and general categories of software are described. Information about open source software, a concept that is finding some support in healthcare, and software copyright are also included. To those who have never used a computer, or whose experience is limited, facing one may seem intimidating. Yet, there are many features, which when learned can be applied across all genres of software. It is these topics that are explored in Chapter 4. The last chapter in this section, Chapter 5, examines the technology behind the scenes of computer networks.

Introduction to Nursing Informatics: Managing Healthcare Information

Learning Objectives

After studying this chapter you will be able to:

1. Describe some of the forces inside and outside healthcare that are driving a move toward a greater use of informatics.

2. Define nursing informatics.

3. Distinguish between the computer and informatics.

4. Explain the need for all nurses to have basic skills in informatics.

5. Analyze the effects of informatics on healthcare.

6. Interpret the need for nurses to be computer fluent and information literate to today's healthcare environment.

Key Terms

American Association of Colleges of Nursing (AACN)
Aggregated Data
American Nurses Association (ANA)
Biosurveillance
Computerized Provider Order Entry (CPOE)
Data
Decision Support Systems
Deidentified Data
Electronic Health Record (EHR)
Electronic Numerical Integrator and Computer (ENIAC)
Evidence-Based Care
Genomics
Healthcare Informatics
Health Information Technology (HIT)

Informatics
Information Technology
Information Literacy
Institute of Medicine (IOM)
Listserv
National League for Nursing (NLN)
Nursing Informatics
President's Information Technology Advisory Committee (PITAC)
Problem-Oriented Medical Record (POMR)
Problem-Oriented Medical Information System (PROMIS)
Protocols
Real Time
Secondary Data
Standardization

"In attempting to arrive at the truth, I have applied everywhere for information, but in scarcely an instance have I been able to obtain hospital records fit for any purposes of comparison. If they could be obtained, they would

enable us to decide many other questions besides the ones alluded to. They would show subscribers how their money was being spent, what amount of good was really being done with it, or whether the money was not doing mischief rather than good." (Nightingale, 1859)

 Informatics Introduction

What is **informatics**? Isn't it just about computers? Taking care of patients is nursing's primary concern, not thinking about computers! These are not unusual thoughts for nurses to have. Transitions are always difficult, and a transition to using more technology in managing information is no exception. This use of **information technology** in healthcare is known as informatics, and its focus is information management, not computers. Whether nursing uses informatics effectively or not will determine the quality of future patient care as well as the future of nursing.

Information is an integral part of nursing. Think about your practice for a minute. When you are caring for patients, what besides the knowledge that nursing education and experience has provided do you depend on to provide care? You need to know the patient's history, medical conditions, medications, laboratory results, and more. Could you walk into a unit and care for a patient without this information? How this information is organized and presented to you affects the care that you can provide as well as the time you spend finding it.

The old way is to record and keep the information for a patient's current admission in a paper chart. Today, with several specialties, consults, medications, laboratory reports, and procedures, the paper chart is inadequate. A well-designed information system, developed with you and for you, can facilitate finding and using information that you need for patient care. Informatics skills enable you to participate in and benefit from this process. Informatics does not perform miracles; it requires an investment by you, the clinician, to assist those who design information systems

so the systems are helpful and do not impede your workflow.

If healthcare is to improve, it is imperative that there be a workforce that can innovate and implement information technology (AHIMA & AMIA, 2006). There are two roles in informatics: the informatics specialist and the clinician who must use health information technology. This means that in essence every nurse has a role in informatics. Information, the subject of informatics, is the structure on which healthcare is built. Except for purely technical procedures (of which there are few if any), a healthcare professional's work revolves around information. Is the laboratory report available? When is Mrs. X scheduled for surgery? What are the contraindications for the prescribed drug? What is Mr. Y's history? What orders did the physician leave for Ms. Z? Where is the latest x-ray report?

An important part of healthcare information is nursing documentation. When information systems are designed for nursing, this documentation can also be used to expand our knowledge of what constitutes quality healthcare. Have you ever wondered if the patient for whom you provided care had an outcome similar to others with the same condition? From nursing documentation, are you easily able to see the relationship between nursing diagnoses, interventions, and outcomes for your patients? Without knowledge of these chain events, you have only your intuition and old knowledge to use when making decisions about the best interventions in patient care. Because observations tend to be self-selective, this is often not the best information on which to base patient care. Informatics can furnish the information needed to see these relationships and to provide care based on actual patient **data**.

If Florence Nightingale were with us today, she would be a champion of the push toward more use of healthcare information technology. Information in a paper chart essentially disappears into a black hole after a patient is discharged. Because we can't easily access it, we can't learn from it and use it in patient care.

This realization is international. Many countries, especially those with a national health service, have long realized the need be able to use information buried in charts. Tommy Thompson (Thompson, 2004), the then U.S. Secretary of Health and Human Services, in a talk at the May 6, 2004, Health Information Technology Summit said that "the most remarkable feature of this 21st-century medicine is that we hold it together with 19th-century paperwork. This is just inexcusable. And it has to change."

In the United States, this statement was backed up with the introduction of bills in the U.S. Congress and the creation of the **President's Information Technology Advisory Committee (PITAC)**, all of which call for greater use of informatics. In 2004, the president also called for "widespread adoption of interoperable **electronic health records (EHRs)** within 10 years, as well as the establishment of the position of National Coordinator for Health Information Technology" (Office of the National Coordinator for Health Information Technology, 2004). In the first report from this office, a strategic plan was announced "to guide the nationwide implementation of **HIT (Health Information Technology)** in both the public and private sectors." The strategic plan formulated four goals, all of which will affect nurses and nursing. They are as follows:

1. Inform clinical practice with use of EHRs. The strategies for achieving this goal are
   a. Provide incentives for EHR adoption
   b. Reduce risk of EHR investment
   c. Promote the diffusion of EHR in rural and underserved areas
2. Interconnect clinicians so that they can exchange health information using advanced and secure electronic communication. The strategies for achieving this goal are
   a. Encourage regional collaborations that reflect the needs and goals of the region
   b. Develop a national health information network
   c. Coordinate federal health information systems

3. Personalize care with consumer-based health records and better information for consumers by
   a. Encourage the use of personal EHRs
   b. Enhance informed consumer choice by providing information about clinicians and institutions
   c. Promote use of telehealth systems
4. Improve public health through advanced **biosurveillance** methods and streamlining the collection of data for quality measurement and research. This requires the collection of detailed clinical information and will be accomplished by
   a. Unify public health surveillance architectures by making the systems able to exchange information
   b. Streamline quality and health status monitoring to provide the ability to look at quality at the point of care and in **real time**
   c. Provide tools to accelerate research and dissemination of evidence into clinically useful products, applications, and knowledge

To fulfill these goals, information, which is the structure on which healthcare is built, can no longer be managed with paper. If we are to provide **evidence-based care**, the mountains of data that are hidden in medical records must be made to reveal their secrets. Bakken (2001) told us that there are five components needed to provide evidence-based care: 1) **standardization** of terminologies and structures used in documentation, 2) the use of digital information, 3) standards to permit healthcare data exchange between heterogeneous entities, 4) the ability to capture data relevant to the actual care provided, and 5) competency among practitioners to use this data. All of these are part of informatics.

Information is a capital good with a value the same as labor and materials (National Advisory Council on Nurse Education and Practice, 1997). The financial health of organizations depends on effective and efficient information management. Today, healthcare organizations are waking up to the fact that how information is handled and processed has a great effect on both the outcomes for those who purchase services and the economics of healthcare. Manual recording and filing of information are inadequate to manage today's healthcare information. We have made some attempts to use technology to manage information, but these efforts often fall short as a result of our inexperience in grasping the schemes of where information originates, how it is used clinically and administratively, and how it can be used to improve practice.

The complexity of today's healthcare milieu, added to the explosion of knowledge, makes it impossible for any clinician to remember everything needed to provide high-quality patient care. Additionally, healthcare consumers today want their healthcare providers to integrate all known relevant scientific knowledge in providing their care. We have passed the time when the unaided human mind can perform this feat: Modern information management tools are needed as well as a commitment by healthcare professionals to change practices when more knowledge becomes available.

Information Overload: Informatics at Your Service

Informatics is about managing information. The tendency to relate it to computers comes from the fact that the ability to manage large amounts of information was born with the computer and progressed as computers became more powerful and commonplace. It is, however, human ingenuity that is the crux of informatics. The term "informatics" originated from the Russian term "informatika" (Sackett & Erdley, 2002). A Russian publication, *Oznovy Informatiki* (Foundations of Informatics), published in 1968 is credited with the origins of the general discipline of informatics (Middle East Technical University, n.d.). At that time it was described within the context of computers. "Medical informatics" was the first term used to identify informatics in healthcare. It was defined as the information technologies

that are concerned with patient care and the medical decision making process. Another definition stated that medical informatics is complex data processing by the computer to create new information. As with many healthcare enterprises, there was debate about whether "medical" referred only to informatics focusing on physician concerns, or if it refers to all healthcare disciplines. Increasingly, it is seen that other disciplines have a body of knowledge separate from medicine, but part of healthcare, and the term **healthcare informatics** is becoming more commonly used. In essence, informatics is the management of information, using cognitive skills and the computer.

HEALTHCARE INFORMATICS

Healthcare informatics focuses on managing information in healthcare. It is an umbrella term that describes the capture, retrieval, storage, presenting, sharing, and use of biomedical information, data, and knowledge for providing care, problem solving, and decision making (Shortliffe & Blois, 2001). The purpose is to improve the use of healthcare data, information, and knowledge in supporting patient care, research, and education (Delaney, 2001). The focus is on the subject, information, rather than the tool, the computer. The distinction is not always obvious as a result of the need to master computer skills to enable one to manage this information. The computer is used in acquiring, organizing, manipulating, and presenting the information. It will not produce anything of value without human direction in how, when, and where the data is acquired, how it is treated, interpreted, manipulated, and presented. Informatics provides that human direction.

NURSING INFORMATICS

Healthcare has many disciplines, thus it is not surprising that healthcare informatics has many specialties of which nursing is one. **Nursing informatics** is also a subspecialty of nursing which the **American Nurses Association** (ANA) recognized in 1992, with the first informatics certification examination being given in the fall of 1995 (Newbold, 1996). Nursing informatics has as its focus managing information pertaining to nursing. Specialists in this area look at how nursing information is acquired, manipulated, stored, presented, and used. Informatics nurses work with practicing nurses to identify the needs of nurses for information and support, and with system developers in the development of systems that work to complement the practice needs of nurses. Nursing informatics specialists bring to system development and implementation a viewpoint that supports the needs of the clinical end user. The objective is an information system that is not only user friendly for data input, but presents the clinical nurse with needed information in a manner that is timely and useful. This is not to say that nursing informatics stands alone, it is an integral part of the interdisciplinary field of healthcare informatics, hence related to and responsible to all the healthcare disciplines.[1]

DEFINITIONS OF NURSING INFORMATICS

The term "nursing informatics," was probably first used and defined by Scholes and Barber in 1980 in their address that year to the MED-INFO conference in Tokyo. There is still no definitive agreement on exactly what the term nursing informatics means. As Simpson once said (Simpson, 1998), defining nursing informatics is difficult because it is a moving target. The original definition said that nursing informatics was the use of computer technology in all nursing endeavors: nursing services, education, and research. (Scholes & Barber, 1980) Another early definition that followed the broad definition of Scholes and Barber was written by Hannah, Ball & Edwards (1994). They defined nursing informatics as any use of information technologies in carrying out nursing functions. Like the Scholes and Barber definition, these definitions focused on the technology and could be interpreted to mean any

use of the computer from word processing to the creation of artificial intelligence for nurses as long as the computer use involved the practice of professional nursing.

The shift from a technology orientation in definitions to one that is more information oriented started in the mid 1980s with Schwirian (Staggers & Thompson, 2002). She created a model to be used as a framework for nursing informatics investigators (Schwirian, 1986). The model consisted of four elements arranged in a pyramid with a triangular base. The top of the pyramid was the desired goal of the nursing informatics activity and the base was composed of three elements: 1) users (nurses and students), 2) raw material or nursing information, and 3) the technology, which is computer hardware and software. They all interact in nursing informatics activity to achieve a goal. The model was intended as a stimulus for research.

The first widely circulated definition that moved away from technology to concepts was from Graves and Corcoran (Staggers & Thompson, 2002). They defined nursing informatics as "a combination of computer science, information science and nursing science designed to assist in the management and processing of nursing data, information and knowledge to support the practice of nursing and the delivery of nursing care" (Graves & Corcoran, 1989)(p. 227). This definition secured the position of nursing informatics within the practice of nursing and placed the emphasis on data, information, and knowledge (Staggers & Thompson, 2002). Many consider it the seminal definition of nursing informatics.

Turley (Turley, 1996), after analyzing previous definitions, added another discipline, cognitive science, to the base for nursing informatics. Cognitive science emphasizes the human factor in informatics. Its main focus is the nature of knowledge, its components, development, and use. Goossen (1996), thinking along the same lines, used the Graves and Corcoran definition as a basis and expanded the meaning of nursing informatics to include the thinking that is done by nurses to make

---

[1] The nursing informatics subspecialty will be explored in more detail in Chapter 18.

knowledge-based decisions and inferences for patient care. Using this interpretation, he felt that nursing informatics should focus on analyzing and modeling the cognitive processing for all areas of nursing practice. Goossen also stated that nursing informatics should look at the effects of computerized systems on nursing care delivery.

The first ANA definition in 1992 added the role of the informatics nursing specialist to the Graves and Corcoran definition. The 2001 ANA definition stated that nursing informatics combines nursing, information and computer sciences for the purpose of managing and communicating data, information, and knowledge to support nurses and healthcare providers in decision making (American Nurses Association, 2001). Information structures, processes, and technology are used to provide this support. In the latest ANA Scope and Standards this definition was reiterated, albeit in slightly different wording (American Nurses Association, 2008), with the addition of wisdom to the data, information, and knowledge conceptual framework. This most recent definition emphasized again that the goal of nursing informatics is to optimize information management and communication to improve the health of individuals, families, populations, and communities.

Staggers and Thompson (2002), who believe that the evolution of definitions will continue, pointed out that in all of the current definitions, the role of the patient is under emphasized. Some early definitions included the patient, but as a passive recipient of care. With the advent of the Internet, more and more patients are taking an active role in their healthcare. This factor changes not only the dynamics of healthcare, but permits a definition of nursing informatics that recognizes that patients as well as healthcare professionals are consumers of healthcare information and that patients may be participating in keeping their medical records current. Staggers and Thompson also pointed out that the role of the nurse as an integrator of information has been overlooked and should be considered in future definitions.

Despite these definitions, the focus of much of today's practice informatics is still on capturing data at the point of care and presenting it in a manner that facilitates the care of an individual patient. Although this is a vital first step, when designing patient care information systems, thought needs to be given to **secondary data** analysis, or analysis of data for purposes other than for which it was originally collected. Using **aggregated data**, or the same piece(s) of data, for example, outcomes of a given intervention for many patients, you can make decisions based on actual patient care data. Understanding how informatics can serve you as an individual nurse, as well as the profession, puts you in a position to work with informatics specialists to make data needed to improve patient care retrievable.

Forces Driving Toward More Use of Informatics in Healthcare

The ultimate goal of healthcare informatics is a lifetime EHR with **decision support systems**. These records will include standardized data, permit consumers to access their records, and provide for secondary use of healthcare data. President Bush set a goal of 2014 for every American to have an EHR; however, there are many issues that must be addressed before this becomes a reality.

NATIONAL FORCES

Federal efforts behind a move to EHRs include not only the creation of PITAC but also efforts to standardize data. The **Institute of Medicine (IOM)**, an independent body that acts as an adviser to the U.S.[2] government to improve healthcare, has completed several reports aimed at improving healthcare, all of which foresee a large role for information technology (IT). The IOM report *Health Professions*

---

[2] See Chapter 16 for more information on U.S. government efforts.

Education: A Bridge to Quality (Greiner & Knebel, 2003) includes informatics as a core competency required of *all* healthcare professionals. In the report *Crossing the Quality Chasm: A New Health System for the 21st Century*, IT is seen as an important force in improving healthcare. Some of the IT themes in this report are a national information infrastructure, computerized clinical data, the use of the Internet, clinical decision support, and evidence-based practice integration (Staggers, 2004).

NURSING FORCES

Nursing too has recognized the need for informatics. In 1962, before the term informatics was coined, Dr. Harriet Werley recognized the value of nursing data and insisted that the ANA make research about nursing information a priority. Although there were many articles written about informatics in the intervening years and the journal *Computers in Nursing*[3] was started as a mimeograph sheet in 1982, few nurses realized the value of and need for informatics. In 1993, the National Center for Nursing Research released the report *Nursing Informatics: Enhancing Patient Care,* which set six program goals for nursing informatics research: 1) to establish a nursing language (useful in computerized documentation), 2) develop methods to build clinical information databases, 3) determine how nurses give patient care using data, information and knowledge, 4) develop and test patient care decision support systems, 5) develop workstations that provide nurses with needed information, and 6) develop appropriate methods to evaluate nursing information systems (Pillar & Golumbic, 1993).

In 1997, the Division of Nursing of the Health Resources and Services Administration convened the National Advisory Council on Nurse Education and Practice. They produced the National Informatics Agenda for Education and Practice. One of their recommendations was to include core computing and nursing informatics concepts in nursing curricula (National Advisory Council on Nurse Education and Practice, 1997). This report made five recommendations: "1) Educate nursing students and practicing nurses in core informatics content, 2) Prepare nurses with specialized skills in informatics, 3) Enhance nursing practice and education through informatics projects, 4) Prepare nursing faculty in informatics, and 5) Increase collaborative efforts in nursing informatics."(p. 8). The **American Association of Colleges of Nursing's (AACN)** list of core competencies includes many recommendations in the area of information and healthcare technologies (American Association of Colleges of Nursing, 1998) such as the use of information and communication technologies, the use of ethics in the application of technology, and the enhancement of one's knowledge using information technologies.

The ANA has been another force moving nursing toward effectively using informatics. Starting in 1994 with two documents, *Standards of Practice for Nursing Informatics* and *The Scope of Practice for Nursing Informatics*, the association has since combined these documents. The third edition, which is greatly expanded, was released in 2008. Within ANA there are two committees whose work concerns informatics, the Committee for Nursing Practice Information Infrastructure (CNPII) and the National Information and Data Set Evaluation Center (NIDSEC).

The current shortage of nurses in many countries, including the United States and Canada, is another driving force. A report from the Maryland Statewide Commission on the Crisis in Nursing (Womack, Newbold, Staugaitis, & Cunningham, 2004) examines technology's role in addressing the nursing shortage and makes many recommendations. Evidence is accumulating that well-designed documentation systems can improve the nursing working environment (Baldwin, 2002) by eliminating much of nursing's paper work. As

---

[3] Now named *CIN: Computers Informatics Nursing* and since 1984 a full-fledged journal.

such informatics can maximize nursing productivity, increase the quality of patient care, and improve the work environment infrastructure (Covington, Koszalka, Newbold, & Womack, 2004).

The latest move toward improving the integration of informatics into nursing education and practice is the Technology, Informatics, Guiding Educational Reform (TIGER) initiative. This group originated after several years of planning with a two-day invitation-only conference starting October 30, 2006. Their objective is to make nursing informatics competencies part of every nurse's skill set, with the aim of making informatics the stethoscope of the 21st century (Dulong & HIMSS Nursing Task Force, 2007). They are working to ensure that nursing can be fully engaged in the digital era of healthcare by ensuring that all nurses are educated in using informatics, empowering them to deliver safer, high-quality, evidence-based care.

OTHER DRIVING FORCES

Healthcare is an information-intensive industry, yet most healthcare providers often consider the management of their information as an onerous, unappreciated task (Korpman, 1990). Poorly organized and implemented documentation systems tend to hinder the process of finding and using the information one needs to provide high-quality care. Add to that time requirements for documentation, the frequent need to enter data in duplicate or even triplicate, time spent trying to locate patient records, and missing reports, and the reasons for dissatisfaction become clear.

Patient Safety

Patient safety is a primary concern and one that drives many informatics initiatives. At least 10 patient safety databases use aggregated healthcare data to identify safety issues. Most, such as the National Nosocomial Infections Surveillance System from the Centers for Disease Prevention and Control (CDC) and the National Database of Nursing Quality

Indicators from ANA are voluntary, but two, the vaccine adverse event report system from the CDC and Food Drug Administration (FDA) are mandatory (Bakken, 2006).[4]

Some other informatics implementations that focus on safety include bar coding for medication administration and **computerized provider order entry** (CPOE). A well-designed CPOE system not only can prevent transcription errors, but when combined with a patient's record it can also flag any condition that might present a hazard or would need additional assessment. Clinical decision support systems that provide clinicians with suggested care information or remind busy clinicians of items easy to forget or overlook are also being pushed to improve patient safety.[5]

Costs

Healthcare costs are also driving the move to informatics. One example is the Leapfrog Group. Upset by the rising cost of healthcare, in 1998 a group of chief executives of leading corporations in the United States met to discuss how they could have an influence on its quality and affordability (Leapfrog Group, 2007a). They were spending billions of dollars on healthcare for their employees, but lacked a way of assessing its quality or comparing healthcare providers. The Business Roundtable provided the initial funding and this group took the name "Leapfrog Group" in November 2000. This move was given further impetus by the 1999 IOM report *To Err Is Human* that reported up to 98,000 preventable hospital deaths and recommended that large employers use their purchasing power to improve the quality and safety of healthcare.

Today the Leapfrog Group is also supported by the Robert Wood Johnson Foundation, Leapfrog members, and others. Their mission is to improve the safety, quality, and affordability

---

[4] Providing the data for these reports is not possible without standardization of data, a topic that will be further investigated in Chapters 16 and 17.

[5] CPOE will be further discussed in Chapter 20 and decision support systems in Chapter 21.

of healthcare by encouraging the availability of the information necessary for consumers to make informed healthcare decisions and the use of incentives and rewards to promote high-value healthcare (Leapfrog Group, 2007b). They have four current missions: 1) promote the use of CPOE systems to reduce medication errors, 2) encourage consumers and healthcare purchasers to select hospitals with extensive experience and good outcomes for certain high-risk surgeries, 3) promote the staffing of intensive care units (ICUs) with intensivists, or doctors with special training in the care of ICU patients, and 4) assessing hospitals' progress on the National Quality Forum–endorsed safe practices. Efforts toward this last goal are met by collecting data voluntarily submitted by hospitals and posting this information on a Web site (http://www.leapfroggroup.org/cp) where consumers can check the outcomes of hospitals in their areas for selected procedures. Members of the Leapfrog Group also educate their employees about patient safety and the importance of comparing healthcare providers. They will offer financial incentives to their covered employees for selecting care from hospitals that meet their standards. Healthcare providers without information systems will have a difficult time in providing the information that these healthcare buyers demand and could see themselves losing patients.

As healthcare informatics moves to solve these problems, the need for interdisciplinary, enterprise-wide, information management becomes clearer. The advances of information technology coupled with the evolution of the EHR will create a steady progression to this end. Integration, however, is not without its perils. Any discipline that is not ready for this integration may find itself lost in the process. For nursing to be a part of healthcare informatics, all nurses must become familiar with the value of nursing data, how it can be captured, the terminology needed to capture it, and methods for analyzing and manipulating it. True integration of data from all healthcare disciplines will improve patient care and the patient experience, as well as enabling economic gains.

The Information Management Tool: Computers

In 1850, it was possible for all the medical knowledge known to the Western world to be put into two large volumes making it possible, for one person to read and assimilate all this information. The situation today is dramatically different. The number of journals available in healthcare and the research that fills them have increased many times over. Even in the early 1990s, if physicians read two journal articles a day, by the end of a year they would be 800 years behind in their reading (McDonald, 1994). A healthcare clinician may be expected to know something about 10,000 different diseases and syndromes, 3,000 medications, 1,100 laboratory tests and the information in the more than 400,000 articles added to the biomedical information each year (Davenport & Glaser, 2002). Additionally, current knowledge is constantly changing: one can expect much of their knowledge to be obsolete in five years or less.

In healthcare, the increase in knowledge has led to the development of many specialties such as respiratory therapy, neonatology, and gerontology, and subspecialties within each of these. As these specialties have proliferated and spawned the development of many miraculous treatments, healthcare has too often become fractionalized, resulting in difficulty in gaining an overview of the entire patient. The pressure of accomplishing the tasks necessary for a patient's physical recovery usually leaves little time for perusing a patient's record and putting together the bits and pieces so carefully charted by each discipline. Even if time is available there is simply so much data, in so many places, that it is difficult to merge the data with the knowledge that a healthcare provider has learned, as well as with new knowledge needed to provide the best patient care. We are drowning in data but lack the time and skills to transform it to useful information or knowledge.

The development of the computer as a tool to manage information can be seen in its history. The first information management task "computerized" was numeric manipulation. Although not technically a computer by today's terminology, the first successful computerization tool was the abacus, which was developed about 3000 BC. Although when one developed skill, real speed in these tasks was possible, the operator of the abacus still had to mentally manipulate data. All the abacus did was store the results step by step. Slide rules came next in 1632, but like the abacus required a great deal of skill on the part of the operator. The first machine to add and subtract by itself was Blaise Pascal's "arithmetic machine," built in 1542. The first "computer" to be a commercial success was Jacquard's weaving machine built in 1804. Its efficiency so frightened workers at the mill where it was built that they rioted, broke apart the machine, and sold the parts. Despite this setback, the machine proved a success because it introduced a cost-effective way of producing goods.

The difference and analytical engines, early computers designed by Charles Babbage in the mid 19th century, although never built, laid the foundation for modern computers (Analytical Engine, 2007). The first time that an automatic calculating machine was successfully used was in the 1900 census. Herman Hollerith (who later started IBM) used the Jacquard loom concept of punch cards to create a machine that enabled the 1900 census takers to compile the results in one year instead of the 10 (Herman Hollerith—Punch Cards) required for the 1890 census. The first computer by today's perception was the **Electronic Numerical Integrator and Computer** (ENIAC) built by people at the Moore School of Engineering at the University of Pennsylvania in partnership with the U.S. Government. When completed in 1946, it consisted of 18,000 vacuum tubes, 70,000 resistors, and 5 million soldered joints. It consumed enough energy to dim the lights in an entire section of Philadelphia (Moye, 1996). The progress in hardware since then is phenomenal; today's "Palmtop" computers have more processing power than ENIAC did.

Computers and Healthcare

The use of computers in healthcare originated in the late 1950s and early 1960s as a way to manage financial information. This was followed in the late 1960s by the development of a few computerized patient care applications (Saba & Erdeley, 2006). Some of these hospital information systems included patient diagnoses and other patient information as well as care plans based on physician and nursing orders. Because of the lack of processing power then available, these systems were unable to deliver what was needed and never became widely used.

EARLY HEALTHCARE INFORMATICS SYSTEMS

One of the interesting early uses of the computer in patient care was the **Problem-Oriented Medical Information System** (PROMIS) begun by Dr. Lawrence Weed at the University Medical Center in Burlington, VT (McNeill, 1979) in 1968. The importance of this system is that it was the first attempt at providing a total, integrated system that covered all aspects of healthcare, including patient treatment. It was patient oriented and used as its framework the **problem-oriented medical record** (POMR). The unit featured an interactive touch screen and was known for fast responsiveness (Problem-Oriented Medical Information System, n.d.). At its height, it consisted of over 60,000 frames of knowledge.

PROMIS was designed to overcome four problems that are still with us today: lack of care coordination, reliance on memory, lack of recorded logic of delivered care, and lack of an effective feedback loop (*PROMIS: The Problem-Oriented Medical Information System*, 1980). The system provided a wide array of information to all healthcare providers. All disciplines recorded their observations and plans, and related them to a specific problem. This broke down barriers between disciplines, making it possible to see the relationship between conditions, treatments, costs, and outcomes. Unfortunately, this system did not have wide acceptance. To embrace it meant a change in the structure of healthcare, something that did not begin to happen until the 1990s, when managed care in all its variations reinvigorated a push toward more patient-centered information systems, a push that is continuing as you read this.

Another early system that became functional in 1967 and is still functioning, is the Help Evaluation Logical Processing (HELP) system developed by the Informatics Department at the University of Utah School of Medicine. It was first implemented in a heart catheterization laboratory and a post open heart intensive care unit. It now is hospital wide and operational in many hospitals in the Intermountain Healthcare system (Gardner, Pryor, & Warner, 1999). This is not only a hospital information system, but integrates a sophisticated clinical decision support system that provides information to clinical areas. It was the first hospital information system that collected data for clinical decision making and integrated it with a medical knowledge base. It is well accepted by clinicians and has demonstrated that a clinical support system is feasible and that it reduces healthcare costs without sacrificing quality.

PROGRESSION OF INFORMATION SYSTEMS

As the science of informatics has progressed, there have been changes in information systems. Originally computerized clinical information systems were process oriented. That is, they were implemented to computerize a specific process, for example, billing, order entry, or laboratory reports. This led to the creation of different software systems for different departments, which unfortunately could not share data, creating a need for clinicians to enter data more than once. An attempt to share data by integrating data from disparate systems is a difficult and sometimes impossible task. Even when possible, the results are often disappointing and can leave negative impressions of computerization in users' minds. These barriers are being slowly overcome with the introduction of data standards, both in terminology and in **protocols** for passing data from one system to another.

Newer systems, however, are organized by data and are designed to use the same piece of data many times, thus requiring that the entry be made only once. The primary design is based on how data is gathered, stored, and used in an entire institution rather than on a specific process such as pharmacy or laboratory. For example, when a medication order is placed, the system can have access to all the information about a patient including his diagnosis, age, weight, allergies, and eventually **genomics**, as well as the medications he is currently taking. The order and patient information can also be matched against knowledge such as what drugs are incompatible with the prescribed drug, the dosage of the drug, and the appropriateness of the drug for this patient. If there are difficulties, the system can deliver warnings at the time the medication is ordered instead of requiring clinician intervention either in the pharmacy or at the time of administration. Another feature in a data-driven system is the ability to make the same information available to the dietician planning the patient's diet and the nurse providing patient care and doing discharge planning, thus enabling a more complete picture of a patient than one that would be available when separate systems handle dietetics and nursing.

Evidence-based practice will result not only from research and practice guidelines, but also from unidentifiable (data minus any patient identification) aggregated data from actual patients. It will also be possible to see how patients with a given genomics react to a drug, thus helping the clinician in prescribing drugs. This same aggregated data will help clinicians make decisions by providing information about treatments that are most effective for given conditions, replacing the current system, which is too often based on "what we have always done" rather than empirical information. These systems will use computers that are powerful enough to process data so that information is created "on the fly," or immediately when requested. Systems that incorporate these features will require a new way of thinking. Instead of having all one's knowledge in memory, one must be comfortable both with needing to access information and with changing one's practice to accommodate the new knowledge.

Computerization will affect healthcare professionals in other ways. Some jobs will change focus. As nurses we may find that our job as a patient care coordinator has shifted from transcribing and checking orders to accessing this information on the computer. To preserve our ability to provide full care for our patients, and as an information integrator for other disciplines, we will need to make our information needs known to those who design the systems. To accomplish this we all need to be aware of the value of both our data and our experience and to be able to identify the data we need to perform our job, as well as to appreciate the value of the data that others and we add to the healthcare system.

Benefits of Informatics

The information systems described above will bring many benefits to healthcare. These benefits can be seen in the ability to create and use aggregated data, prevent errors, ease working conditions, and provide better healthcare records.

FOR HEALTHCARE IN GENERAL

One of the primary benefits of informatics is that data that was previously buried in inaccessible records becomes usable. Informatics is not just about collecting data, but about making it useful. When data is captured electronically in a structured manner, it can be retrieved and used in many different ways, both to easily assimilate information about one patient and as aggregated data. Aggregated data is the same piece or pieces of data for many patients. Table 1-1 shows some aggregated data for postsurgical infections sorted by physician and then by the organism. Because infections for some patients are caused by two different pathogens in Table 1-1, you see two entries for some patients, however, this is all produced from only one entry of the data. With just a few clicks of a mouse, this same data could be organized by unit to show the number of infections on each unit. This is possible because data that is structured as in Table 1-1 and standardized can be presented in many different views.

When aggregated data is examined, patterns can be seen that might otherwise take several weeks or months to become evident, or might never become evident. When patterns, such as the prevalence of infections for

TABLE 1-1 • *Aggregated Data*					
First Name	**Last Name**	**Unit**	**Surgery**	**Physician**	**Pathogen**
Charles	Babbage	3 West	Cholecystectomy	Black	*E. coli*
Jack	Of All Trades	4 West	Appendectomy	Black	*Strep*
George	Washington	4 West	Tonsillectomy	Black	*Strep*
John	Wayne	2 East	Herniorrhaphy	Greene	*E. coli*
Gloria	Swanson	2 East	Cholecystectomy	Greene	*E. coli*
Gloria	Swanson	2 East	Cholecystectomy	Greene	*Strep*
Susan	Anthony	3 West	Tubal ligation	Jones	*Strep*
Alexander	Hamilton	2 East	Cholecystectomy	Smith	*E. coli*
Florence	Dayingale	4 West	Hysterectomy	Smith	*E. coli*
Abigail	Adams	2 East	Herniorrhaphy	Smith	*Staph*
Johnny	Appleseed	3 West	Open reduction, left femur	Smith	*Staph*
Davey	Jones	3 West	Transurethral resection	Smith	*Staph*
Alexander	Hamilton	2 East	Cholecystectomy	Smith	*Strep*
Florence	Dayingale	4 West	Hysterectomy	Smith	*Strep*

Note: Fictitious patient names are used here to help in understanding the concept; real secondary data should be unidentifiable.

E.coli, Escherichia coli; Staph, Staphylococcus; Strep, Streptococcus.

Dr. Smith emerge (Table 1-1), investigations into what these patients have in common can begin. Caution, however, should be observed. The aggregated data in Table 1-1 are insufficient for drawing conclusions; the data only serves as an indication of a problem and clues to where to start investigating. Aggregated data is a type of information or even knowledge, but wisdom says that it is incomplete.[6] If this data were shared outside of an agency, or with those who don't need to have personal information about a patient, it would be **deidentified**, that is, there would be no patient names and probably no physician names. Deciding who can see what data is one of the current issues in informatics.

Informatics through information systems can improve communication between all healthcare providers, which will improve patient care as well as reduce stress. Additional benefits for healthcare include making the storage and retrieval of healthcare records much easier, quicker retrieval of test results, printouts of needed information organized to meet the needs of the user, and fewer lost charges as a result of easier methods of recording charges. The computerization of administrative tasks such as staffing and scheduling also saves time and money.

BENEFITS TO THE NURSING PROFESSION

Each healthcare discipline will benefit from its investment in informatics. In nursing, informatics will not only enhance practice, but also allow nursing science to develop (Fitzpatrick, 1988). Informatics will improve documentation and, when properly implemented, can reduce the time spent in documentation. It is believed by many nurses that they spend over 50% of their time doing paperwork (Womack et al., 2004). Entering vital signs both in nursing notes and on a flow sheet, wastes time and invites errors. In a well-designed clinical documentation system, this data will be entered once, retrieved, and presented in many different forms to meet the needs of the user.

Paper documentation methods create other problems such as inconsistency and irregularity in charting as well as the lack of data for evaluation and research mentioned above. An electronic clinical information system can remind users of the need to provide data in areas apt to be forgotten and provide a list of terms that can be clicked to enter data. The ability to use patient data for both quality control and research is vastly improved when documentation is complete and electronic.

Despite Florence Nightingale's emphasis on data, for much of nursing's history, nursing data has not been valued. It is either buried in paper patient records that make retrieving it economically infeasible or, worse, discarded when a patient is discharged, hence unavailable for building nursing science. With the advent of electronic clinical documentation, nursing data can be made a part of the EHR and become available to researchers for building evidence-based nursing knowledge. The recent Maryland report on the use of technology to address the nursing shortage demonstrated that informatics can be used to improve staff morale and patient care (Womack et al., 2004). For example, paper request forms can be eliminated, work announcements can be more easily communicated, the time for in-services can be reduced, and empty shifts can be filled using Internet software.

In understanding the role and value that informatics adds to nursing, it is necessary to recognize that the profession is not confined to tasks, but that it is cognitive. Providing the data to support this is a joint function of nursing informatics and clinicians. Identifying and determining how to facilitate its collection is an informatics skill that all nurses need.

Nursing Informatics Competencies and Information Literacy

The need to manage complex amounts of data in patient care demands that nurses, regardless of specialty area, have informatics skills (Gaumer, Koeniger-Donohue, Friel, & Sudbay, 2007; Nelson, 2007; Wilhoit, Mustain, &

---

[6] Aggregated data will be further discussed in Chapter 10.

King, 2006). Informatics skills require basic computer skills as one component (Staggers, Gassert, & Curran, 2002). A recent survey of hospital administrators in three states in the southeastern United States revealed that one of the competencies that they wanted from nurses dealt with the use of the computer (Uttley-Smith, 2004). This supports an earlier study by Gravely, Lust, & Fullerton (1999) that found that 83% of hospital recruiters indicated the importance of computer skills. Another skill needed for proficiency in informatics is **information literacy**. Both these skills have also been identified by the ANA and **National League for Nursing** (NLN) as necessary for evidence-based practice.

COMPUTER FLUENCY

The 20th century was described as the information age; the present century will be the information processing age, that is, the use of data and information to create more information and knowledge (University of Minnesota Duluth, 2006). The term "computer literacy" is used broadly to mean the ability to perform various tasks with a computer. Given the rapid changes in technology and in nursing, perhaps a better perspective on computer use can be gained by thinking in terms of computer fluency rather than literacy. The term "fluency" implies that an individual has a lifelong commitment to acquiring new skills for the purpose of being more effective in work and personal life (Committee on Information Technology Literacy, 1999). This necessitates a goal of gaining sufficient foundational skills and knowledge to enable one to independently acquire new skills. Thus, computer literacy is a temporary state, whereas computer fluency involves being able to increase one's ability to effectively use a computer when needed.

A perusal of **Listserv**[7] archives in informatics reveals periodic requests for instruments to measure the computer competency of staff.

[7] A Listserv is an email discussion list that has participants who discuss various aspects of a topic such as informatics.

Unfortunately, there is little agreement on specific competencies needed, let alone an instrument to measure this, but there is a consensus that it involves a positive attitude toward computers, knowledge and understanding of computer technology, computer hardware and software skills, and the ability to visualize the overall benefits to nursing from this technology (Hobbs, 2002). Simpson (1998) pointed out the need for nurses to master computers to avoid extinction. A computer is a mind tool that frees us from the mental drudgery of data processing, just as the bulldozer frees us from the drudgery of digging and moving dirt. Like, the bulldozer, however, the computer must be used intelligently or damage can result.

Given the forces moving healthcare toward more use of informatics, it is important for nurses to learn the skills associated with using a computer for managing information. Additionally, knowing how to use graphical interfaces and application programs such as word processing, spreadsheets, databases, and presentation programs is as an important an element in a professional career as mastering technology skills (McCannon & O'Neal, 2003). Just as anatomy and physiology provide a background for learning about disease processes and treatments, computer fluency skills are necessary to appreciate more complex informatics concepts (McNeil & Odom, 2000) and for learning clinical applications (Nagelkerk, Ritolo, & Vandort, 1998).

Ronald and Skiba (1987) were the first to look at computer competencies required for nurses. In the late 1990s and early part of this century this issue was revisited, but the focus became the use of computer skills as part of informatics skills (McCannon & O'Neal, 2003; McNeil et al., 2003; Pew Health Professions Commissions, 1998; Staggers, Gassert, & Curran, 2001; Staggers et al., 2002; Uttley-Smith, 2004). One of the more thorough studies is by Staggers, Gassert, and Curran (2001). They defined four levels of informatics competencies for practicing nurses. The first two pertain to all nurses, the last two to informatics nurses.

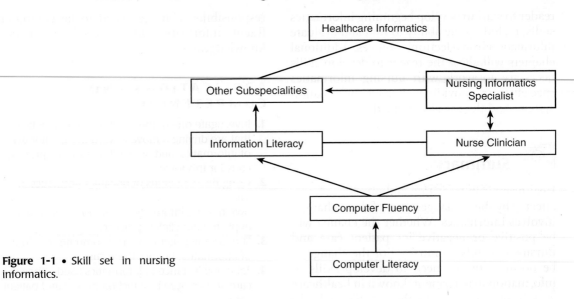

Figure 1-1 • Skill set in nursing informatics.

▼ The beginning nurse should possess basic information management and computer technology skills. Accomplishments should include the ability to access data, use a computer for communication, use basic desktop software, and use decision support systems.

▼ Experienced nurses should be highly skilled in using information management and computer technology to support their major area of practice. Additional skills for the experienced nurse include being able to make judgments on the basis of trends and patterns within data elements and to collaborate with nursing informatics nurses to suggest improvements in nursing systems.

▼ The informatics nurse specialist should be able to meet the information needs of practicing nurses by integrating and applying information, computer, and nursing sciences.

▼ The informatics innovator will conduct informatics research and generate informatics theory.[8]

[8] A Word document containing the complete list of the levels and competencies is available at http://www.nurs.utah.edu/informatics/competencies.htm or from the book Web page at http://dlthede.net/Informatics/Competencies2008.doc).

INFORMATION LITERACY

Information literacy, or the ability to know when one needs information and how to locate, evaluate, and effectively use it (National Forum on Information Literacy, 2004) is an informatics skill. Although it involves computer skills, like informatics, it requires critical thinking and problem solving. Information literacy is part of the foundation for evidence-based practice and provides nurses with the ability to be intelligent information consumers in today's electronic environment[9] (Jacobs, Rosenfeld, & Haber, 2003).

The level of computer fluency needed by nurses to be both information literate and informatics capable in their practice is what is expected of any educated nurse (see Figure 1-1). In this book, the chapters addressing basic computer skills will emphasize concepts that promote the ability to learn new applications. These chapters provide information underlying the use of informatics in professional life both on and off a clinical unit, and to adapt to changes in technology. In future chapters these principles will be built upon to allow the

[9] Information Competency will be discussed in Unit III.

reader to start to develop beginning informatics skills, including the ability to find and evaluate information from electronic sources. Additional chapters will allow the reader to develop skills necessary to work with nursing informatics specialists in providing effective information systems and the use of nursing data.

Summary

Healthcare is in transition and nursing is being affected by these changes. Part of these changes involves informatics. Whether the change will be positive or negative for patient care and nursing depends on nurses. For the change to be positive, nurses need to develop skills in information management, known in healthcare as informatics. To gain these skills, a background in both computer and information literacy skills is necessary.

As knowledge continues to expand logarithmically, data and information can no longer be managed solely by the human mind. The use of tools to aid the human mind has become mandatory. Although healthcare has been behind most industries in using technology to manage its data, there are many forces, both at the governmental and private levels that are working to change this. With these pressures, healthcare informatics is rapidly expanding. There are many subspecialties in informatics, of which nursing is one. Embracing informatics will allow nurses to assess and evaluate practice just as a stethoscope allows the evaluation and assessment of a patient.

The use of computers in healthcare started in the 1960s, mostly in financial areas, but with the advance in computing power and the demand for clinical data, computers are being used more and more in clinical areas. With this growth has come a change in focus for information systems from providing solutions for just one process, to an enterprise-wide patient-centered system that focuses on data. This new focus provides the functionality that allows one piece of data to be used in multiple ways. To understand and work with clinical systems, as well as to fulfill other professional responsibilities, nurses need to be computer fluent, information literate, and informatics knowledgeable.

APPLICATIONS AND COMPETENCIES

1. Investigate one of the forces outside healthcare that are driving a move toward the greater use of informatics, and briefly discuss some pros and cons for this force.
2. Using the definitions of nursing informatics in this chapter or from other resources, create your own nursing informatics definition that would apply to your clinical practice.
3. Support the statement: "The computer is a tool of informatics, but not the focus."
4. Take one instance of informatics used in healthcare and analyze its effect on nurses and patient care.
5. List reasons why every nurse needs to have informatics skills.
6. The results of the Delphi Study by Staggers, Gassert, & Curran (2002) are available at http://www.nurs.utah.edu/informatics/competencies.htm (or from the book Web page at http://dlthede.net/Informatics/Competencies2008.doc) as a Word document. Download the list and rate yourself for each of the competencies. Select one for which you need to improve your skills and design a plan for reaching competency.
7. Analyze all the information beyond your immediate knowledge that you need and use in caring for one of your patients on just one shift. Where does this information originate? When do you need it for care? How do your obtain it? How do you use it?
8. Write one or two few paragraphs on how you now think a practicing nurse can use computer fluency and information literacy to advance in a career. Save this and at the end of this book, compare it with how you then see these two skills affecting a nursing career.

REFERENCES

AHIMA & AMIA. (2006). *Building the workforce for health information transformation*. Retrieved November 11, 2008, from http://www.ahima.org/emerging_issues/Workforce_web.pdf

American Association of Colleges of Nursing. (1998). *The essentials of baccalaureate education*. Washington, DC: American Association of Colleges of Nursing.

American Nurses Association. (2001). *Scope and standard of nursing informatics practice* (No. 1-55810-166-7). Washington, DC: American Nurses Publishing.

American Nurses Association. (2008). *Nursing informatics: Scope and standards of practice*. Silver Spring, MD: American Nurses Association.

Analytical Engine. (2007, October 1). Retrieved November 11, 2008, from http://en.wikipedia.org/wiki/Analytical_engine

Bakken, S. (2001). An informatics infrastructure is essential for evidence-based practice. *Journal of the American Medical Association*, 8(3), 199–201.

Bakken, S. (2006). Informatics for patient safety: A nursing research perspective. *Annual Review of Nursing Research*, 24, 219–254.

Baldwin, F. D. (2002, March). Making do with less. *Healthcare Informatics*, 40, 37–38.

Committee on Information Technology Literacy. (1999). *Being Fluent with information technology*. Washington, DC: National Academy Press.

Covington, B., Koszalka, M. V., Newbold, S. K., & Womack, D. (2004, July 22). *Technology's role in addressing Maryland's nursing shortage: Innovations and examples*. Paper presented at the Summer Institute in Nursing Informatics 2004, Baltimore, MD.

Davenport, T. H., & Glaser, J. (2002). Just-in-time delivery comes to knowledge management. *Harvard Business Review*, 80(7), 107–111.

Delaney, C. (2001). Health informatics and oncology nursing. *Seminars in Oncology Nursing*, 17(1), 2–6.

Dulong, D., & HIMSS Nursing Task Force. (2007, April 23). *The T.I.G.E.R. Update: Facilitating collaboration among participating organizations to achieve the TIGER vision*. Retrieved November 11, 2008, from http://www.himss.org/handouts/TIGER_PhaseII_Collaboratives.pdf

Fitzpatrick, J. (1988). Nursing: How do we know, what do we do; and how can we enhance nursing knowledge and practice. In N. Daly & K. J. Hannah (Eds.), *Proceedings of the Third International Symposium on Nursing Use of Computers and Information Science* (pp. 58–65). St. Louis, MO: C. V. Mosby.

Gardner, R., Pryor, T. A., & Warner, H. R. (1999). The HELP hospital information system: update 1998. *International Journal of Medical Informatics*, 54(3), 169–118.

Gaumer, G. L., Koeniger-Donohue, R., Friel, C., & Sudbay, M. B. (2007). Use of information technology by advanced practice nurses. *Computers, Informatics, Nursing: CIN*, 25(6), 344–352.

Goossen, W. T. F. (1996). Nursing information and processing: A framework and definition for systems analysis, design and evaluation. *International Journal of Biomedical Computing*, 40(3), 187–195.

Gravely, E. A., Lust, B. I., & Fullerton, J. T. (1999). Undergraduate computer literacy: Evaluation and intervention. *Computers in Nursing*, 17(4), 166–170.

Graves, J. R., & Corcoran, S. (1989). The study of nursing informatics. *Image: Journal of Nursing Scholarship*, 21, 227–231.

Greiner, A. C., & Knebel, E. (Eds.). (2003). *Health professions education: A bridge to quality*. Washington, DC: National Academy Press.

Hannah, K. J., Ball, M. J., & Edwards, M. J. A. (1994). *Introduction to nursing informatics*. New York: Springer-Verlag.

Herman Hollerith—Punch Cards. (n.d.). Retrieved November 11, 2008, from http://inventors.about.com/library/inventors/blhollerith.htm

Hobbs, S. D. (2002). Measuring nurses' compute competence: an analysis of published instruments. *Computers, Informatics, Nursing: CIN*, 20(2), 63–73.

Jacobs, S. K., Rosenfeld, P., & Haber, J. (2003). Information literacy as the foundation for evidence-based practice in graduate nursing education: A curriculum-integrated approach. *Journal Professional Nursing*, 19(5), 320–328.

Korpman, R. A. (1990). Patient care automation the future is now: Introduction and historical perspective, part 1. *Nursing Economics*, 8(3), 191–193.

Leapfrog Group. (2007a). *How & why Leapfrog started*. Retrieved November 11, 2008, from http://www.leapfroggroup.org/about_us/how_and_why

Leapfrog Group. (2007b, February). *Leapfrog fact sheet*. Retrieved November 11, 2008, from http://www.leapfroggroup.org/about_us/leapfrog-factsheet

McCannon, M., & O'Neal, P. V. (2003). Results of a national survey indicating information technology skills needed by nurses at time of entry into the work force. *Journal of Nursing Education*, 42(8), 327–340.

McDonald, M. D. (1994, March/April). Telecognition for improving health. *Healthcare Forum Journal*, 18–21.

McNeil, B. J., Elfrink, V. L., Bickford, C. J., Pierce, S. T., Beyea, S. C., Averill, C., et al. (2003). Nursing information technology knowledge, skills, and preparation of student nurses, nursing faculty, and clinicians: A U.S. survey. *Journal Nursing Education*, 42(8), 341–349.

McNeil, B. J., & Odom, S. K. (2000). Nursing informatics education in the United States: Proposed undergraduate curriculum. *Health Informatics Journal*, 6, 32–38.

McNeill, D. G. (1979). Developing the complete computer-based information system. *Journal of Nursing Administration*, 9(11), 34–46.

Middle East Technical University. (n.d.). *Introduction to medical informatics*. Retrieved November 11, 2008, from http://www.ii.metu.edu.tr/~ion535/demo/lecture_notes/week1/week1-4.html

Moye, W. T. (1996, January). *ENIAC: The Army-sponsored revolution*. Retrieved November 11, 2008, from http://ftp.arl.army.mil/~mike/comphist/96summary/

Nagelkerk, J., Ritolo, P. M., & Vandort, P. J. (1998). Nursing informatics: The trend of the future. *Journal of Continuing Education in Nursing*, 29(1), 17–21.

National Advisory Council on Nurse Education and Practice. (1997). *A national informatics agenda for nursing education and practice*. Retrieved October 3, 2007, from Full report at ftp://ftp.hrsa.gov// bhpr/nursing/nireport/NIFull.pdf

National Forum on Information Literacy. (2004). *Forum overview*. Retrieved November 11, 2008, from http://infolit.org/

Nelson, R. (2007). U.S. Hospitals need staffing makeover. *American Journal of Nursing*, 107(12), 19.

Newbold, S. K. (1996). The informatics nurse and the certification process. *Computers in Nursing, 14*(2), 84–86.

Nightingale, F. (1859). *Notes on hospitals.* London: John W. Parker and Son.

Office of the National Coordinator for Health Information Technology. (2004, November 9). *Health IT strategic framework executive summary.* Retrieved November 11, 2008, from http://www.hhs.gov/healthit/executivesummary.html

Pew Health Professions Commissions. (1998). *Recreating health professional practice for a new century: The fourth report of the Pew Health Professions Commission.* San Francisco, CA: Pew Health Professions Commission. Retrieved November 11, 2008, from http://www.futurehealth.ucsf.edu/ pdf_files/recreate.pdf

Pillar, B., & Golumbic, N. (Eds.). (1993). *Nursing informatics: Enhancing patient care.* Betheseda, MD: National Center for Nursing Research, U.S. Department of Health and Human Services.

Problem-Oriented Medical Information System. (n.d.). Retrieved November 11, 2008, from http://encyclopedia.thefreedictionary.com/Problem-Oriented%20Medical%20Information%20System

PROMIS: The Problem-Oriented Medical Record System. (1980). Unpublished manuscript.

Ronald, J., & Skiba, D. (1987). *Guidelines for basic computer education in nursing.* (No. NLN Pub No 41-2177). New York: National League for Nursing.

Saba, V. K., & Erdeley, W. S. (2006). Historical perspectives of nursing and the computer. In V. K. Saba & K. A. McCormick (Eds.), *Essentials of nursing informatics* (4th ed., pp. 9–27). New York: Mc-Graw Hill.

Sackett, K. M., & Erdley, W. S. (2002). The history of health care informatics. In S. Englebardt & R. Nelson (Eds.), *Healthcare informatics from an interdisciplinary approach* (pp. 453–477). St. Louis, MO: Mosby.

Scholes, M., & Barber, B. (1980). Towards nursing informatics. In D. A. D. Lindberg & S. Kaihara (Eds.), *MEDINFO: 1980* (pp. 7–73). Amsterdam, Netherlands: North Holland.

Schwirian, P. (1986). The NI pyramid—A model for research in nursing informatics. *Computers in Nursing, 4*(3), 134–136.

Shortliffe, E. H., & Blois, M. S. (2001). The computer meets medicine: Emergence of a discipline. In E. H. Shortliffe & L. E. Perrault (Eds.), *Medical informatics: Computer applications in healthcare* (pp. 3–40). New York: Springer-Verlag.

Simpson, R. (1998). The technologic imperative: A new agenda for nursing education and practice, part 1. *Nursing Management, 29*(9), 22–24.

Staggers, N. (2004). Assessing recommendations from the IOMs quality chasm report. *Journal of Healthcare Informatics Management, 18*(1), 30–35.

Staggers, N., Gassert, C. A., & Curran, C. (2001). Informatics competencies for nurses at four levels of practice. *Journal of Nursing Education, 40*(7), 303–316.

Staggers, N., Gassert, C. A., & Curran, C. (2002). A Delphi study to determine informatics competencies for nurses at four levels of practice [Research]. *Nursing Research, 51*(6), 383–390.

Staggers, N., & Thompson, C. B. (2002). The evolution of definitions for nursing informatics: A critical analysis and revised definition. *Journal of the American Medical Informatics Association, 9*(3), 255–261.

Thompson, T. G. (2004, May 6). *Health information technology summit.* Retrieved November 11, 2008, from http://www.hhs.gov/news/speech/2004/040506.html

Turley, J. (1996). Toward a model for nursing informatics. *Image: Journal of Nursing Scholarship, 29*(4), 309–313.

University of Minnesota Duluth. (2006, July 17). *Computer literacy homepage.* Retrieved November 11, 2008, from http://www.d.umn.edu/student/loon/acad/ComputLit.html

Uttley-Smith, Q. (2004). Competencies needed by new baccalaureate graduates. [Research]. *Nursing Education Perspectives, 25*(4), 166–170.

Wilhoit, K., Mustain, J., & King, M. (2006). The role of frontline RNs in the selection of an electronic medical record business partner. *Computers Informatics Nursing: CIN, 24*(4), 188–195.

Womack, D., Newbold, S. K., Staugaitis, H., & Cunningham, B. (2004, January). *Technology's role in addressing Maryland's nursing shortage: Innovations & examples.* Retrieved November 11, 2008, from http://maryland.nursetech.com/F/NT/MD/nursingInnovations2004.pdf or http://www.vocera.com/pef/NursingInnovations2004.pdf

Meet the Computer

Learning Objectives

After studying this chapter you will be able to:

1. *Recognize computer characteristics.*

2. *Explore ways to overcome computer anxiety.*

3. *Differentiate uses for various types of computers.*

4. *Describe battery capabilities.*

5. *Distinguish between the various forms of computer storage.*

6. *Identify uses in healthcare for computer peripherals.*

7. *Identify nosocomial infection hazards with computers in the clinical area.*

8. *Apply good ergonomic principles for computer use.*

9. *Define selected computer terms.*

Key Terms

American Standard Code for Information Interchange (ASCII)
Backward Compatibility
Bit
Black Hat Hacker
Boot
Bug
Bus
Byte
Case Sensitivity
Chip
Clock Speed
Cold Boot
Central Processing Unit (CPU)
Cracker
Data Dump
Disk Wiping
Docking Station
Driver
File
Firewire
Flash Drive

Flash Memory
Forward Compatibility
Hacker
Hard Disk
Hertz
Jaz Disk
Logical
Mainframe
Minicomputer
Motherboard
Object
Parallel Port
Peripheral
Physical
Port
Serial Port
Server
Thin Client
Universal Serial Bus (USB) port
Videotext terminal
Warm boot
White Hat Hacker
Zip disk

Introducing the use of a stethoscope precedes learning how to listen to heart and lung sounds. To be effective in using the stethoscope, a clinician needs to know when to use the bell and when to use the diaphragm. In the same way, it is imperative to have some understanding of how and when to use the tool of informatics, the computer.

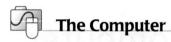

The Computer

A complete computer system is the integration of human input and information resources using hardware and software. In computer terms, hardware refers to objects such as disks, disk drives, monitors, keyboards, speakers, printers, mice, boards, **chips**, and the computer itself. Software includes programs that give instructions to the computer that make the machine useful. Information resources are data that the computer manipulates. Human input refers to the entire spectrum of human involvement, including deciding what is to be input and how it is to be processed as well as evaluating output and deciding how it should be used. In this chapter, we look at the computer, and in the next, at software.

COMPUTER MISCONCEPTIONS

When computers were new, there were many fears and misconceptions about using them. Some of these were computers can think, computers require a mathematical genius to use, and computers make mistakes (Perry, 1982). Today there are other misconceptions, perhaps born of familiarity, which can be dangerous to users.[1] It is important to understand that computers cannot think, and they are not smart. Incidents like the one in which Deep Blue (the nickname given to an IBM computer specially designed to play chess) won a chess game against world champion Garry Kasparov led to such misperceptions. Consider the game of

chess. Although there are many possible combinations, there are a given set of moves, rules, and goals that make it a perfect stage to display the potential of computers. Deep Blue is a very powerful computer, capable of quickly analyzing hundreds of millions of possible moves and responding according to rules (known as algorithms) that were part of the software that beat Kasparov. It made use of these qualities to beat Kasparov. It did not use thinking in the human sense.

The thought that only mathematical geniuses can use computers, although just as false, continues to flourish. This belief is linked to the development of the first computers as a means to "crunch numbers," or process mathematical equations. Hence, in colleges and universities, many computer departments are still housed in, or closely related to, the departments of mathematics. It did not take experts long to translate the mathematical concepts into everyday language, an accomplishment that made the computer available to everyone, regardless of level of proficiency in math.

The last myth, that computers make mistakes, makes it a wonderful excuse for human error. This was well illustrated by a cartoon in the early 1990s that showed a man saying, "It's wonderful to be able to blame my mistakes at the office on the computer, I think I'll get a personal computer." Computers act on the information they are given. As one humorist said, "Computers are designed to DWIS, or Do What I Say." As many a user will tell you, they resist with great determination any inclination to DWIM, or "Do What I Mean!" Unlike a colleague to whom you only need to give partial instructions because the person is able to fill in the rest, a computer requires complete, definitive, black-and-white directions. Unlike humans, computers cannot perceive that a colon and semicolon are closely related, and in many cases, a computer believes that an uppercase letter and a lower case letter are as different as the letter A from the letter X. This is known as **case sensitivity**. There are no "almosts" with a computer.

---

[1] Computer security will be discussed in Chapter 5.

COMPUTER CHARACTERISTICS

A computer accomplishes many things that are impossible without it. When programmed properly, it is superb in remembering and processing details, calculating accurately, printing reports, facilitating editing documents, and sparing users many repetitive, tedious tasks, which frees time for more productive endeavors. Remember, however, that computers are not infallible. Being electronic, they are subject to electrical problems. Humans build computers, program them, and enter data into them. For these reasons, many situations can cause error and frustration. Two of the most common challenges with computers are "glitches" and the "garbage in, garbage out" (GIGO) principle . That is, if data input has errors, then the output will be erroneous.

Anyone, who had been using a computer when it crashed or "went down" may have experienced a guilty feeling that she or he did something wrong. If the person actually did create the crash, unless she or he were purposely engaged in something destructive, that person did not cause the crash; she or he just found a flaw in the system that was inadvertently created by the programmer(s).[2] There are times, however, when crashes occur for seemingly no reason. Computers, regardless of their manufacturer, will at some time, for unknown reasons, perform in a totally unexpected manner (Perry, 1982). This is as true today as when computers were new. The good news is that this is much less apt to happen despite the complexity of today's computers.

---

[2] Given the complexity of programming, it is not unusual to find "bugs" or glitches in a new system. You may have experienced a problem when a new information system was installed at your place of work. If you should be the unfortunate one who discovers a bug, you can help the programmers to correct it by carefully communicating the actions you took that preceded the problem (as far as you can remember), and the exact result. If an error number was presented on the screen, be sure to include this in your communication. Finding the problem is usually harder than fixing it. The hardest mistakes to fix are those that cannot be recreated.

OVERCOMING COMPUTER ANXIETY

The attitudes people have toward computers range from complete dislike and frustration to curiosity and excitement. Although the mass media and personal acquaintances convey both perceptions, people seem to remember the negative points more clearly. As with all new experiences, becoming acquainted with a computer or learning a new computer application can produce anxiety. When computers in healthcare were fairly new, many studies were done that looked at the attitude of nurses toward computers (Focus, 1995; McBride & Nagle, 1996; Simpson & Kenrick, 1997). Today, these studies look at the attitudes and anxiety toward the electronic health record (Chan, 2007; Dillon, Blankenship, & Crews, 2005). It is highly likely that the same type of anxieties were present when the general population found it necessary to learn to drive. There are, however, no known studies of this phenomena dating from that time (Box 2-1).

Addressing these fears takes time for both a trainer and the individual experiencing the fears. One-on-one sessions for the person affected may be necessary and save time in the long run by preventing frantic calls to the help center. Studies show that the learning patterns of those afraid of computers can be improved by treating the bodily symptoms of anxiety and providing distracting thought patterns (Bloom, 1985). Techniques, such as teaching relaxation methods before starting any hands-on training, often helps, as does giving the anxious trainee something to repeat internally such as, "You're in control, not the computer."

Other helpful techniques include recognizing and accepting fear. One method is to have trainees check off from a list of possible feelings (e.g. panicky, lost, curious) those that they are feeling, a practice that can help them face their fears. Inherent in all these terrors is the fear of failure and of looking incompetent in front of their peers. This may be especially evident in people who see themselves as having a high degree of competence in their profession and to whom people look for answers. Therefore, placing themselves in a learning

Box 2-1 • Computer Anxiety

Overcoming Computer Application Anxiety

My great-great grandmother rode a horse, but was afraid of a train. My great-grandmother rode the train, but was afraid to drive a car. My grandmother drove a car, but was afraid to fly. My mother flies in an airplane, but is afraid of computers. I use a computer, but am afraid to ride a horse. . . .

What we fear is often what we are unfamiliar with, or something with which we have had a bad experience. It is not unusual to be unfamiliar with computers, and it is quite possible that some of you have had a less than pleasant encounter with a computer application. Unpleasant experiences with computers are often related to a lack of meaningful help when trying to figure out how to accomplish a task. Not too long ago documentation for software provided information about a function, but neglected to say how to perform it. Fortunately, today's online documentation has progressed to a point where it is much more helpful.

Another thought that can impede one in using a computer fully is a fear that one will break the computer. In truth, it is very difficult to break a computer. Unless of course you dump a cup of coffee or other liquid on it, throw it out of the window, or hit it with a baseball bat.* At times, everyone has been tempted to do at least one of these things. Computers can be frustrating! Breaking the computer or erasing an entire system by means that do not involve physically attacking it, such as by pressing a key, is not something users can do accidentally. In the rare instance that the computer should "crash", it is NOT the user who has created the problem. It is the software (or hardware) producers who have failed to produce a robust system. Creating good software involves trying to anticipate all the various ways that a user could act when she or he misunderstands what is required and providing error traps to assist the user in these instances. An error trap is a programming sequence that responds to erroneous keystrokes or actions with feedback that gives information about the difficulty and how to correct it.

Not knowing what to do when using a computer is where we all begin. This also occurs when we learn a new program, or when we need to learn a new version of an existing program. We stumble and make false starts as we learn new things. We were not born knowing how to walk, read, or write. Yet today, we can do all these things because we learned how. In the same way, anyone who wants to can learn to use a computer. Just as you made many false starts learning to do any

* There was one frustrated owner who, forgetting that the computer was inhuman, or maybe because of it, shot his computer dead. He put four bullets into the hard drive and one into the monitor whereupon he was taken to a mental hospital for observation. (Simpson & Kenrick, 1997).

situation can be very threatening to their self-image.

If you are calling your information services (IS) department for help, it is sometimes difficult to understand what you are being told. One remedy for this is to say, "I just don't get it. Could you please explain it like you were talking to your non-computer-using mother?" We all tend to downgrade the knowledge that we possess, believing that others also possess this knowledge, which causes us to provide explanations that are unclear. IS department personnel are just as susceptible to this condition as nurses are when we talk with our patients.

TYPES OF COMPUTERS

The progress in computers is measured by generations, each of which grew out of a new innovation (Table 2-1). Computer sizes vary from supercomputers intended to process large amounts of data for one user at a time to small palmtop computers. Each type has its niche in healthcare. However, it is becoming increasingly difficult to classify the different types of computers, because smaller ones take on the characteristics of their bigger brothers as the amount of space needed for processing lessens.

of the aforementioned, when you are learning to use a computer you will not always accomplish your - objectives on the first or even the third try.

One source of frustration in using computers is their lack of ability to discriminate shades of gray. With a computer, an action you perform either produces the desired result or it does not. This behavior, however, is no different than that of other technologies with which you are familiar. If you are in an elevator and push the number five, the elevator will stop at the fifth floor whether you really wanted to go to the fifth floor or not, even when you realize you made a mistake and push six for the sixth floor. This exactness, however, produces a machine of great predictability, which is the same characteristic that makes the computer functional. A given command produces a given function. Period! Almost is not a computer parameter.

When you think of learning to use a computer, think of trial and error. It is this process that produces the knowledge and competency that you are seeking. If you perform an action and what you expected to have happen does not, observe what has happened. Then try again. It may be necessary to use one of the help systems available to you before you gain your goal. **Try to look at your situation as though you made a discovery, not a mistake.** This of course is not the model of learning with which most of us are familiar (Simpson, 1996). Prior experience has led us to fear mistakes and regard them as a sign of failure.

Educational experience has often conditioned us to expect a teacher to impart the knowledge we need to function. In learning to use a computer, didactic information can only give a small part of the picture. As thinking human beings, we need to apply this information by actively experimenting, observing the results of our experimentation, and reflecting on what actually happens.

Also, try to remember that as humans we cannot open our heads and have information or skills poured in. We have to work at learning. Senge (1994) tells us that real learning occurs only when we struggle with feeling incompetent and ignorant. You need to accept the fact that you will make many discoveries before you feel comfortable. And that you will feel frustrated at times. A good rule of thumb to follow is to take a break when frustration threatens to disable you. Many problems are solved when an individual takes a break and lets the subconscious work. When your frustration level gets high, take a break and remember that you have learned to ride a bike and drive a car, both potentially far more dangerous to your health than using a computer. You can also learn to drive a computer.

REFERENCES

Senge, P. (1994). *The fifth discipline: The art and practice of the learning organization.* New York: Currency Double Day.

Simpson, R. (1996). Creating a true learning organization. *Nursing Management., 27*(4), 18,20.

TABLE 2-1 ● *The Five Generations of Computers*		
Generations	**Dates**	**Innovation**
1	1940–1956	Vacuum tubes
2	1956–1963	Transistors
3	1964–1971	Integrated circuits
4	1971–present	Microprocessors
5	Present and beyond	Artificial intelligence, which can produce voice recognition and responses to natural language. Powerful chips that are stronger.

Webopedia. *The five generations of computers.* Retrieved November 12, 2008, from http://www.webopedia.com/DidYouKnow/Hardware_Software/2002/FiveGenerations.asp

Supercomputers

Technically, supercomputers are the most powerful type of computer, if power is judged by the ability to do numerical calculations. Supercomputers can process hundreds of millions of instructions per second. They are used in applications that require extensive mathematical calculations, such as weather forecasts, fluid dynamic calculations, and nuclear energy research. Supercomputers are designed to execute only one task at a time; hence, they devote all their resources to this one situation. This gives them the speed they need for their tasks.

Mainframes

The first computers were large, often taking up an entire room. They were known as **mainframes** and were designed to serve many users and run many programs at the same time. These computers formed the backbone of many hospital information systems. Users used what were technically called **videotext terminals**, but often referred to as "dumb terminals." A videotext terminal consisted of a display screen, keyboard, and modem or device that connected it to the mainframe. Information was entered on the keyboard and transmitted to the mainframe, which was located somewhere else, often in the basement in a secure, temperature-controlled room. Any processing done to the information was done by the mainframe, which returns the results to the screen of the videotext terminal. This is why you still find the IS departments in the basement of hospitals.

Minicomputers

As computers became more powerful, their size was reduced. The same work done by a mainframe became amenable to being accomplished on what was termed a **minicomputer**. Minicomputers were like mainframes (i.e., they were multiuser machines that originally served videotext terminals), but they were smaller and less costly. Unlike larger mainframes, they did not require a special temperature-controlled room and were useful in situations with fewer users. As computers started to be built in many sizes, it became impossible to classify one as a mainframe or another as a minicomputer; these terms are seldom used today.

Servers

The functions served by mainframes and minicomputers today are performed by computers of varying sizes, which are referred to as **servers**. The functions performed by servers and their powers are as varied as the needs of the users. These functions vary from servers that operate in the mainframe/videotext format especially in hospital information systems to those that are just a repository for **files** (a user-created item) that are "served" to users who have software that does the processing on their personal computer (PC). Some servers in the middle of this continuum may also store the programs that a user needs and provide them as needed by the user.

Thin Clients

Thin clients are today's version of the videotext terminal. These are computers without a hard drive and with limited, if any, processing power. Besides costing much less, thin clients do not need to be upgraded when new software is made available because they do not contain any applications. Because they do no processing, older PCs can function in this capacity instead of being retired.

Personal or Single-User Computers

PCs are designed for one individual to use at a time. PCs are based on microprocessor technology that enables manufacturers to put an entire processing (controlling) unit on one chip, thus permitting the small size. When PCs were adopted in business, they freed users from the resource limitations of the mainframe computer and allowed data processing staff to concentrate on tasks that needed a large system. Today, although capable of functioning without being connected to a network, in businesses including healthcare, PCs are usually connected or networked to either other PCs or servers. They still process information, but when networked, they can also share data.

In information systems, PCs often replace the old videotext terminal and handle the tasks of entering and retrieving information from the central computer or server, although thin clients may be used for this purpose instead. When a full PC is available on the unit, personnel can use application programs such as word processing. PCs are available in many different formats such as a desktop or tower model, laptops, and tablet computers.

Desktop and Towers. The original PC was a desktop model. You are probably familiar with these. They were placed horizontally on a desk and a monitor was placed on top of them. As the use of computers became more common, users were reluctant to give up desk space to their computer, and computers that stood upright, known as towers, were developed. With these, only the monitor needed was on the desk, while the computer itself stood on the floor, often under the desk.

Laptops/Notebooks. As computer usage became popular, people found that they needed the files and software on their computer to accomplish tasks away from their desks. The first computer that made this practical was really more transportable than portable. Developed in the 1980s, it was about the size of a desktop and had a built-in monitor. Toward the end of the 1980s, the transportables were replaced by true portables: laptops, or computers small enough to fit on one's lap. As technology continued to place more information on a chip, laptops became smaller. They are now referred to as notebook computers. Some healthcare organizations use notebook computers for point-of-care (POC) data entry at the bedside or anyplace where care is delivered.

Notebook computers do have some drawbacks. The screen is usually smaller than the one in a desktop, and the resolution may not be as crisp. Keyboards are also smaller. The mouse, or pointing and selecting device, can be a button the size of a pencil eraser in the middle of the keyboard, or a small square on the user end of the keyboard, or a small ball embedded in the keyboard. Some users

purchase **docking stations** for their notebook computers. The computer can be placed in the docking station (may be called a port replicator, or notebook extender), which is connected to hardware such as a larger monitor, keyboard, and regular mouse. This enables the user to have access to these devices when at their desk, but makes it easy to remove the computer and enjoy its portability, albeit, without the hardware connected to the docking station.

Other Mobile Computers. Again, as the processing power and storage capacity of computers increased, there was a demand for mobile computers that were more versatile than laptops. The subnotebook and tablet computer are some of these as are personal digital assistants (PDAs).[3]

Batteries

One thing that all portable electronic devices share is a need for a rechargeable battery. Keeping batteries charged in healthcare agencies can be a difficult process. Selecting the right battery and caring for it properly will increase the battery life and length of time it will power a device. This time is related not only to the care a battery receives but also to the type, size, and age of the battery. As batteries age, they lose the ability to retain a full charge (Buchmann, 2005b). There are several types of batteries: nickel–cadmium, nickel–metal hydride, lead–acid, and lithium ion. With the exception of the lead–acid battery, any of these can be found in mobile computing devices (Buchmann, 2005c).

NICKEL-BASED BATTERIES

The nickel–cadmium batteries were the first batteries used in laptops and can still be found in some laptops. They are relatively heavy and need to be fully discharged occasionally[4] to

---

[3] See Chapter 19 for a full discussion of mobile computers and computing and their uses in healthcare.

[4] Do not, however, fully discharge these batteries with every use because it puts undue stress on the battery.

avoid decreasing the usage time. This need is a result of crystalline formation on their cells, which decreases the length of time the battery can be used. Their life can be extended if they are fully discharged once every three months. They are useful where extended temperature range will be experienced and long life is needed. The nickel–metal hydride battery, an outgrowth of the nickel–cadmium battery, may be found in mobile phones and laptop computers. Although at first it was thought that it did not suffer from the same memory problem as the nickel–cadmium battery, it has been found to have this problem too, although to a lesser degree.

LITHIUM ION BATTERIES

The trend today is toward lithium ion batteries. These batteries have a typical life span of two to three years because of loss of capacity through cell oxidation, although they are continually being improved (Buchmann, 2005b). These batteries respond better if they are only partially discharged, and frequent full discharges are avoided. To maintain the battery life, charge the battery more often or use a larger battery. A lithium ion battery must have a protection circuit to shut off the power source when it is fully charged (Buchmann, 2005a). Overheating may result if this is not present and can cause batteries to explode. Since about 2003, the search for cheap batteries has produced a flood of counterfeit batteries that do not have this protection. This is why manufacturers advise customers to buy only approved batteries.

BATTERY SELF-DISCHARGING

If you have ever used a laptop, you may have noticed that after it has been unplugged for a while, the battery charging light comes on when you plug the computer into an electrical outlet. This is a result of self-discharge, from which all batteries suffer (Buchmann, 2005b). Interestingly, it is highest right after charge. The nickel-based batteries lose 10% to 15% of capacity in the first 24 hours after charge,

which levels off to 10% to 15% a month. Lithium ion batteries self-discharge only about 5% in the first 24 hours and then 1% to 2% in a month. Higher temperatures will increase the self-discharge rate which doubles roughly with every 18°F (10°C) rise in temperature. Leaving the battery in a hot car will create a noticeable energy loss.

PC Systems

Desktop and laptop computers consist of at least three components: a display screen, a keyboard for entering data, and the system components generally housed in a rectangular box often referred to as the **CPU** (**central processing unit**). These parts provide the input, processing, and output functions needed by a computer.

Computers, whether mobile or stationary, need a continuous nonvariable supply of power. Their operation can be affected by a power surge. Although the power surge may be generated by the electrical company, in some homes this can occur when a large electrical device such as an air conditioner comes on. To protect against this, all computers come with some degree of built-in surge protection. When this protection is inadequate, the **motherboard**, or heart of the computer, may be damaged. For this reason, it is a good idea to use a separate, high-quality surge protector. No surge protector, however, will protect from a lighting strike. Some users elect to unplug their computer and monitor altogether during thunderstorms.

PROCESSING COMPONENTS

The processing part of a computer consists of a motherboard, a CPU, **bus**, and cards.

Motherboard

The motherboard determines the type of computer and power supply that the computer can support. It's the main circuit for a microcomputer. The motherboard typically contains the CPU, the basic input–output system (BIOS), memory, and connections to all ports, expansion slots, disks, and all input-output devices. It contains the chip[5] that is the microprocessor or, on a PC, the CPU.

CPU/Microprocessor

The CPU is the heart or brains of the computer; it controls what the computer does. Some computer types such as supercomputers or mainframes may have many CPUs. PCs, however, have a single CPU that consists of a single chip called a microprocessor. The CPU consists of an arithmetic logic unit (ALU), a control unit, and some memory registers. The ALU performs all arithmetic and logical operations such as calculating a formula or comparing two items. The control unit directs the flow of information in the computer. It can be thought of as a combination traffic officer and switchboard. It gets instructions from memory, interprets them, directs them, and makes certain they are properly executed. It performs these operations in nanoseconds (one billionth of a second) so that to a user the results appear instantaneous.

These chips, smaller and thinner than a baby's fingernail, come in different varieties. They may be referred to by manufacturer and number or name (e.g., Pentium Intel Current, Athlon AMD Pentium, and Celeron Intel.). All chips with the same number or name are not the same, however. Differences may include power management modifications for battery-run computers or the speed at which the chip accomplishes its tasks. The processing speed is referred to as the **clock speed** of the computer. The clock speed determines how often a pulse of electricity "cycles" or circulates through the circuits, hence how fast information is processed. The more cycles per given time period, the greater the processing speed will be. Clock speed is measured in **hertz**, which is one cycle per second. Computers today are capable of speeds in the gigahertz (Ghz) range (one billion hertz).

---

[5] A chip is a small box with prongs to enable it to be attached to the motherboard, which is the key to making the computer work.

The speed of processing is also affected by what is called "word size." This is not related to a word as we know it in reading, but to the number of **bits** that a computer processes at one time. If a CPU processes 16 bits of information at a time, it is said to be a 16-bit computer, and its word size is 16 bits. A computer that processes 32 bits of information at one time is a 32-bit computer and has a word size of 32 bits. The 32-bit computer, of course, is faster than the 16-bit computer.

The Bus

The speed with which the computer returns results is affected not only by the speed of the CPU but also by the speed and width of a device called a bus. Like a bus one sees on a highway, a computer bus is a mode of transportation for data. Physically, a bus is a collection of wires that transmits data from one part of a computer to another, such as from the CPU to the main memory. It also transmits information about where the data should go. Like a CPU, the bus is measured by the number of bits it transfers at one time and the speed of this transfer.

Cards

Many of the functions that a computer performs are regulated by cards that are inserted into slots on the motherboard. These cards, which like the motherboard are printed circuit boards, are used for things such as the video display, network connections, and expansion.

How a Computer Works With Data

A computer does all its work on the basis of whether electronic circuits are on or off. In giving information to the computer, these conditions are represented by a one (1) if the circuit is on and a zero (0) if it is off. Because only 1s and 0s are used, the data are said to be binary system data. The decimal system with which we are familiar is base 10, that is, we start expressing our numbers by reusing the last numbers in multiples of 10, e.g., the number 11 reuses the 1 from the 10 and adds the 1, 20 reuses the 2 and adds numbers zero to nine, etc. In a binary system, which is base 2, numbers are reused starting with 3. Besides the binary system, two other numbering systems may be seen in computers: octal or base 8, and hexadecimal, which is base 16.

BITS AND BYTES

The amount of data that can be represented by one circuit is formally called a binary digit and is usually referred to as a bit. Bits hold only one of two values: 0 or 1. They are the smallest unit of information that a machine can hold. When eight of these bits are combined, there is enough memory, or on-off switches, to represent a letter, number, or other character. This amount of memory is called a **byte**.

ASCII

To make it possible for data to be exchanged between computers, standards were set very early in the evolution of the computer for how the on-off switches in a byte would be used for each character. The standard for PCs is the **American Standard Code for Information Interchange** (ASCII). Under this system, each character on the keyboard is represented by a number.

MEMORY

To work with data, to store it, and report it to users, computers need two types of memory: temporary and permanent. Temporary memory is what the computer uses to hold program instructions and data that are being created, edited, or used by a user. Anything temporary that the memory contains is deleted when the computer is turned off, unless it is a permanent resident on the computer such as software, or saved by the user when it is something the user created. Permanent memory is not really permanent in the sense that it cannot be changed or lost, but is a form of storage. It is the way that software and the file[6] users create using the software are preserved for future use.

---

[6] A file is anything that a user creates on a computer and saves.

Temporary Memory (Primary Memory)

This is the memory that is available to you for the software you use and the files you create. A file is anything that you create on a computer, including a word-processed document or a Microsoft PowerPoint® presentation. There are two types of primary memory. One is the memory that you the user have access to for the software you are using and the files that you create and is called random access memory (RAM). The second type is preprogrammed and unchangeable by the user and is known as read-only memory (ROM).

Read-Only Memory. The first type of memory, ROM, can only be read by the computer; no information can be written to it and no information can be erased or deleted from it. The users' only awareness of ROM may be when they see information flashing on the screen when the computer is turned on. The information in ROM is written to a chip before it is installed at the factory. It has no relationship to programs installed by a user or any data that a user creates on the computer. The set of instructions it contains are part of the processor of the computer. ROM is used to store critical programs that all computers need, such as the program that **boots** (starts) the computer. The BIOS, built-in software that determines what the computer can do without accessing any additional software, is usually found on a ROM chip. The last instruction that the BIOS executes is to look for an operating system[7] and install it.

Random Access Memory. RAM is the working or primary memory of the computer. It is temporary, or what is termed "volatile," and everything in it is lost when the computer is turned off unless it has been stored or saved. RAM is the memory area, where the software that is stored on a drive, often the main internal storage device of the computer known as a hard drive, is put when you ask to use a program

---

[7] Operating systems will be discussed in Chapter 3. An operating system is software that has the overall control of a computer, that is, it determines what software can be used.

such as a word processor, or a Web browser. RAM also stores the files on which you are working. When you close the program, it is erased from memory, but not from its storage place. To preserve the files that you create using a program, you must save the file before closing it or the program, or shutting down the computer.

When you open a program or a file, you are not removing it from its storage place but asking that a copy of the program or file be placed in RAM for your use. The original, however, remains on the storage device unless you give a command to delete it. What is not in storage, however, is any change you make to a file after it has been saved. That is, if you retrieve a file from storage and make changes to it, what is in storage is the file that was there when you retrieved it or last saved it. Thus, you must re-save a file for it to reflect what is currently in RAM. What does not need to be resaved is the application program because you have generally not changed it, but just used it. In the rare instance that you have made any changes to the program itself, such as changed what it contained on the top of the screen, you will be asked if you want to save these changes. If you like your changes, click Yes.

The amount of RAM that is needed depends on how the computer will be used. If all a computer will be used for is accessing the Web and perhaps a little word processing, it will need only enough RAM to accommodate the operating system's requirements and the applications. Users who routinely keep several programs open at once will want more than the minimum amount of RAM. When the RAM is inadequate to the tasks it is being called on to do, the computer slows down. This is caused by the computer having to exchange parts of the application that are in RAM with the parts that are on a disk that are now needed. Because this exchange is slower than the immediate access that RAM provides, the program slows down. Graphical programs such as picture-editing programs require a lot of RAM; hence, those who wish to use a computer for this purpose will want as much RAM as possible. Because the amount of RAM that a computer can access is dependent on the processor, one needs to have this information before deciding which computer to buy. A good rule of thumb is to buy as much RAM as the processor in the computer will support.

Cache. Cache, which is pronounced "cash," is a special high-speed storage mechanism that permits rapid access to frequently used data. It may be an independent storage device, or a reserved section of main memory. Cache is often used by hard drives, CPUs, and Web browsers. You may have heard the term "cache" in connection to your Web browser's memory or history of recently viewed pages. Two types of caching are commonly used in PCs: memory caching and disk caching. In memory caching, a special high-speed static RAM known as SRAM contains the data. In disk caching, the hard drive's hardware disk buffer stores the most recently accessed data from the disk. When there is a need to access data from the disk, the computer first checks the disk cache, because retrieving data from the disk cache is faster than from the disk.

Measurement of Memory

The measurement of memory of any type is based on the byte, or the amount of memory required to store one character such as the letter "L." It is expressed by placing prefixes in front of the word byte that denote increments of approximately 1000. A kilobyte is 1024 bytes, whereas a megabyte is more than 1 million bytes. Although the prefixes in Table 2-2 are from the decimal system, the words they create

TABLE 2-2 ● *The Bytes*	
Name	**Number of Bytes**
Kilobyte	1024
Megabyte	1,048,576
Gigabyte	1,073,741,824
Terabyte	1,099,511,627,776
Petabyte	1,125,899,906,842,624
Exabyte	1,152,921,504,606,846,976
Zettabyte	1,000,000,000,000,000,000,000 (approx.)
Yottabyte	1,000,000,000,000,000,000,000 (approx.)

do not represent numbers divisible by 10 because the amounts are translations from the binary numbering system. The same prefixes are used to describe the number of hertz or the measurement of the computer's clock speed. Thus a GHz would be 1,073,741,824 hertz or cycles per second.

"Permanent" or Secondary Memory

Secondary memory provides a form of permanent storage for a computer. This type of storage is permanent only in that the user determines whether or not this data will be retained. Except for files in ROM, a user can delete any data in secondary memory. For many programs and users, this type of storage is on the computer's **hard disk**, (a large storage device internal to PCs). For those who might be concerned that they would accidentally delete an application program from the hard disk, be assured that this action requires a great deal of effort and is very unlikely to be done accidentally. Additionally, a copy of any application programs on the computer should either be on another storage mechanism that is not attached to the computer, or available from the Internet. Many devices are used to provide storage. They employ either magnetic or optical methods of storing data.

Magnetic Storage. Magnetic storage takes advantage of the on-off capacity for bytes that a computer uses and stores information by making the polarity of a magnetic field positive for the 1 or "on" bytes and negative for the 0 or "off" bits. Audio and videotape are examples as are some of the various disks and diskettes used for storing computer data.

Tape Drive. Tape is the least expensive medium for storage and is still used, particularly where large storage capacities are needed. The disadvantage to tape as secondary memory is that, like tape in a tape recorder, it is accessed sequentially versus the random access of diskettes. Thus, to read a specific block of data, it is necessary to read all the preceding blocks, making tapes too slowly for general-purpose storage. Tapes have a storage size from a few hundred kilobytes to hundreds of gigabytes.

On the plus side, a fast tape drive can transfer as much as 120 megabytes per second. In the late 1970s and early 1980s, tape drives were used on PCs, but because of their disadvantages they were replaced by diskettes.

Magnetic Disks. Magnetic disks store information in a magnetized format. Lower–storage capacity magnetic diskettes consist of a core of a plastic sheet, whereas larger-capacity disks often have a glass or aluminum core. No matter what material is used to create the core, the base is covered with a thick coating of a magnetizable substance. When in use, the material in this coating is organized so that each bit of information is represented as either magnetized (on) or not magnetized (off). Because magnetizable material is used, the disk can be remagnetized (i.e., rewritten) many times.

Before being used, a magnetic disk needs to be formatted. Formatting puts the magnetic covering of the disk into a pattern so that the operating system with which it will be used can send or retrieve information from it. This process creates what is called a FAT, an acronym for file allocation table. The FAT is the portion of the disk that contains the table of contents of the disk, which is used to locate requested information.

Disks are used in what are called disk drives. This drive contains a "read/write" head and a mechanism that can rapidly spin the disk. As the disk is spinning, the read/write head finds the location of the requested information by using the FAT and retrieves the information in the form of bits that are either "on" or "off."

Diskettes. The original "floppy diskettes" were 8 inches in diameter and used on dedicated word processors. When the first PCs arrived, 5¼-inch diskettes were the norm, although very early PCs used tape drives for storage. These diskettes were a thin sheet of material with a magnetic center and were quite floppy! By the 1990s this type of diskette was being replaced by a firm 3½-inch disk. Each of these progressions was accompanied by an increase in the amount of information (measured in

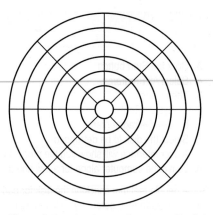

Figure 2-1 • Anatomy of a magnetic disk.

Disks are made up of tracks and sectors that create areas on the disk that can be labeled. The "address" of a file in the FAT table is recorded according to the labels given to the sectors.

Large drives may have several layers formatted in this manner.

bytes) that the disk could hold. Figure 2-1 shows the structure of a magnetic diskette.

Diskettes are not an integral part of a computer and can be stored away from the computer. To read and/or write information to them requires that they be inserted into the disk drive, which is generally a slot in the front (on the side of a laptop) of the computer into which the disk can be inserted.

Magnetic storage on diskettes is subject to being corrupted, that is data can be made unretrievable, by another magnetic field. Although the storage mechanisms used today are fairly reliable, if you are using a magnetic disk (and this holds true for video tapes too), it is advisable to store them where they are safely away from items such as televisions, ringing telephones, or any electrical device. It is the magnetic field that these items create that can corrupt a disk. Hard drives, however, are not easily demagnetized without a very strong magnet such as a laboratory degausser (Keizer, 2004). The biggest advantage of magnetic storage devices is that they can be written to and rewritten to many more times than optical storage devices. See Box 2-2 for information about maintaining a hard disk.

Hard Drive

What is called a hard drive is a large capacity storage disk. Hard drive storage capacity in today's PCs is measured in gigabytes, but one expects to see terabyte storage in PC hard drives in the not too distant future. On home PCs

and many that are found in agencies[8], a hard drive, which is internal to the computer, is installed. Usually named "C:" this drive contains the operating system. Users often install the software that they have purchased on this hard drive, although some will use a program from another source. External hard drives or storage devices measured in gigabytes that can be connected to the computer when desired are also available. These external hard drives are often used for backing up information on the computer. Like their smaller counterparts, all hard drives need to be formatted for use with the operating system. Information is stored on them in the same method as on smaller disks. They are, however, much more stable than diskettes.

Zip/Jaz Drives. Before optical disk storage or external hard drives became economically available, the need for storage of information that exceeded the capacity of diskettes led to the development of both **Zip disks** and **Jaz disks**. Both were developed by the Iomega Corporation. Zip disks could hold about 100 or 250 megabytes of information, while a Jaz disk was capable of containing two gigabytes of data. This was in contrast to the 720 kilobytes that a double-sided 3½-inch diskette could hold. Neither of these storage mechanisms are used much today.

---

[8] Some agencies will install what look like PCs, but are more like thin clients. Or, if they are PCs, they may access all program applications from the network server rather than the hard disk.

Box 2-2 • Maintaining a Hard Disk

As you continually use your hard drive, saving, deleting, saving again a file, the access to files on the hard drive slows down. This occurs because the FAT saves files in those sectors you see in Figure 2-1, but often a file size exceeds the size of the sector (technically known as clusters). When that happens, the FAT looks for the next vacant sector on the disk and makes a note of where on the disk the next part of the file is located. This creates files that are fragmented, or files with parts stored randomly around the disk.

When we request that a file be retrieved, the FAT tells the read/write head on the disk drive where on the disk to find the file. When it has to keep moving around the disk to find all the parts of a file, or to save one, these processes slow down. To put the disk back into a condition in which all parts of all files are contiguous, a process known as defragging the disk should be done periodically. How often depends on the type of use as well as the size of the hard drive.

To make this task easy on Microsoft Windows® computers, a program called Disk Defragmenter (a coincidence no doubt) exists that performs this task. This process can take an hour or several hours depending on both the size of your disk and how long it has been since you last used this accessory. To access this program in Windows XP®:

1. Close all programs that are running, including your screen saver.
2. Delete any unwanted programs or files.
3. Click the Start button.
4. Select All Programs.
5. Then select:
   a. System Tools
   b. Disk Defragmenter
6. Select the disk to be defragged.
7. A user interface will show you the progress.
8. Leave the computer alone for a few hours.

Some people feel that checking the disk for bad sectors should be performed before trying to defrag the disk. To do this:

9. Close all programs.
10. Click the Start button.
11. Select Computer (or My Computer).
12. Right click the disk you wish to check.
13. Click Properties.
14. Click the Tools tab.
15. Click Check Now under Error-checking.

The Windows Vista® operating system automatically defrags the disk on a set schedule as well as looks for and repairs bad sectors. If you wish to do this manually:

1. Click the Windows logo in the lower left corner:
2. Click Computer in the right column.
3. Right click the disk you wish to check.
4. Select Properties.
5. Click the Tools tab and make your choice.

Flash Drive. A flash drive is a flash memory storage device that plugs into a universal serial bus (USB) port. One can think of it as both the drive and the disk in one, although the similarity ends there. Flash memory is memory that can be erased and reprogrammed in units termed "blocks." It differs from the more common type of erasable memory by erasing and rewriting these blocks in a "flash" from which its name is derived (Collins & de Silva). Disks write and rewrite using individual bytes. Flash drives are popular because they are rewritable, can hold up to several gigabytes of information, and are small, fast, reliable, relatively inexpensive per byte, and portable. They are also easily lost!

One caution with flash drives, including card readers for cameras: Unlike other non-temporary memory, a flash drive is the drive and disk in one small piece of hardware. Consequently, the power that they need is derived from the computer itself. Although they can be inserted into a USB port with the computer on, they should be removed with more thought and never in the middle of being written to or reading from them. The safest way to remove them is to right click the Safely Remove Disk icon in the lower right corner of the screen (if it is not visible, click the "<" at the end of the icons. Then follow the steps in Figure 2-2.

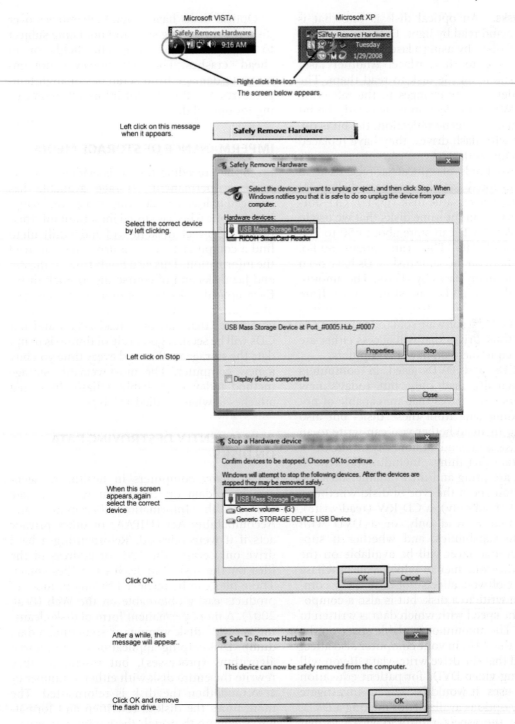

Figure 2-2 • Safely removing a flash drive.

Optical Disks. An optical disk is one that is written to and read by light. Data are recorded on optical disks by using a laser to burn microscopic pits onto the surface. Another laser beam is shone on the disk to read them. The pits are detected by changes in the reflection pattern. When a reflection is detected, the bit is on; when there is no reflection, the bit is off. Together with flash drives, they have replaced diskettes for storage.

The two kinds of optical storage used in computers today are the compact disk (CD) and the digital versatile disk (DVD). CD storage originated on the same disks that we use in audio disks. A CD can store about 650 to 700 megabytes of data. They can contain audio, video, or both on the same disk. CDs have been replaced in many cases by DVDs. The amount of data that a DVD can store varies from 4.7 gigabytes to almost 10 gigabytes depending on the disk. Most software sold today is on a CD or DVD; thus, drives that will access either are standard equipment on newer computers.

The CDs and DVDs used in computers were originally read only, but today's new computers have drives that are capable of not only reading data from these disks but also writing to them. Whether you can write to an optical disk is dependent not only on the drive but several other things, including the type of disk you are using and the available software. Information about the type of disk, whether a CD-ROM (read only), a CD-RW (read/write), a DVD that is read only, or a DVD with read/write capabilities, and whether it supports a double layer will be available on the label of the container in which you purchase the disk. Software affects not only if the computer can write to a disk, but is also a component of the speed with which data is written to the disk. The amount of available space on the disk and the RAM in your computer also affect the speed that the drive writes data. If you will be burning video DVDs for patient education or other uses, it would be wise to investigate the many options available for making a DVD, including the aspect ratio and video format that are available in the help feature for Windows Vista®.

Optical disks have several advantages over diskettes, including size, and not being subject to corruption from magnetic fields or to "head" crashes. They are, however, not immune to damage from scratches or high temperatures. See Box 2-3 for information on caring for optical disks.

IMPERMANENCE OF STORAGE MEDIA

From the preceding text, it is evident that the type of "permanent" storage available has changed in less than 20 years and is still changing. Anyone who has stored important information on a 3½-inch diskette will find it difficult to find a computer that has a drive that can read the information. This also holds true for the Zip and Jaz disks and of course the 5¼-inch disks. Even optical disks are not immune to this type of obsolescence. In the not too distant future, computers that can only read DVDs and not CDs will be seen. A good rule of thumb is to update the storage media used every time you buy a new computer. The most versatile storage method today is probably a flash drive that attaches to what is called a USB port.

PERMANENTLY DESTROYING DATA ON DISKS

Today many computers in healthcare agencies have data on them that would violate the Health Information Portability and Accountability Act (HIPAA) or other privacy acts if it were released. Reformatting a hard drive only erases the FAT, or address of the files on the disk, but leaves the files intact. These files can be retrieved by any number of products easily obtainable on the Web (Beal, 2007). A more permanent form of disk cleansing is called **disk wiping**, or sometime a **data dump**. Disk-wiping applications use different algorithms (processes), but essentially they rewrite the entire disk with either a number or zero, and then the disk is reformatted. The more times the disk is rewritten and formatted, the more thorough the wiping process is. A government's standard (DoD5330.33M), which provides medium security, requires

---

Box 2-3 • Caring for Optical Disks

DO:

1. Keep the disks clean.
   a. Clean with a clean cotton cloth by wiping from the center to the outer edge, not around the disk which can cause scratches.
   b. Use isopropyl alcohol or methanol or CD/DVD cleaning detergent for stubborn dirt.
2. Handle the disk by the center hole, or the edges. Some disks are two sided so be careful of both sides.
3. Put the disk back in a hard plastic case as soon as you eject it from the computer.
4. Store the disk:
   a. Upright like a library book.
   b. In moderate temperatures.
   c. Away from smoke or other air pollutants.
   d. Out of sunlight.
5. Label the plastic case containing the disk, not the disk.
6. Realize that the length of time before data is corrupted on an optical disk is directly proportional

to the conditions under which it is stored and the quality of the disk.

7. Update the storage mechanism with every new computer.

DO NOT:

8. Attach an adhesive label to the disk. The adhesive in the label can corrupt data within a few months.
9. Write on or scratch either side of the disk with any object. Pens or pencils scratch the surface and solvent-based markers may dissolve the protective layer.
10. Expect data on an optical disk to last longer than five years.

REFERENCE

Smith, J. (2008). *Computer basics: Storage optical disks.* Retrieved November 12, 2008, from http://www.jegsworks.com/Lessons/lesson6/lesson6-9.htm

---

three repeats of a two-step process. Each time the process is performed, two passes are made; first the drive is overwritten with ones, and then with zeros. After the third time, a government-designated code of 246 is written on the drive, which is verified by a final pass using a read-verify pass.

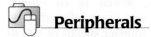

Peripherals

A **peripheral** is any external device such as a keyboard, monitor, or mouse, which is connected to the computer. Because they are external in desktops, it is easy to see that these are peripherals. On laptops, however, the connection of keyboards and monitors is internal. In general, peripherals are the devices that allow inputting of data to a computer and outputting of information from a computer. Besides these obvious peripherals, there are many others such as printers (output) and scanners (input) that allow humans to use computers. See Appendix A (on thePoint) for a description of all input

devices. Although the CPU would happily complete any instructions it received without any visible output, users generally want some type of output, such as what is seen on a monitor or video screen (see Appendix B on thePoint for a description of all output devices). There are also devices that both input and output information to a computer such as the port to which a printer is connected. (See Appendix C on thePoint for a description of all devices that serve both input and output functions.)

DIGITAL CAMERAS

Digital cameras are finding a place in healthcare for purposes such as recording the healing progress of wounds. Text descriptions cannot compare with a picture in letting clinicians and patients see healing progress.

SCANNERS

Scanners take a picture of a document and then allow users to save this as a file. Unless there is character recognition software available, any text that is scanned will be in a picture format and uneditable. Additionally some healthcare agencies are inputting clinical records to electronic health records by scanning free text. Even when character recognition software is used to translate the words in the "picture" to text, the result needs to be checked for accuracy. Further, unless the form that is scanned is especially designed for scanning, this free text is unstructured and not easily used for reporting information from data.

CLINICAL MONITORS

Clinical monitors can be part of a network and monitored at a central location. They can also be programmed to provide alarms, either at the central station or to individual pagers, when the monitor shows something beyond the norm. Clinical monitors whether attached to a network, or not, can allow patient data such as that produced by cardiology or fetal monitors to be directly input to a computer. The advantage of computerized clinical monitoring is that it allows one person to monitor many patients at once as well as provide notification of problems. It should never be allowed to reduce nurse–patient interaction.

 ## Connecting Peripherals

A peripheral is connected to a computer through a **port**.[9] Although today the USB port is the de facto standard for PCs, in the past there were other types of ports such as **serial and parallel**. (See Appendix B for a description.) Computers manufactured in the last few years do not have serial or parallel ports.

USB PORT

A USB port or universal serial bus is a standard that was originally created to connect phones to PCs in the mid-1990s ("Everything USB . . . We Mean Everything!"). Lately, it has become the standard port for connecting peripherals[10] to PCs. These ports are a thin slot, about half inch by one fourth of an inch, which are found on the sides of laptops and on the front of newer desktops or towers. The port is designed with a solid piece in one part, usually the top, so that USB device can only be inserted one way.

The original USB port was capable of transmitting data at only 12 megabits (Remember, it takes 8 bits to form a byte, which is required to transfer one letter) per second, which made it useful for only mice and keyboards ("Everything USB . . . We Mean Everything!"). This easy connection method, however, created a revolution that resulted in devices such as flash drives, external hard drives, and webcams, which needed faster transmission speeds. This need was met by a new standard, the USB2.0 port, which transmits information at 480 megabits per second. The USB connection has largely replaced older serial and parallel connectors.

FIREWIRE

Firewire originated in the mid-1980s as a high-speed data transfer method for Macintosh internal hard drives (Nathanael, 2006). Apple presented this technology to the Institute of Electrical and Electronics Engineers (IEEE) who in December 1995 released IEEE 1394, which is an official Firewire standard. It was often referred to as Firewire 400 and had transfer speeds of 100 to 400 megabits per second. In April 2002, the IEEE released a new standard for Firewire 800, which can theoretically transfer data at up to 3.2 gigabits per second.

Although its speed is faster than USB ports, it is impractical for low-bandwidth devices. This fact, together with the knowledge that only Macintoshes include Firewire ports by

---

[9] The term port is also used for networking connections. Internet connection ports are all internal to the computer.

[10] Docking station connections are one exception to this rule.

default, has kept it out of the mainstream. Because of its superior ability to transfer uncompressed video from digital camcorders, it is now found in all modern digital camcorders. Most digital cameras, however, still use USB to transfer images because USB ports are today standard equipment on computers.

Infrared Port

An infrared (IR) port is a connection on a computer that uses IR signals to wirelessly transmit information between devices such as a PDA and a computer. It has a range of about 5 to 10 feet. Most handheld devices have the capability to communicate via IR ports that allow the device to directly interface with another device to exchange data.

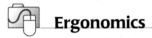

Ergonomics

Ergonomics is the science of designing a work environment so that it is convenient to use and does not prove injurious to health. Although it is an important consideration for preventive health, it is too often overlooked when setting up computer hardware. This despite the fact that using a keyboard injures more workers in the United States than any other workplace tool (Bailin, 1995)! Even nurses who do not spend all day at the computer are affected. One study from a Scandinavian journal, reported by Nielsen and Trinkoff (Nielsen & Trinkoff, 2003) found that some nurses, even those who use a computer less than four hours a day, had a 32% prevalence of upper arm repetitive stress injury, 60% of which was carpal tunnel syndrome.

Healthcare agencies, which should be very concerned about preventing injuries associated with any repetitive activity such as typing, could save money by focusing more on ergonomics. Computers are supposed to facilitate data recording, not impose additional burdens on healthcare personnel. Those planning a system should walk a day in the shoes of a user or several days in the shoes of several users before making firm decisions about computer placement. Asking staff nurses and other clinical computer users to participate in determining computer workstation design is another way of improving ergonomics (Nielsen & Trinkoff, 2003).

Unfortunately, few studies have been done on nursing use of computers with most research concentrating on seated workstations (Nielsen & Trinkoff, 2003). Some simple things could improve the work environment of nurses who document with or otherwise use computers. For nurses who are on their feet all day, if they are to chart at the point of care, they need a way to be able to sit while using the computer. If the computer is also used by those standing, an adjustable computer stand could be employed so that a user who is standing does not have to stoop. Additionally, if the computer is fixed at a height for users who are standing, a stool should be provided for the nurse who uses the computer extensively. Touch screens and light pens may be ideal for quick entry, but for extended entries, they are very tiring to the arm. Providing dual means of entry may solve this situation. Resolution of a screen is also important. The higher the resolution, the easier the screen is on the eyes. It is also important to prevent glare on the screen. In situations where this is impossible, it is possible to purchase screen filters that will cut down the glare.

More thought also needs to be given to how a workstation is designed for those who will use a computer for more than four hours a day. Consideration needs to be given to the posture the user will be forced to adopt. The best chairs have adequate support for the outward curve of the lumbar spine and the inward curve of the thoracic spine. Studies have shown that a 100 to 110 reclined position is better than an upright posture (Cornell University Ergonomics Web, 2007). The feet should be flat on the floor, or a footrest should be provided (Figure 2-3). Wrists, knuckles, and the top of the forearm should fall into a straight line while typing (Bailin, 1995). To promote circulation to the lower arm and hand, the elbow angle should be open. Both of

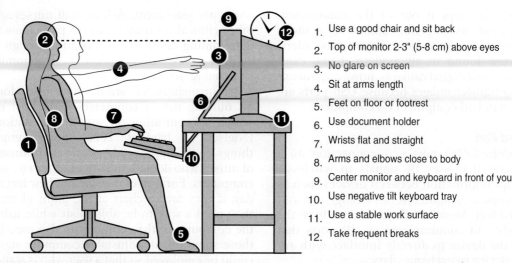

1. Use a good chair and sit back
2. Top of monitor 2-3" (5-8 cm) above eyes
3. No glare on screen
4. Sit at arms length
5. Feet on floor or footrest
6. Use document holder
7. Wrists flat and straight
8. Arms and elbows close to body
9. Center monitor and keyboard in front of you
10. Use negative tilt keyboard tray
11. Use a stable work surface
12. Take frequent breaks

Figure 2-3 • Ideal computer posture. (Reprinted with permission of Professor Ann Hedge. From a class project of the DEA651 class of 2000. Found at http://ergo.human.cornell.edu/dea6512k/ergo12tips.html)

these can be accomplished with a negative tilt keyboard (Cornell University Ergonomics Web). The monitor should be placed directly in front of the user to avoid neck twisting. Studies have found that the best position for the monitor is for the center of the screen to be about 17.5 degrees below eye level and about an arm's length away. The ideal placement of a mouse is on a flat, movable mouse platform positioned one to two inches above the numeric keypad. An excellent checklist for workstation design can be found at http://www.osha.gov/SLTC/etools/ computer-workstations/checklist.html

Laptops, under most use conditions, violate all ergonomic requirements for computers (Cornell University Ergonomics Web, 2004). This is caused by the connection between the keyboard, screen, and computer. It the computer rests on a table, the keyboard will be too high for proper arm positioning. If the computer is lower, the monitor placement may require that the head be tilted forward for use. For these reasons, if a laptop is your primary computer, to provide more ergonomic working conditions you should invest in a docking station. If you carry the laptop and all the required accessories such as spare battery, power cord, or external drive weighing 10 pounds or more, consider a wheeled carrying case.

Infection Control

Computers, particularly keyboards, have become commonplace in healthcare settings and are easily contaminated with potentially pathogenic microorganisms (Rutala, White, Gergen, & Weber, 2006). Many studies have demonstrated the presence of these organisms, not only in healthcare agencies but also on a nurse's home computer (Neely, 2002). These studies also demonstrated that these organisms can be spread to patients. Although hand-washing before touching a keyboard or any other computer part can help, all computer peripherals in a room should be routinely cleaned with a solution recommended by infection control personnel. If possible, engineering the physical environment to prevent contamination should also be done.

Computerese

Many computer-related terms are used in discussion, instruction, and advertising. Although they are not strictly hardware terms, they can often be confusing. If one watches a computer when it has just been turned on, one will see different types of information flashing across the screen. This information is produced by what is called the "booting" process. **Booting** refers to all the self-tests that a computer performs and the process of retrieving, either from the BIOS or a disk, the instructions necessary to allow the user to start using the computer. The term "reboot" means to restart the computer. A **warm boot** is restarting the computer without turning it off, a selection that is offered when one elects to start turning off the computer. A **cold boot** is starting the computer when the power is completely off. Avoid cold boots if you can, because the jolt of electricity received each time the computer is turned on may shorten its life span. Warm boots are often used when a computer freezes or crashes. It erases information in RAM, which often eliminates memory conflicts that may have caused the problem. These conflicts can be caused by different programs trying to store data in the same location. If a warm boot fails to notify the programs that it is time to stop fighting for the same space and give control back to the user, the machine must be turned off for a cold boot.

A **bug** is a defect in either the program or hardware that causes a malfunction. It may be as simple as presenting the user with a blood pressure chart when a weight chart was requested, to a more serious defect that causes the entire system to crash.

Compatibility refers to whether programs designed for one chip will work with an older or newer chip, or whether files created with one version of a program will work with another version of the same program. Most computer chips and software are **backward compatible**, that is, they will work with older versions of a program or files created with an older version of a program. Some are not, however, **forward compatible**, or the situation in which an older program does not recognize files created by a newer version of the same program. This is particularly true of spreadsheets, databases and presentation programs.

A **driver** is a software program that allows data to be transmitted between the computer and a device that is connected to the computer. Drivers are generally specific to the brand and model of the device. They may come with a new peripheral, or can often be downloaded from the vendor's Web site.

Although the term **hacker** originally meant a person who enjoyed learning about computer systems and was often considered an expert on the subject, mass media have turned it into a term to refer to individuals who gain unauthorized access to computer systems for the purpose of stealing and corrupting data. The original term for such a person was **cracker**. Today, differentiations may be made by using the term **white hat hacker** for a person who uses his or her computer knowledge to benefit others. **Black hat hacker** is the term used for those who use their computer skills maliciously.

When used with a computer the terms **logical** and **physical** refer to where data are located in the computer. The physical structure is the actual location, whereas a logical structure is how users see the data. For example, when a user requests information about laboratory tests, he or she may see the indications for the test, the normal values, the cost of a test, and the patient's test results. Although this information may be presented as one screen, which is a logical structure, different pieces will have been retrieved from different files in different locations, which is the physical structure of the information.

Another potentially confusing computer term is **object**. Although the more common use of the term "object" is for a physical entity, or at least a picture on the screen, to a computer, an object is anything the computer can manipulate. That is, an object can be a letter, word, sentence, paragraph, piece of a document, or an entire document. Objects can be nested, that is, a word is an object nested within a sentence object. A paragraph is an object that is contained in a document. When an object is selected, clicking the right mouse button presents a menu of properties of that object that can be changed.

Summary

Understanding how computers function forms the background for a beginning understanding of informatics. Computers are devices, which, although we may anthromorphize them, are still inanimate objects. Computers do not think; they need explicit instructions and are incapable of interpreting gray areas. This is not to say that gifted programmers cannot make one think a computer is behaving in a seemingly human manner.

Like informatics, computers have many different types and parts. When all these parts function together along with human interventions, the results benefit healthcare. Regardless of size, all computers possess some given parts, a CPU, memory, storage devices, and ways to both enter and retrieve data. How many and how much of each of these parts a computer needs depends on the function the computer is intended to serve and often the depth of the owner's pocketbook. Understanding the function of each of these parts allows nurses to creatively and effectively use a computer both professionally and personally.

Computers, however, are not without their hazards in healthcare. Their parts, particularly mice and keyboards, are capable of harboring pathogenic microorganisms, which have been known to create infections in patients. Data that they can contain could create harm if it became known; hence, computers that will need to be discarded must have their internal storage devices thoroughly wiped before being released.

APPLICATIONS AND COMPETENCIES

1. A friend tells you that the defeat of Gary Kasparov by Deep Blue indicated that computers can think. How would you respond?
2. You need to help a colleague, who is afraid of computers, learn to use one. Outline a plan to help this person reduce his or her anxiety.
3. Identify the battery type in a healthcare device and plan how the battery life can be prolonged in a clinical situation.
4. To what uses would you put a digital camera in a healthcare situation?
5. List disadvantages to scanning free text into an electronic health record.
6. In a clinical area with which you are familiar, identify situations that may lead to nosocomial infections. Propose a plan to lower the chances of occurrences of these infections.
7. Evaluate a computer workstation for ergonomic factors and propose a plan to ameliorate any difficult areas.
8. What steps would you suggest to overcome the negatives of clinical monitoring systems that allow many patients to be monitored at a central location?
9. Define the following in relationship to computers:
   a. Hacker
   b. Backward compatibility
   c. Logical
   d. Physical
   e. Warm boot
   f. Port
   g. Object
   h. Case sensitivity
   i. Disk wipe
   j. Docking station

REFERENCES

Bailin, J. (1995). *Ergonomics & computer injury: FAQs.* Retrieved November 12, 2008, from http://www.netsci.org/Science/Special/feature01.html

Beal, V. (2007, January 12). *How to completely erase a hard disk drive: Tips to avoid data theft when donating a computer system.* Retrieved November 12, 2008, from http://www.webopedia.com/DidYouKnow/Computer_Science/2007/completely_erase_harddrive.asp

Bloom, A. J. (1985). An anxiety management approach to computer phobia. *Training and Development Journal, 19*(1), 90–94.

Buchmann, I. (2005a). *Choosing the right battery for wireless communications (BU37).* Retrieved November 12, 2008, from http://www.batteryuniversity.com/parttwo-37.htm

Buchmann, I. (2005b). *The secrets of battery runtime (BU31).* Retrieved November 12, 2008, from http://www.batteryuniversity.com/parttwo-31.htm

Buchmann, I. (2005c). *What is the best battery?* Retrieved November 12, 2008, from http://www.batteryuniversity.com/partone-3.htm

Chan, M. F. (2007). A cluster analysis to investigating nurses' knowledge, attitudes, and skills regarding the clinical management system. *Computers, Informatics, Nursing: CIN, 25*(1), 45–54.

Collins, S., & de Silva, J. (November 23). *Flash memory.* Retrieved November 12, 2008, from http://searchstorage.techtarget.com/sDefinition/0,sid5_gci212130,00.html

Cornell University Ergonomics Web. *Ideal typing posture: Negative slope keyboard support.* Retrieved November 12, 2008, from http://ergo.human.cornell.edu/AHTutorials/typingposture.html

Cornell University Ergonomics Web. (2004, October 16). *5 Tips for using a laptop computer.* Retrieved November 129, 2008, from http://ergo.human.cornell.edu/culaptoptips.html

Cornell University Ergonomics Web. (2007, March 16). *Ergonomic Guidelines for Arranging a Computer Workstation—10 steps for users.* Retrieved November 12, 2008, from http://ergo.human .cornell.edu/ergoguide.html

Dillon, T. W., Blankenship, R., & Crews, T., Jr. (2005). Nursing attitudes and images of electronic patient record systems. *Computers, Informatics, Nursing: CIN, 23*(3), 139–145.

Everything USB. . . We mean everything! Retrieved November 12, 2008, from http://www.everythingusb.com

Focus. (1995). The impact of computer anxiety and computer resistance on the use of computer technology by nurses. *Journal of Nursing Staff Development, 11*(3), 172–175.

Keizer, G. (2004). *Busting the biggest PC myths* [Electronic version at http://www.pcworld.com/article/id,116572-page,1/article.html retrieved on November 12, 2008]. *PC World.*

McBride, S. H., & Nagle, L. M. (1996). Attitudes toward computers: A test of construct validity. Stronge and Brodt's Nurses' Attitudes Toward Computerization (NATC) questionnaire. *Computers in Nursing, 14*(3), 164–170.

Nathanael. (2006). *Firewire vs. USB: A comparison.* Retrieved November 12, 2008, from http://www.directron.com/firewirevsusb.html

Neely, S. (2002). Basic microbiologic and infection control information to reduce the potential transmission of pathogens to patients via computer hardware. *Journal of the American Medical Informatics Association, 9*(5), 500–508.

Nielsen, K., & Trinkoff, A. (2003). Applying ergonomics to nurse computer workstations: Review and recommendations. *Computers, Informatics, Nursing: CIN, 21*(3), 150–157.

Perry, W. E. (1982). *Survival guide to computer systems.* Boston, MA: CBI Publishing Company.

Rutala, W. A., White, M. S., Gergen, M. F., & Weber. D. J. (2006). Bacterial contamination of keyboards: Efficacy and functional impact of disinfectants [Electronic version]. *Infection Control Hosptial Epidemiology, 27*(4), 372–377.

Simpson, G., & Kenrick, M. (1997). Nurses' attitudes toward computerization in clinical practice in a British general hospital. *Computers in Nursing, 15*(1), 37–42.

CHAPTER 3

Software: Information Management

Learning Objectives

After studying this chapter you will be able to:

1. Describe features of operating systems.

2. Apply basic features of Microsoft Windows™ operating system.

3. Differentiate application software.

4. Define a computer algorithm.

5. Explain the importance of user groups.

6. Differentiate the various types of software copyright.

Key Terms

Active Window
Algorithm
Application Program
Code
Computer Crash
Disk Operating System (DOS)
Flow Chart
Freeware
Graphical User Interface (GUI)
Groupware
Mouse
Office Suites

Open Source
Operating System
Palm Operating System
Point and Click
Quick Launch Bar
Shareware
Software
Software Piracy
Speech Recognition
Task Bar
Title Bar
Windows Vista
Windows XP

The computer, despite all its parts, will do nothing but act as an expensive paperweight unless it is told what to do. These instructions, which allow us to manage data and information, come in the form of **software**, or computer programs. Many kinds of software exist. Basically, software manages either the computer system itself or information. Software that manages the computer system includes two overall items: those programs and utilities that reside in read-only memory (ROM), which enable the computer to boot, and system software. This latter category includes the **operating system** that controls the computer and the utilities that allow the user some control over that operating system. Software that manages user information is known as **application programs**. Application programs include information systems in healthcare agencies and off-the-shelf generic applications that can perform a variety of tasks. Examples of the latter include the many **office suites** such as Microsoft Office®, Corel WordPerfect Office®, and Lotus SmartSuite®. **Speech recognition** software that can convert spoken words to text is another type of application program. There are also software packages that allow users to organize and edit photos, create graphics including animation, create learning packages, and many other tasks.

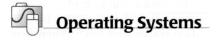 ## Operating Systems

Hands down, the most important program on your computer is the operating system. It coordinates input from the keyboard with output on the screen, responds to **mouse** clicks, heeds commands to save a file, retrieves files, and transmits commands to printers and other peripheral devices. It is the software platform on top of which all application programs run. Application programs are written to work with a specific operating system. Thus, the operating system that you select determines which applications you can run. Personal computers (PCs) today and most notebooks use a version of Microsoft Windows®. The Apple Macintosh® uses a different operating system, as do larger computers. The operating system on personal digital assistants (PDAs), or handhelds, varies, but most today use the Windows CE operating system, although some handhelds still use the **Palm operating system.**

The operating systems for large servers, such as those that control hospital information systems, have large responsibilities and powers (Webopedia, 2002). They must act like a traffic cop – making sure that different programs and users do not interfere with one another, as well as accept, store, and retrieve data. They are also responsible for ensuring that unauthorized users cannot access the system. In this chapter we will concern ourselves only with operating systems and software that one is likely to encounter on a PC.

DOS

Early PCs used the **DOS** operating system, which is an acronym for **disk operating system**. Although it could refer to any operating system, the term "DOS" came to mean the operating system developed by Microsoft® for PCs. DOS was text based, and it required users to remember a set of commands such as Delete, Run, Copy, and Rename. Unlike today's operating systems, DOS allowed only one program at a time to be operational. Transferring information between programs was difficult and time consuming, as was creating anything that was not text.

GRAPHICAL USER INTERFACES (GUI)

In a **graphical user interface** (GUI – pronounced "gooey"), users no longer had to remember esoteric commands. Instead commands are entered by "pointing and clicking." Pointing and clicking refers to moving a mouse,[1] which moves the screen mouse pointer in the direction that the mouse is moved. When the mouse pointer is in the desired location, the user taps (clicks) the left mouse button. GUIs are oriented to this **point and click** method of giving commands and to icons or small pictures instead of words.

GUIs were designed by the Xerox Corporation's Palo Alto Research Center in the 1970s (Webopedia, 2004). Because they required more CPU power and a high-quality monitor, which were then prohibitively expensive, they were slow to be accepted. It was the Apple Macintosh that first employed them,

---

[1] A device that behaves like a mouse does not always resemble the typical external mouse. On laptops it may be a small eraser type device in the middle of the keyboard, or a rectangular pad at the base of the keyboard with buttons beneath it. On this type of touch pad, tapping the pad after the mouse pointer is on the desired selection will evoke the command just as if the user had clicked the left mouse button.

followed in the late1980s by PCs. Most health-care agencies use PCs with Windows, thus this book will concentrate on that computer and operating system. Many home computers are Macintoshes, although the exact implementation of commands will not translate most of the principles and features that are discussed in this chapter, and others that address PCs will also be useful with that type of computer.

Microsoft Windows® Operating System

Because GUIs are easy to use, most healthcare information systems use a GUI operating system, usually a version of Microsoft Windows. For this reason, as well as the computer fluency demanded of healthcare professionals, it is appropriate to review some basics of using Windows. When a PC is turned on and finishes booting (often a three- to five-minute process!), the screen that appears is called the desktop. The desktop has icons representing many of the application programs that are installed on the computer. Below these icons is the name of the application that the icon represents. When "clicked" (putting the mouse pointer on the icon and left clicking), the program the icon represents will open.

OPENING A PROGRAM IN A PC

As with all things with Microsoft Windows®, there are several ways to start a program when using a PC. Clicking the icon on the desktop, mentioned earlier, is often used when the computer is first turned on. If an icon for the desired program is not on the desktop, the user should click the Start button, then click All Programs and click the name of the program on that list. The Start button, so called because it "starts" processes, in the lower left corner of the screen, is located in the lower left corner of the screen. In **Windows Vista®**, the start button is the Windows logo surrounded by a blue circle. Some programs that are together in a suite such as Corel Office®, Lotus SmartSuite®, or Microsoft Office® may require that the folder containing all of them

be opened, then the program selected from the secondary menu contained in the folder. In XP, this will be indicated by a black triangle mark pointing to the right. In Vista, a container for more programs will be the folder icon as seen in Figure 3-1. In either case, clicking the container will show the programs with that folder, and you can make your selection from there.

WORKING WITH A PROGRAM IN A PC

Once a program is opened, you will see the work screen, which may look like any of those in Figure 3-2. The choices on the menu bar can be clicked for a menu of features classified by that choice. If you are using Microsoft Word 2007®, the menu bar is replaced with tabs, which when clicked have icons for the features classified under that tab.[2] When first starting to use a new application program, or a major update, using Help to find the feature you want is often necessary.

All programs will have a symbol, which represents the mouse pointer, the shape of which may vary according to the task and the program. In some cases it can be changed by the user. In word processing software it is often a vertical "I" bar; in spreadsheets it may be a large plus sign; and in a presentation or graphics program, an arrow. Although many choices on the top of the screen may be represented by icons, if you rest the mouse pointer on an icon, after a few seconds words describing what the icon will open will appear.

MULTIPLE WINDOWS

One of the advances of GUIs over DOS included the ability to have multiple programs open at the same time and to easily move data between them. This makes it possible to copy a graph from a spreadsheet into a word processing document, or a graphic from PowerPoint into a spreadsheet or word processing document.

Closing Files and Programs

In the context of a PC, the term "windows" may refer to the operating system or to the

---

[2] There will be more about these choices in Chapter 4. In this chapter we are just looking at an overview.

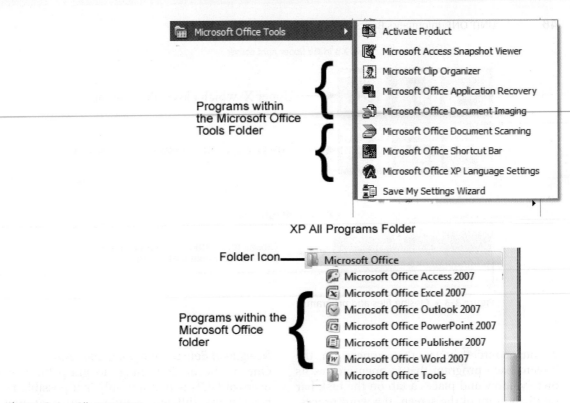

XP All Programs Folder

Programs within the Microsoft Office Tools Folder

Folder Icon

Programs within the Microsoft Office folder

Vista All Programs Folder

Figure 3-1 • All programs folders.

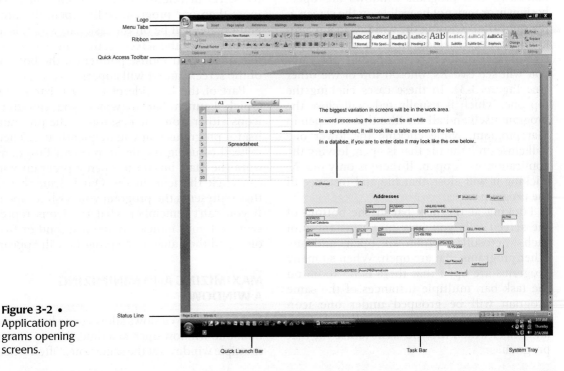

Figure 3-2 • Application programs opening screens.

Two X's in the upper right corner

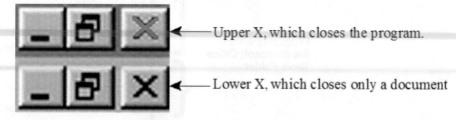

Upper X, which closes the program.

Lower X, which closes only a document

One X in the upper right corner

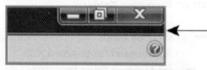

Closes this instance of the program
and the file within that program

Figure 3-3 • Closing files and programs.

various content boxes that appear on the screen. Each program that is open creates its own window and places a tab on the **task bar** on the bottom of the screen. If a word processor and a spreadsheet program are open simultaneously, two program windows are open; both may or may not be visible on the screen at the same time. Closing the window in any program involves clicking on an X in the upper right corner of the screen. In some programs you will see two Xs, one on top of the other (see Figure 3-3). In these cases clicking the top one, which is usually red, will close the program itself and all the files that are open in that program, while clicking the lower one will close only the file that is open, leaving the application itself open. If there is only one X, clicking it will close that file and instance of the program.

Looking at the task bar at the bottom of the screen tells you how many instances of each Microsoft program are open, and any other programs that are open. When so many programs are open that there is no room on the task bar, multiple instances of the same program will be grouped under one icon meaning that you will have to click that tab and select which file you wish to use for that program.

Navigating Between Programs and Files

One of the hardest things to grasp for new users of GUIs is that not only is it possible to have many different windows open at one time, but using this option is an aid to productivity. As mentioned earlier, when you have more than one program or file open, the program name will be on the task bar, which is at the bottom of the screen. If this line is not visible, place your mouse pointer on the bottom of the screen, and it will appear.

Part of the left side of the task bar is the **Quick Launch bar** to which you can drag icons either from the desktop or the program list for programs that you frequently use. Then instead of using the desktop or All Programs from the Start button to open a program you can click the icon in the Quick Launch bar that represents the program you wish to open. If you can't remember what the icons represent, rest your mouse pointer a second or two on it and the name of the program will appear.

MAXIMIZING AND MINIMIZING A WINDOW

Not only does Windows allow you to have more than one window open at a time, it lets you see multiple windows at the same time. Often when

When this icon is seen in the upper right corner of the screen, it indicates that the document is **maximized**. Clicking on it will minimize the document.

When this icon is seen in the upper right corner of the screen, it indicates that the document is **minimized**. Clicking on it will maximize the document.

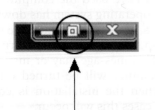
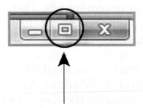

Click this button to make Window smaller or minimize the Window

Click this button to make Window fill entire screen or maximize the Window

Figure 3-4 • Maximizing and minimizing a window.

you open a program, you will see that it does not take up the entire screen. You may even see another program, or the desktop behind it. In this format, the window is said to be "minimized." This holds true whether it takes up almost the entire screen or is reduced to just the **title bar** (see Figure 3-4). You can maximize it by clicking the square in the upper right corner of the screen and minimize it by clicking the 3D square that replaces the original square when the window is maximized.

In a minimized format, you can place your mouse pointer on the sides of the window until it becomes a double-edged arrow ($\leftrightarrow$), then drag the side to change the size of the window. To move a window, place the mouse pointer in the title bar, or the top line of the window that has the name of the program and often of the file itself, and drag the window wherever you want it. If the windows overlap, the window that is the **active window**, or the window in which you are working, will be on top. Clicking in a window makes it the active window. If the windows are side by side, the active window is the one where the mouse pointer is, although sometimes the title bar will be a little darker in color in the active window. Placing windows side by side or one on top of the other can be very useful when working on two files

in the same program, or needing to synchronize files from different programs.

ACCESSORIES AND UTILITIES

Operating systems usually come with some utilities and built-in software. Certain utilities are helpful with disk maintenance, such as the disk utilities ScanDisk and Disk Defragmenter discussed in Chapter 2. Additional accessories such as Paint, a simple drawing program, allow a user to create drawings or various shapes, such as circles, squares, or triangles, in any of the colors available in the program. Also available are writing accessories such as Notepad, a product that is useful in creating files in ASCII (American Standard Code for Information Interchange), which is a format that can be read by many different programs.

EASE OF ACCESS

Given the prevalence of computers in today's society, and the increasing use that is being made of the Web for patient empowerment,[3] nurses need to be aware of the various options available

---

[3] See Chapter 15 for more information about facilitating computer use for patients with disabilities.

for helping those with disabilities to use computers. Both Apple Computers and Microsoft maintain pages that provide information about the various options to assist those whose disabilities present problems with using computers. Some examples of the adjustments that can be made with both **Windows XP®** and Vista® are changing how items on the screen are displayed, a screen magnifier, and an option to provide visual warnings for system sounds. There are also many options for changing how the keys on a keyboard work as well as the way the mouse behaves. In Windows XP, information about making these changes is available from the Accessibility Wizard; Windows Vista has an Ease of Access choice on the classic view of the Control Panel (accessible from the Start button). There is even a narrator that will read each character that is entered when using Microsoft Office Products. Microsoft's Web site at http://www.microsoft.com/enable/provides links to information about using these utilities in addition to tutorials and guides to accessibility options for many disabilities including dexterity problems. Apple Computer maintains a similar site for Macintosh users at http://www.apple.com/accessibility/

EXITING WINDOWS

In the earlier sections we have discussed how to close a file on which you are working, and how to close a program. Before shutting down a computer, it is necessary to exit Windows. Although invisible to users, Microsoft Windows, like all operating systems, actually works very hard behind the scenes to provide its many functions, as do many of the application programs. To do this, application programs and Microsoft Windows have to have easy access to specific information. Often, this is accomplished by creating files on the hard disk of the information that the application needs to use. These files are temporary and unknown to the users. They are created, changed, and deleted as users change what they are doing. Before quitting Windows, the application programs need to be able to shut these files down. If users do not exit all programs and close Microsoft

Windows properly, these temporary files are left on the disk and can cause problems as well as fill up your hard disk. To exit Windows and shut down your computer, click the Start button in the lower left corner of the screen, select Shut Down from the menu and let the computer go through the shutdown process, which may take a minute or more. If during the time you have used the computer, a program or the operating system has downloaded some updates, you may see a message that files are being updated, please don't turn off the computer. This message may or may not add that the computer will be turned off by the program, when the installation is complete, but in most cases this will occur.

HANDLING MINOR PROBLEMS

As robust as today's computers are, they sometimes get themselves tangled up and, through no fault of the user, refuse to respond to commands. This is most apt to happen to an individual program, not the entire computer. If you are working in a computer laboratory, or on an agency computer, leave the computer alone and notify the laboratory or network manager. If, however, you are home there are some things you can do. If you get a message saying, "This program is not responding" and are asked if you want to shut it down, you have no choice except to say yes. It may or may not shut down. If it does not, this is the time to use what is affectionately referred to as the "three finger salute," because it requires three fingers to execute. To carry it out you press down and hold the Ctrl, Alt, and Delete keys until you get a menu on which one of the choices is to open the task manager (Microsoft Vista) or the task manager itself (Microsoft XP). From there you can locate the offending program and click the End Task button (see Figure 3-5). You may then get still another window telling you that the program is not responding and asking you if you want to end it. You may need to tell it yes more than once! But eventually it will close the program. After letting it rest for a few minutes, you can then restart that program if you wish.

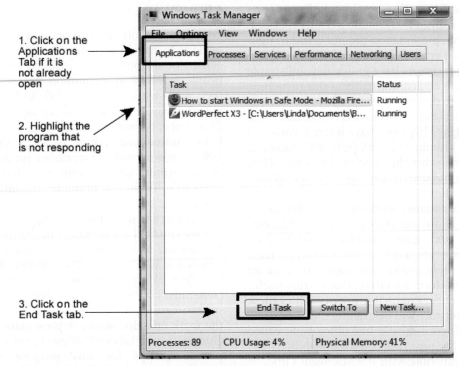

1. Click on the Applications Tab if it is not already open

2. Highlight the program that is not responding

3. Click on the End Task tab.

Figure 3-5 • Closing a nonresponding program.

The biggest drawback is that when a program **crashes**, you will lose whatever you have not saved, which is a reason to save continually as you work! However, most of today's programs will do a backup save every 10 or 15 minutes, a time that you can set in the preferences. After a program crash, when you reopen the program you will be told that it did not close properly last time and be asked about files that were open and not saved. The best approach is to look at each one and match with what you have on disk to see which is the latest version, the backup or the one you can retrieve from the disk.

On rare occasions, the above approach does not work, and the computer seems bent on doing its own thing with absolutely no regard for what you want. No matter what you do, you can't seem to get its attention. Those who program operating systems, knowing that despite all their efforts occasionally this can happen, have provided an out. To turn off a nonresponding computer, press the power button (yes, the power button on the CPU)

and hold it down until the computer turns off! If you are using an older laptop, you may need to remove the battery for a minute to cut off its power. After that you can restart the computer, and it will probably be back to normal! Beyond this, see your guru!

Application Programs

There are many different types of software application programs. You are probably familiar with a hospital information system, and possibly even programs that access the Web, or browsers, which are all application programs. There are many others that can improve your productivity professionally and personally. Word processors, spreadsheets, presentation programs, and databases form the bulk of professional use, whereas displaying, organizing, and printing photos are one of the main leisure uses of computers. There are many different software packages for any of these functions. Three vendors offer proprietary office suites that contain a word processor, spreadsheet, presentation program, and in their professional version, a relational database.[4]

Word processors have grown beyond simple text creation and editing to being able to include graphics in a document and produce pamphlets. Spreadsheets have many uses for tasks that focus on numbers. They even have limited statistical features, although a full-featured statistical package will serve this function far better. They are sometimes used as databases (Sewell, 2006), but unless the user needs only a simple database, a relational database works far better. Relational databases allow users to track, summarize, manipulate, and gain knowledge from data. Presentation programs allow users to create computer slide shows, although care must be taken to produce something that is truly useful to an audience. Productive use of each of these types of software will be examined in a separate chapter. There is also a free office suite called Open Office.org (http://www.openoffice.org/) that is compatible with the Microsoft Office™ products. The two other proprietary office suites, Corel™ and Lotus™, will also create files that are compatible with Microsoft Office products. There are several photo editing and printing packages, some come with a digital camera, others are proprietary, such as Adobe Photoshop™, and some are even free, such as Picasa (http://picasa.google.com/).

SOFTWARE FOR COMPUTER-TO-COMPUTER COMMUNICATION

As soon as computers could store information, the desire to share this information between computers arose. It was, however, the development of a standard method of computer communication and production of inexpensive modems that made this interaction available to the general public. This software includes email and networking packages.[5]

---

[4] Corel™, Microsoft™, and Lotus™. The Lotus Office Suite comes complete with a relational database in its regular version.

[5] Computer-to-computer communication software is examined in Chapters 5 and 6.

GROUPWARE

Groupware is software that permits two or more persons to have a meeting, work on a file together, or do both. It is designed to facilitate people involved in a common task to achieve their goals without meeting face to face. These meetings can be synchronous, or asynchronous. This category was introduced in 1989 when Lotus introduced Lotus Notes™ (Woolley, 1996), an outgrowth of an earlier product used on the mainframe. The term as currently used refers to software that promotes not only group discussion, but an array of activities such as scheduling and document sharing.

One can find a wide range in the features in groupware, as well as the definitions. Wikis, which are user-created information sites, are one type of groupware as is text messaging. Generally, however, the term refers to a more sophisticated product in which users share the work on a document or presentation. Both Google™ and Yahoo™ allow users to create private groups for this purpose without charge. There are also many proprietary products. Some of these products allow the meeting coordinator to show a screen that all see, some also allow the use of cameras. A quick search with a Web search engine will find many such programs.

SPEECH RECOGNITION

Speech, or voice, recognition in the context of computer input,[6] is the ability of a computer to recognize spoken words and translate them into printed text. This must not to be confused with understanding what is said; that is a function of a field called natural language processing (Webopedia, 2007). With the increased power of computers and improved microphones, voice recognition systems have greatly improved since the early days when using one could be an exercise in frustration. The two types of voice recognition are discrete and continuous speech processing. Discrete speech processing, which is not used much today, requires the speaker to

---

[6] Voice recognition can also refer to the forensic voice recognition.

say one word at a time, pausing briefly after each word. In continuous speech processing, the user can speak at a normal rate, although speaking distinctly is necessary.

In the past, systems required the user to train the program extensively to understand the spoken word. The training consisted of the user repeating those words the computer would be required to understand, until the word was recognized as spoken by that person. Some systems today are capable of recognizing the spoken word from different people without this special training, but for optimal use of more than a few phrases, all require some training (Seymour, 2001). The accuracy of voice software is also affected by the quality of the microphone used for voice input.

Speech recognition has received a welcome reception in the field of medical transcription. To meet this need, and because the vocabulary used is quite different from everyday use, several companies have introduced systems that have a large built-in vocabulary that focus on a specific field, such as radiology. No matter how good a speech recognition program is, proofing the result is very necessary.

Microsoft made speech recognition software available as an accessory that could be downloaded with Service Pack 1 for Windows XP™. (See http://www.microsoft.com/windows xp/using/setup/expert/moskowitz_02september 23.mspx for how to do this.) With Vista, it is an integral part of the operating system and is an accessory, although you may have to use the Help and Support options to find it. With training, it can provide good speech recognition. It is useful, however, only with Microsoft products.

Installing Software

Installing a legal copy of software, after the computer hard drive is set up for use, is usually quite easy. A good rule of thumb to follow is to first close all other applications before installing something new. After that, insert the disk that the program is on and follow the screen directions. At one point you will have to check a box, indicating that you accept the licensing agreement. Unless you are very versed in file and disk anatomy, it is best to let the program decide into what folder (named container on a disk) it will install itself, and select the usual installation process. In Windows Vista, you must have administrator privileges to do the installation, a process that can prevent programs that would harm the computer from installing themselves without user knowledge. On laboratory or agency computers, you will probably not be allowed to install any program on the computer. This protects the agency against illegal software and software that could interfere with the network system.

Creating Software

Software is created using a programming language, of which there are many. There are also different levels of languages. These levels depend on the degree to which the language approaches "natural language" – the higher the level, the closer to regular language. The drawback is that as the level of the language increases the flexibility of the language decreases. The lowest level, machine language, communicates directly with the zeros and ones that represent bits. The next level, assembly language, uses cryptic names instead of numbers to translate commands to the machine language. Level three, or the so-called high-level languages, includes such well-known languages as COBOL, FORTRAN, and Basic. Fourth-level languages are designed for a specific purpose. Structured query language (SQL) is a fourth-level language designed specifically to query relational databases. Ultimately, no matter which level language is used or which language a program is written in, it must be translated to machine language in a process called compiling.

Computer software works by taking a user's commands and quickly providing the computer with a detailed step-by-step set of instructions in such a manner that the computer can understand and comply. These instructions are called **code**. Before a single line of code is written, it is necessary to define the

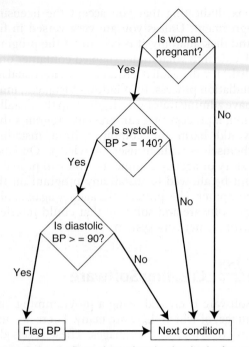

Figure 3-6 • A flow chart that is the basis for an algorithm.

problem the computer is to solve and develop a **flow chart** of instructions. From this flow chart, a detailed set of instructions can be developed and turned into code. These instructions are known as an **algorithm**. A flow chart in computer programming is like a flow chart used to model any process. It is a pictorial representation of the process or project being planned with decision points. Flow charts provide people with a common understanding of the process. Figure 3-6 shows an example of a flow chart.

As a healthcare professional, a nurse may be called on to assist in defining a problem or testing the proposed solution. Defining a problem with enough accuracy and detail so that the computer can be used to solve it is a difficult task. A simple problem such as asking the computer to flag vital signs that require nursing attention requires attention to many details. First, the nurse needs to determine the limits of normal. This may sound easy until the nurse remembers that in some cases, a

temperature elevated by 2.25°F may not be of any concern. In the same way, the nurse also must define "normal" pulse and respiration rates and blood pressures. To do this, the nurse must come up with a set of rules or algorithms stating what readings need flagging under which conditions.

This information is then programmed using "if-then-else" statements that tell the computer what to do if a certain condition exists. In the situation in Figure 3-6, an if/then statement would be part of the code for each of the decisions depicted. When one considers the many variables that impinge on clinical decisions, it becomes easy to see why humans must always evaluate computer output. Evaluation is helped if the nurse knows what limits were placed on each variable. In this example, the user would want to know that the computer flags the blood pressure for a pregnant woman only when the systolic exceeds 140 mm Hg and diastolic 90 mm Hg. Because it is highly unlikely that every condition can be programmed, it is imperative that computer users not rely solely on computer output for determining anomalies. There is no substitute for critical thinking by a perceptive healthcare professional. Common sense and expert intuition will *never* be replaced by a computer.

Open Source Software

Open source software is software that is copyrighted, but whose source code is available to anyone who wants it. The idea behind this is that when the source code is available, many programmers, who are not concerned with financial gain, will make improvements to the code and produce a more useful, bug-free product (Beal, 2005). This concept is based on using peer review to find and eliminate bugs, a process that is unfortunately absent in many proprietary programs. Open source grew in the technological community as a response to proprietary software owned by corporations.

User Groups

When learning to use any software, sources of help can be extremely useful. Whether using a book, teacher, or other source of instruction, questions arise for which answers are not readily available. One excellent source of help is a user group, which is a gathering of people who meet regularly for the purpose of sharing information about a given topic. There are user groups for PC application programs and hospital information systems. User group members range from novices to those who make a living as consultants for the program. The level of formal organization varies with the size and purpose of the group. Most user group meetings have an agenda that includes both a question-and-answer session and a presentation by a member or invited guest on some aspect of the group's focus.

There are few geographic areas today in the United States that do not have a computer user group for PCs or Macintoshes. In large cities, there may be one umbrella group with smaller significant interest groups (SIGs) that meet independently to learn more about a specific program. For more information about user groups and how to find a group, see the Web site for the Association of Personal Computer User Groups at http://www.apcug.org, or call a local computer store. Computer stores usually have information on the groups in the area. In fact, they may even be the sites for meetings.

Information system user groups for health information systems are of two types: internal and external. An internal group consists of users of a system within a given institution, whereas an external group has members from healthcare institutions all over the country (or even the world). Like other software user groups, they share experiences both positive and negative. If a nurse from each unit is not a member of a user group for the information system in his or her institution, nurses are missing opportunities to improve the program so that it serves nursing better, be a powerful advocate for nursing, and learn shortcuts for using the information system which can be shared with colleagues.

Software Program Copyright

When selling software, many vendors believe that the users are not buying the software, but instead buying a license to use it. In this thinking, breaking the shrink-wrap means the user agrees to the conditions of the license. These licenses generally state that the software cannot be sold or given away without the permission of the vendor and that the vendor cannot be held responsible for any problems the software might cause the computer. Depending on the vendor, users may be told that they can install the software on only one computer, or in some cases, on more than one computer if only one copy will be used at a time.

Today, installing most proprietary software such as Microsoft Office Suite™ requires the user to register the software – a process that generally requires the user to be connected to the Internet (online). During installation, one must enter a number that may be called the serial number, product key, or some other designation, which can be found either on the installation disks, or the envelope in which the software disk came. The program then checks to see if the program has been registered before, and if not, allows the installation to go forward. Some products that allow trial periods will give the user a chance to either register after a given number of days, or when it is installed if the product is already purchased. In any case, keep a record of these numbers in case they are needed at a later date. Product numbers may be matched to a number in the BIOS. Should the hard disk crash, the software can be easily reinstalled on a new disk on that computer if the user still has the registration information.

Today, given the ease with which programs can be checked to see if they are legitimate, pirated software is more a problem than illegal installations of legitimate software. Most problems are from countries outside the Western world. The Fourth Annual Business Software Report found that for every $2 spent on legitimate software, $1 was lost to pirated software, but that this ratio was reversed in some countries (Business Software Alliance, 2007). In 1992, Congress passed the Software Copyright Protection Bill, which raised software piracy from a misdemeanor to a felony (Nicoll, 1994). Penalties of up to $100,000 for statutory damages and fines of up to $250,000 can be levied for this crime, plus the people responsible can be sentenced to a jail term of up to five years.

Healthcare and educational organizations are not immune from prosecution. One western university paid $130,000 to the Software Publishers Association when it was found to have illegal software in a laboratory. A hospital in Illinois was fined about $161,000 when they were found engaging in unauthorized software duplication ("Chicago hospital caught pirating," 1997). Organizations without an enforced software oversight policy are possible candidates for investigation. To want to spend less for software is always tempting, but beware of pirated copies. Besides opening the owners up to lawsuits, jail terms, and economic losses, they can carry viruses that can affect the computer. The Business Software Alliance (BSA) is so serious about pirated software that they provide an online method of reporting software piracy (https://reporting.bsa.org/usa/home.aspx).

Some software is distributed as **shareware**. Software of this type is often found on the Internet. The publishers of shareware encourage users to give copies to friends and colleagues to try out. They request that anyone who uses the program after a trial period pay them a fee. Registration information is included in the program. Continuing to use shareware without paying the registration fee is considered software piracy. In many cases, access to the program may be denied after a given period of time, which will be stated when the program is installed.

Freeware is an application the programmer has decided to make freely available to anyone who wishes to use it. Although it may be used without paying a fee, the author usually maintains the copyright, which, unless the program is open source, generally means a user cannot do anything with the program other than what the author intended. Some freeware programs

available on the Internet are in the public domain and for which the author states that they can be used any way the user desires, including making changes. When users accept software through any channel but a reputable reseller, they should be certain that they know whether the software is proprietary, shareware, freeware, or in the public domain. And, unless the vendor is very well known, download the program file, save it, and use a virus checker to see if the file is carrying a virus before installing it.

Summary

There are many different types of software that are useful in managing information. Yet, it can be said that it is generally of two overall types: software that manages systems and software that allows people to manage information. Systems software consists of utilities and operating systems.

An operating system determines what application software you can use. This software includes not only the operating systems, but also accessories that help you to manage the computer and some other programs such as those that create ASCII text or graphics. There are also programs such as a calendar and a calculator.

Software that allows users to manage information includes many different varieties including computer-to-computer communication, and other special niche programs such as photo editing and speech recognition. There are different vendors for application programs, each of which approaches the task of implementing functions a little differently, but, essentially, all produce the same finished product. Several vendors offer office suites, which consist of a word processor, spreadsheet, presentation package, and database. Office suites from one vendor are designed for the programs they contain to integrate well with each other.

Programming languages can be classified as machine language, assembly, high-level, or fourth-level languages. Machine language consists solely of zeros and ones, whereas assembly language, which is one level higher, uses some word-like characters in its code. Fourth-level languages come the closest to natural language. Writing applications involves defining the problem to be solved and translating that to code.

Although there is some open source and free software, most of the software used is proprietary and copyrighted. Using a copy of a proprietary program for which a user does not hold a license is software piracy. Shareware is software that can be tried for free, but a registration fee should be paid if it is regularly used. Only freeware can be used without cost.

APPLICATIONS AND COMPETENCIES

1. Identify the current operating system on the computer you are using.
2. Identify the application software that is available on that computer.
3. Practice maximizing, minimizing, and dragging a window.
4. Open two or three application programs and navigate between them.
5. Write down as many rules as you can think of that define when deviations, either more or less than the normal temperature of 98.6°F (37°C), are cause for action by a nurse.
6. Create a flow chart of the steps for giving a PRN medication. Use a diamond shape for a decision, a rectangle for a process, and a parallelogram for data.

7. A friend gives you a CD-ROM with a program on it for you to install. What things should you consider before doing so?
8. You wish to install a program that you have at home on your computer at work. What things need to be considered?

REFERENCES

Beal, V. (2005, September 26, 2008). *All about open source*. Retrieved November 15, 2008, from http://www.webopedia.com/DidYouKnow/Computer_Science/2005/open_source.asp

Business Software Alliance. (2007). *2006 piracy study*. Retrieved November 15, 2008, from http://w3.bsa.org/globalstudy//upload/2007-Global-Piracy-Study-EN.pdf

Chicago hospital caught pirating. (1997, January). *Healthcare Informatics*, 20.

Nicoll, L. H. (1994). Modern day pirates: Software users and abusers. *Journal of Nursing Administration*, 24(1), 18–20.

Sewell, J. P. (2006). Getting the most from your software: Using excel as the poor man's database. *Computers, Informatics, Nursing*, 24(1), 13–17.

Seymour, J. (2001). *The truth about speech recognition*. Retrieved November 15, 2008, from http://www.pcmag.com/article2/0,1759,262680,00.asp

Webopedia. (2002, January 4). *Operating system*. Retrieved November 15, 2008, from http://www.webopedia.com/TERM/o/operating_system.html

Webopedia. (2004, May 17). *Graphical user interface*. Retrieved November 15, 2008, from http://www.webopedia.com/TERM/G/Graphical_User_Interface_GUI.html

Webopedia. (2007, September 28). *Voice recognition*. Retrieved November 15, 2008, from http://www.webopedia.com/TERM/v/voice_recognition.html

Woolley, D. (1996). *Choosing conferencing software*. Retrieved November 15, 2008, from http://thinkofit.com/webconf/wcchoice.htm

Understanding Computer Concepts: Common Features

Learning Objectives

After studying this chapter you will be able to:

1. Use the right mouse button effectively.

2. Apply computer conventions appropriately.

3. Use the "Help" option to learn to use software features.

4. Select, copy, and move an object on a computer.

5. Use "Save" and "Save As" functions appropriately.

6. Employ file organizational principles.

7. Differentiate between Sleep and Hibernate options.

Key Terms

Alt+
Backwardly Compatible
Clipboard
Context-Sensitive Help
Ctrl+
Default
Dialog Box
Drop-Down Menu
Embed
Function Keys
Hard Return
Hibernate
Icon
Insertion Point
Link
Logical
Menu Tab
Mouse

Multitask
Object
Overtype
Point and Click
Print Screen Key
Rtf File
Scroll Bar
Shift + Tab
Sleep
Status Line
System Tray
Tag
Task Bar
Toolbar
Vertical Bar
Wizard
Word Wrap

Remember the first time you cared for a patient? Everything took a long time and required absolute concentration while you moved through each procedure step by step. After you gained comfort and experience, you were able to adapt procedures to meet individual patient needs because you had developed baseline knowledge that was adaptable to new situations. For example, the first time you measured someone's blood pressure, the procedures involved in wrapping the cuff, pumping up the manometer, placing the stethoscope properly, and slowly releasing the pressure took your total concentration. After some experience, the tasks involved in taking a blood pressure became second nature and you were able to view it as a whole and concentrate on the patient instead of the task. Eventually, you developed the judgment needed to independently decide to take a blood pressure beyond routine assessment. You were now an expert in your approach to blood pressures. When required to learn a new procedure that is related to blood pressures, such as applying an automated blood pressure machine, you easily applied your knowledge to the new task, which shortened the learning curve.

Expanding Your Computer Horizons

This same progression from novice to competent to expert applies to computers. At first, a user may be very concerned about the keystrokes needed to perform each function. As more experience is gained, the tasks are automated and they are used appropriately. When it is necessary to learn a new program or information system, the command of the features that are common to all programs, such as editing text, scrolling the screen, and using the help menu and mouse, makes learning the new program much easier. Without realizing so, users internalize concepts that are transformed into quicker understanding and mastery of other computer tasks. This chapter will explore some of the basic concepts that are needed to get a start on this life-long journey.

THOSE WEIRD KEYS

Computer keyboards have keys on them that are not on a typewriter, such as **Ctrl** (pro-

nounced control) and **Alt**. The top line on the computer has **function keys** such as F1 and F5, which are used to invoke features in software. How they are used varies among application programs, but a universal use for a function key is the help key, F1, which in all Microsoft Window® compatible applications accesses help for the active program. The "Ctrl" and "Alt" keys are often used together with other keys to implement a feature. When you see directions that read **Ctrl+C**, it means that you are to hold down the Ctrl key and while it is down, tap the C, then release both keys. The Alt key works the same way. Sometimes you will see a command such as "Ctrl + Shift + D." Then you hold down both the Ctrl and Shift keys while tapping the "D" key. When you see a plus (+) sign, it means that you are to hold the preceding key(s) down until you have finished the sequence.

Laptops also have a key near the left bottom of the keyboard labeled "FN." This key is used together with a function key to accomplish a task. Which function keys to use in conjunction with the FN key is generally vendor specific, but almost all use FN + F4 to cycle where the screen output is going from the laptop screen to a projector, or to both.

DEFAULT

Default is a word you often see in conjunction with computers. Defaults are properties or attributes that may be changed but are how something will be done unless otherwise specified. For example, when using a word processor, there is a default font and size of the font. Unless these are changed, any text entered will use this font and size. If the default font is Calibri and the font size is 11, but a user needs to use Times New Roman with a font size of 12 and makes those changes, they become the default font for *only* that document. If something different from the default is used frequently, most programs provide a way to change the default so that it will be the default for all documents. They also provide a way to return all settings to the default.

MICE

The basics of **pointing and clicking** have been discussed in Chapter 3, and the varieties of **mice** are available in Chapter 2. There is another item connected with mice. Those for personal computers (PCs) have at least two buttons: the left button that selects objects and the right button that shows features that can be applied to the selected object. Some mice now come with either a scrolling feature that allows you to scroll up and down the screen, others offer the ability to program buttons to perform any feature that you use frequently.

When interpreting the directions on a help screen, or anywhere else, when you see "click the mouse," it means that you should click the left mouse button. Although there are exceptions, generally one left mouse click selects an object, whereas a double click is required to implement a feature or open a program. If the right button is to be clicked, the instructions will specify that. Learning to use a mouse can be trying. There is an excellent video tutorial called "Using the Mouse" that comes with some versions of Microsoft Windows®. You can find it by searching for "use mouse" in the operating system help. If it is not on your computer, you can go to http://windowshelp .microsoft.com/Windows/ en-us/help/cb8832d2- 3cb8-44a5-9636-eef74a92a3c01033.mspx and view it. After viewing this video, to gain practice using the mouse and have some fun, play solitaire, which is one of the games that comes with Microsoft Windows®. Open it by selecting Games from the All Programs Menu. If you are left handed, you can change the mouse so that it can be operated by the left hand (from the Control Panel, in XP select Mouse from Printers and Other Hardware; in Vista select Mouse from the Classic View), but then you would read a click as meaning the right mouse button and a right click as meaning a left mouse button click.

SCROLL BARS

When using most application programs, and even in healthcare information systems, the information that you need may exceed the size of the screen. Most often you will need to scroll down the screen, but in some applications such as spreadsheets or databases, you need to scroll to the right. This is easily accomplished by using either a **scroll box** (also called a **bar**) or the arrowhead on the right side or bottom of the screen. In Figure 4-1 you can see these tools. If you want to scroll down quickly, place your mouse pointer on the vertical scroll bar, hold down the left mouse button, and move the mouse in the direction that you wish to scroll. To scroll one line at a time, point to one of the arrowheads and click once. Holding down the left mouse button while pointing at the arrowhead will also scroll, but more slowly than using the scroll bar. Whether you see a scroll bar or a box is dependent on the amount of information, not on the screen. If you see a scroll bar, you will know that there is information that you cannot see. The size of the box varies with the amount of information that is not visible; the smaller the box, the larger the document, hence the less information visible on one screen. When you are reading a document, where the scroll bar or box is located on the **vertical bar** tells you about how much more of the document is either above or below the screen view. If a screen does not have any scroll bars, it means that what you see on the screen is all there is.

STATUS BAR

In many application programs, a line near the bottom of the screen is the status bar or **status line**. In some programs it may be called the application bar. The status line provides information about the file or document currently in the active window. This information varies among programs and vendors. In many word processors, this line indicates the page of a document, the line of text on that page, or how far from the left margin the **insertion point**[1] is

---

[1] The insertion point used to be called a cursor. With either terminology, it means the place where the next object (remember a character is an object) entered will be placed.

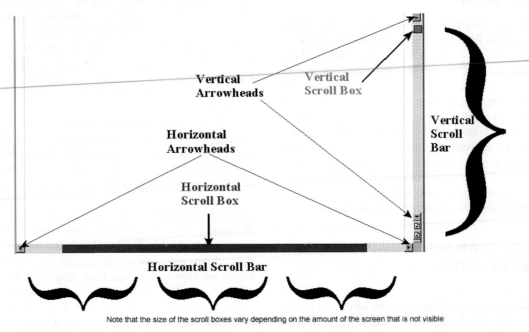

Note that the size of the scroll boxes vary depending on the amount of the screen that is not visible

Figure 4-1 • Horizontal and vertical scroll bars.

located. The status line may also indicate whether the Caps Lock is on or if the user is in Insert mode (any characters entered will make room for themselves) or **Overtype** (a strikeover or typeover status in which entered characters will type over the characters already on the screen) mode. The **task bar** on the bottom of the screen shows an icon for all the programs open at that time. Clicking any of these icons opens the associated window. Figure 3-2 in Chapter 3 shows the status line and program lines.

TOOLBARS

All desktop applications, and even some healthcare information system screens, have **toolbars**. A toolbar is, as the name suggests, a line or bar of tools. The default is to have toolbars at the top of the screen, although provision is usually made to move them for users who would like to have one or all their toolbars on the sides or bottom of the screen. A "ribbon" in Microsoft Word® 2007 is really a toolbar, just a new name for an old feature (see Figure 3-2). Although there are toolbars that are open by default, in programs other than Microsoft Office® 2007, users may choose to have others open or the defaults closed by clicking View on the menu line, toolbars, and checking or unchecking the desired toolbar. Sometimes toolbars are context sensitive, that is, when a feature such as the Outline feature is implemented, a special toolbar is added to those that are visible.

Many users are not happy with the default toolbars, colors of the screen, or other items. These can all be changed. The terminology used to provide this opportunity varies as does the option on the toolbar where it can be found, but when the word "Preferences," "Options," "Settings" or "Customize" is seen, selecting this option will allow making some changes. In XP programs, the most common place to find these options is under Tools. In Office 2007, select Options from the choices displayed when the Office Logo button is clicked.

SYSTEM TRAY

In Figure 3-2 you will also notice a line below the status line. Besides containing the task bar and the quick launch bar from which you can easily open a program, this item on the far right contains icons referred to as the **system tray**. The system tray has objects that generally represent changes that you can make to the system such as the volume of the speakers or your antivirus program. If you place your mouse pointer over an icon in the system tray, a tag will appear telling you what it represents. To access the features in the system tray, you sometimes need to right click the icon.

DROP-DOWN MENUS, DIALOG BOXES, AND MENU TABS

Windows is a very interactive system. Menus, **dialog boxes**, and **menu tabs** offer the ability to easily invoke features. When most off-the-shelf application programs open, you will see a line of menus across the top of the screen. In most application programs from any vendor prior to 2007 versions, when the mouse pointer is placed over a menu choice and the left mouse button clicked, a **drop-down menu** offering a choice of features appears. In the Microsoft Office® 2007 Programs, clicking any of those choices, instead of offering a drop-down box of features, causes a new "ribbon" of icons to appear that represent features that can be implemented. In application programs including most healthcare information systems, items that are not available in the current context are grayed out, that is, appear faded or in gray type. When you see a triangle on a menu item, or on the right bottom of a ribbon group in Microsoft Office 2007 Programs, this indicates that clicking this icon or text menu choice will produce another menu of choices, usually in a drop-down box. In many programs, an ellipsis (. . .) will indicate that a pop-up dialog box, or small window into which you give the computer more information about what you want to do, will appear. Sometimes a dialog box will have menu tabs near the top as you see in Figure 4-2. The tab that is a different color than the rest is the one

that is active. Clicking any of the other tabs will cause a new interactive window to appear. In Figure 4-2, the "Buttons" tab is active.

Many of these conventions are used in healthcare information systems. Making choices from one screen with drop-down menus, tabs, or dialog boxes is easier than going to a new screen. Drop-down boxes can also be used to facilitate data entry by presenting a menu of the usual choices for that entry. For example, a drop-down box is often used when there are fixed choices, such as smoking status or gender, that need to be entered into the system. A drop-down menu using the triangle option may also be used. To illustrate, in an intensive care unit, when users click the black triangle under "tubes," a drop-down list appears, listing all the possible tubes or types of tubes that might be used. Clicking another black triangle, one that indicates drainage, produces a list of possible drainage tubes. The content of these lists is determined by nurses who work in these areas. Good information systems result from a partnership between the nurses who work in an area with those who are involved with designing and implementing the system.

TEXT EDITING

No matter what you are doing with a computer, from entering data into a healthcare information system, writing a paper with a word processor, to entering an address in the location bar of a Web browser, you will be entering and editing text. It is the ability to easily edit that makes writing with a word processor easier; all papers and many memos would be improved with editing after the first draft is completed. Fortunately, all computer programs use similar methods for editing text. A major difference between a typewriter and a computer is that to a computer, a space is a character. It even has its own ASCII (American Standard Code for Information Interchange) representation, the number 32, and is represented in machine language by bits and bytes just as other characters are. Thus, any computer entry that limits the number of characters will count a space as a character. A hard return, or

Tabs ———

The buttons
tab is the
active tab on
this dialog box.

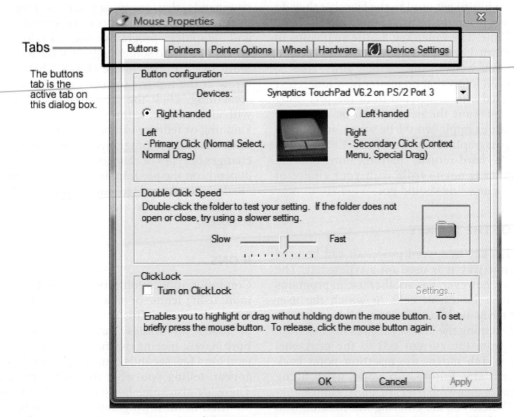

Figure 4-2 • Tabs on a dialog box (Microsoft product screen shot reprinted with permission from Microsoft Corporation).

the action produced by tapping the Enter key, is also counted as a character.

Moving the Insertion Point
Before you can edit text, you need to have your insertion point at the place where you want to edit. There are two ways to do this: using the arrow keys or the mouse. Using either method leaves the underlying text unchanged. Tapping an arrow key will move the insertion point, either line by line with the up and down arrows or character by character with the left and right arrows. To use the mouse, move the mouse pointer to the desired location, left click, and make the needed changes.

Erasing Text
Another universal feature is the use of the delete and backspace keys. When pressed, the backspace key always erases the character to

the insertion point's left, and the delete key erases the character (a hard return is a character) to the insertion point's right. If you need to erase a large portion of text, it may be easier to select the text and then tap the Delete key. To select the text, place the mouse pointer at one end of the text to be deleted and then hold down the Shift key and use the arrow keys or mouse to move to the other end. When the text to be deleted is selected, tap the Delete key. Selected text will always be in a different color than other text.

Word Wrap
Most applications into which text is entered have what is called **word wrap**, or the ability of the computer to "wrap" the entered characters down to the next line when a line has all the characters that it can accommodate. Those who have used typewriters in the past may

take a while to get used to the fact that they do not have to tap the return (Enter) key to create a new line. The Enter key, a little analogous to the return key on a typewriter, is only used when you want to force a new line. That is, when you know that no matter how much text is entered into or deleted from the preceding text, you want the next text to be on a new line. An example would be when you start a new paragraph. This use of the Enter key is called a "**hard return**," hard meaning that the computer is not to trifle with your choice of where a new line should go.

USE OF THE TAB KEY

The Tab key in a word processor can be used the same way it is used on a typewriter. The Tab key, however, has another use in programs that have boxes, or cells to which the user must navigate. In a table, or a cell in a spreadsheet, tapping the Tab key moves the insertion point from the current cell to the next one. **Shift + Tab** moves the insertion point back one cell. This feature also works when filling out boxes on a Web page. In short, almost anyplace where you are entering information into a box or cell, the Tab key can be used to navigate from one cell (box) to either the next or previous one.

UNDO (Ctrl + Z) AND REDO (Ctrl + Y)

There will come a time when after you have completed an action you will realize that this was not what you wanted to do. Two commands that many application programs have, especially word processors, spreadsheets, and graphics programs, are "Undo" and "Redo." To undo something, click the icon that looks like a mirror image of a "C" but has an arrow at the top left (or tap Ctrl+Z). To redo something, click the icon resembling a "C" with an arrow at the top right (or tap Ctrl+Y). Undoing or redoing can be repeated more than once in many programs. The number of changes or types of changes that can be undone depends on the program being used. If you use "Redo," you need to know that this puts changes back in the order in which they were removed.

ICONS

Computer application programs are more and more using **icons**, or small graphical pictures, rather than text. This can be seen in the use of icons for things that were once text. Fortunately, placing the mouse pointer over an icon for a few seconds causes a pop-up label to appear, telling you what the icon represents. There are also some fairly universal icons that are used in most programs. They can be seen in Figure 4-3.

HELP

Feeling comfortable using a computer is often a matter of getting help when it is needed. Classes may provide some beginning skills, but when a user tries to use the functions learned or experiment with new functions,

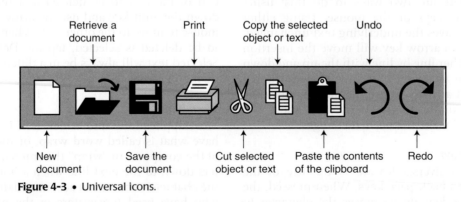

Retrieve a document · Print · Copy the selected object or text · Undo

New document · Save the document · Cut selected object or text · Paste the contents of the clipboard · Redo

Figure 4-3 • Universal icons.

questions often arise. There are many sources of help available; some are on your computer, and others will require access to the Web.

Unfortunately, for most applications available today, printed manuals no longer come with the program, although one is sometimes available for a fee. Instead, users are expected to use the help feature. Although help for basic features is available from information placed on your hard drive when a program is installed, more help is available online. Many programs have a menu option of Help; some use a question mark (?) instead of the word "help." Tapping F1 will access help in any program that works with the Microsoft Windows® operating system.

The appearance of the help screen varies from vendor to vendor. Some programs open up a screen and ask you to enter a search term. Others give you choices through tabs such as contents (generally like a table of contents), index (an index to the contents), and search. The hardest thing may be deciphering what term to enter into the search box to indicate the topic of your search. For some programs, after you select the terms you want, you need to click the button on the bottom of that window that says "Display." For others you can just click "Search."

Using help only works if you know what features the application offers and can ask for help. Books about the software in use are helpful to acquaint you with an application's features. Many texts about popular software products are available; however, there are so many that making a decision about which book to use is a personal decision. Some are written for beginners, whereas others are complete references for a program. Keep in mind that the beginning books are very limited in their coverage of a program's functions. They are helpful when one is first starting to use a program, but it might be more cost-effective in the long run to buy a more complete book. Look at several at a bookstore before making a decision to buy.

Books can be overwhelming in the material presented. If you are learning a program from a book, one suggestion is to work your way through the book until you feel reasonably comfortable with the program. Then using some of the features, create something, referring either to online help or the book when necessary. After becoming a little more comfortable with the program, take the time to peruse the rest of the book, noting what features are available. By knowing what is available, you can plan a document using this information and learn how to implement the feature when you will use it.

Context-Sensitive Help

Many applications today, and this includes healthcare information systems, have what is called **context-sensitive help**. For example, if you are entering vital signs and need help, when you click the Help icon (which may be a question mark in the upper right corner of the screen), the Help screen appears with options for just that feature. This feature can save much time and frustration.

Wizards

Some application programs feature **Wizards**, which take you step by step through executing a task. Wizards can be helpful, but they only cover basic tasks. Depending on them for everything that you need to do with an application will limit what you can do with the program.

Read the Screen

Often the best help is to "read the screen." It sounds obvious, but most of us, when we are coping with learning a new feature, develop tunnel vision and will not see all the choices on the open window. Keep in mind that features are often nested, that is, you need to go through a few options to get to the feature you want. Remember that any rectangle with text or an icon and a triangle pointing down will provide other choices if one clicks that triangle. Many of these drop-down boxes have scroll bars; so scroll up and down before concluding that the feature you want is not available. If you still don't see what you need, look on both the bottom and top of a window; sometimes the needed feature is there, sometimes, especially on Web pages, in very small print.

Other Help

Some healthcare information systems will have printed help attached to the computer. Most also have help desks, which you can call. Application programs for PCs often have a local user group where you can learn more about the program. Whether learning to use an application program or a healthcare organization's information system, it is important that you locate the sources of help available and take advantage of them. Asking for help is a sign that the user is serious about learning to fully use a program, not just get by. Give yourself permission to learn, and ask for help when needed. It is an axiom that most people only use a small percentage of the features that any program has, thus making their job harder.

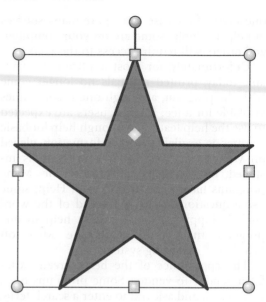

Figure 4-4 • Selected graphical object.

 ### Selecting, Copying, and Moving Objects

Choices on a menu, as well as objects, are selected by moving the mouse pointer over them and clicking, that is, point-and-click. The principle of selecting and clicking is used in all computer applications, not only in menus, but also as they apply to other features. The objects that can be selected vary from application program to application program. Note that the word **object** is applied to anything that is selected. This can be a letter, word, paragraph, page, entire document, cell or cells in a table or spreadsheet, an image, or pieces of that image. Text is selected as described above, and graphical objects are selected by clicking them. When graphical objects are selected, the selected object may show a border with either eight circles on the border, or dots at the corners and a square on each side as seen in Figure 4-4. A selected object may be cut, copied, moved, pasted, or dragged.

When an object is cut, it is removed from where it was and placed in random access memory (RAM) in a space called the **clipboard**. When the object is copied, the object remains where it is, but a copy is placed on the clipboard. From the clipboard, objects are then pasted anywhere the user desires. To paste an object that is on the clipboard, move the mouse pointer or insertion point to the desired location and paste it. There are several ways to paste. A quick method is to hold down the Ctrl (pronounced Control) key and tap the letter "V," or use the Shift + Insert key method. Paste can also be invoked by selecting it from the edit menu or in Microsoft Office® 2007 Programs from the Home tab. In all programs, objects on the clipboard can be pasted many times because they remain on the clipboard until replaced with another object. In Microsoft Office® Programs since 2002, it is possible to place more than one object on the clipboard if the clipboard is open and then select the desired one when ready to paste. Objects on the clipboard can often be pasted into another application program, even one that is not from the same vendor, or open at the time the object is placed on the clipboard. Objects on the clipboard disappear when the computer is turned off.

When any text is highlighted, indicating that it is selected, one can simply type the replacement without deleting the original. For example, if a sentence is selected and the Enter key is tapped, the sentence will disappear and a new line will be entered. (Use the Undo key to get it back!) This principle holds true in any computerized form, or in a Web browser on the address or location bar.

Graphics, or non-text items, such as pictures or photos that can be inserted into word processing programs, spreadsheets, and databases, as well as presentation or graphics programs, can also be copied or moved even in non-graphical oriented programs such as word processors and databases. When a graphical object is selected and the right mouse button clicked, the options presented will be different than those for text. Some of the techniques for working with graphical objects in a presentation program will be addressed in Chapter 8. Tapping the **Print Screen key**, sometimes abbreviated "Prt Sc," will place a copy of the screen on the clipboard. Once on the clipboard, it can be pasted into any program.

Working With Objects That You Create

Remember that we said that an object can be anything, such as a full document, parts of text, or pictures. When you are working on objects, they are only electronic bits in RAM. If the power goes off for some reason or the program crashes and the object has not been converted to a file by saving, it will be lost. This holds true for all computer programs. The only exception may be when entering data into a database. Databases save data as soon as the user leaves the field in which the data was entered. The only thing you need to save in a database is an object such as a form or query that you create[2].

The physical form onto which you save the document will vary depending on what you have available. It may be a diskette, a flash drive, a CD, or a hard drive. To save time, this

Prevent sad faces!
Save frequently.

Figure 4-5 • Save frequently!

chapter will refer to all these physical locations as a disk. The location of the file on the disk is dependent on how the disk is organized and will be explained later in this chapter.

SAVING

Saving a document in any program involves invoking the Save command in one of three ways:

1. Clicking File on the menu line (the logo in the upper left corner in Microsoft Office® 2007) and then Save on the menu.
2. Clicking the disk icon on the toolbar for all applications except Microsoft Office® 2007.
3. Tapping Ctrl+S.

When an object that you have created is saved, a copy of the object as it currently exists in RAM is saved to a disk. When additional changes are made to the object in RAM, these are not recorded on the file on the disk until the document is again saved. Thus, frequent saving keeps users from losing a document in its updated version (see Figure 4-5). More than one person has shed tears because he or she did not follow this rule. A good idea is to get into the habit of tapping Ctrl + S every few minutes.

The first time that an object is saved, the user is asked to name the file into which it will be placed. To make it easier to find the file the next time it is needed, the name chosen should reflect its contents. Names in Microsoft Windows® operating systems since 2002 can have up to 256 characters and include spaces[3]. Some characters may not be used in a file

---

[2] See Chapter 10 for more discussion of saving in a database.

[3] Although files with long file names can exist on most drives, some older CD creation programs will not tolerate a file with a name longer than eight characters, thus creating difficulties if you try to copy to a CD.

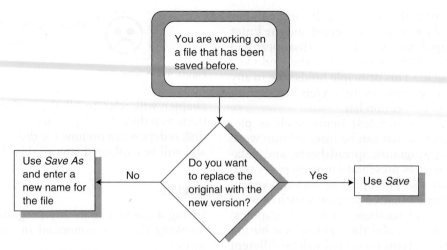

Figure 4-6 • Decision tree for using *Save* or *Save As*.

name (e.g., the hyphen and either slash). Letters and numbers are always safe to use in file names. After the file has been saved the first time, each time it is saved again is a repeat save, that is, the new version of the document replaces the one put on the disk by the previous save. The procedure to do a resave is identical to the first save except you do not need to give the name of the file.

There may be times when you want to preserve the original document but want to use it as a basis for a new document (Figure 4-6). In this case, you should select Save As. Using this option, you give the new file a different name. This choice can be found on the File menu on the menu line or by clicking logo in Microsoft Office® 2007 products. When you do a Save As," you create a separate file. Thus, you now have two files from this document: a copy of the last save plus a copy of the object as it now exists. Beginners sometimes use Save As providing a new name each time they save a document. This often results in confusion when they try to determine which is the current version. As a rule, unless you have a good reason for wanting different copies of a document, do not use Save As.

Sometimes when an object is saved for the first time, after you enter a name for the file, you will receive a message stating that a file by that name already exists. The program also asks whether the existing file by that name

should be replaced. If you say "Yes," the file by that name will be overwritten. Retrieving a file by that name will then retrieve what was saved in the last save. The original file by that name will be forever gone. Thus, unless you know what is in the file on the disk that has that name and do not mind losing that file, you should click "No" and select a different name.

AUTOMATIC BACKUPS

Many programs have a provision for an automatic backup. That is, after a given number of minutes, the computer will back up one's work without a command being given. Although this can be a lifesaver, there are some difficulties associated with it. Automatic backups work best when you are on your own computer, assuming that you have activated the feature to perform automatic backups. One difficulty with depending on this feature is that you may have spent the last 10 minutes creating something that required a lot of work. If the automatic backup time is every 15 minutes and a problem occurs before the next save, you will lose at least some of the work. Although this feature is available in word processing programs, it is not available in all programs. If you are on a computer in a lab, the ability to recover lost files is often not available. There is no substitute for regular saves and re-saves!

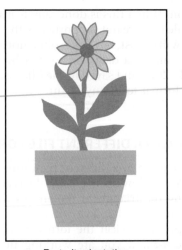

Portrait orientation

Figure 4-7 • Page orientation.

Landscape orientation

PURPOSEFUL BACKUPS OF OBJECTS

Remember that a file that is saved is only zeros and ones on the storage medium. Files on all types of storage material can become corrupted. Smart people save important objects in more than one place. If the object is really important such as a thesis or dissertation, copies of all the needed objects should not only be saved on more than one physical item, but some of these items placed in different geographical locations in case of fire, tornado, or other disasters. This is why backups of healthcare information systems are placed in different geographical locations.

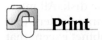 **Print**

Printing is another function that is available for objects that you create with computer programs, as well as items from the Web. Printing a document from a word processor, or for some Web pages, is fairly straightforward because these documents are oriented toward a printed page. However, when printing things such as spreadsheets or databases, or some Web pages, it is easy to forget that a piece of paper has a finite size. It is common with either of those program types to design a docu-ment that is wider than any paper a printer can use. When an attempt is made to print the document, the part that is too wide to fit on one sheet of paper may be completely omitted or it may print on another sheet.

If the document to be printed is not too large, there are two possible ways to solve this problem. One is to change the paper orienta-tion from the default portrait to landscape (Figure 4-7). To do this select Page Setup from the File menu or Orientation from the Page Layout tab in Microsoft Office® 2007 prod-ucts. In landscape orientation, the longer side is horizontal instead of the shorter side. Although this approach can take care of some width problems, it still cannot accommodate all cases. More room can be created by using a font of a smaller point size, but this solution has its limitations in readability. The best solu-tion is to remember paper size when designing any item that will be printed.

 Files

Once an object is saved to disk, it is a file. The file format, or type of file created, is determined by the program that was used to create the doc-ument and save it. Applications from different vendors create files that are often incompatible with other programs, the same applications from other vendors, and even different versions of the same program. Thus, a file created in Corel Word Perfect® may not be able to be opened in Microsoft Word®.

FILE EXTENSIONS

The type of file is usually indicated by an icon before the file name, and a file extension. When you see a list of files, such as when you use the "open file" option, or when using Microsoft Windows Explorer®, the file extension letters may or may not be visible but the icon always will be. Unless you are very familiar with these icons, you may wish to change the default file listings so that these extensions are shown. To learn how to do this, use the help after clicking the Start menu or the Microsoft® logo in Microsoft Vista®. Enter "Show file name extension" into the search box and then follow the directions. Knowing the type of file is always important when you receive a file in an email. If a file extension is unknown to you, go to http://www.sharpened .net/helpcenter/extensions.php and enter the letters into the search box.

BACKWARD COMPATIBILITY

Generally, software is **backwardly compatible**; that is, a newer version will open files created by an older version, but in many cases, the reverse is not true. For example, the file type created by default with Microsoft Office® 2007 applications cannot be opened by Microsoft Office® 2003 products without the use of special software. (You can download this software at http://www.microsoft.com/downloads/ details.aspx?familyid=941B3470-3AE9-4AEE-8F43-C6BB74CD1466&displaylang=en) Lack of backward compatibility, or using software of the same type from different vendors or different versions, is often the cause when recipients of file attachments are unable to open files attached to emails.

When using a later version of the same vendor's product, there is almost always a way to save the file in the format used by the older

version. When this is done, any features in the new file that are not supported by the older program will be lost, but this is often not a problem. For example, a database created by Microsoft Word® 2007 and saved in the Microsoft Word® 2003 format loses any features that are new in Microsoft Word® 2007.

SAVING IN A DIFFERENT FILE FORMAT

To save a file in a different file format with the Save As window open, change the type of file by clicking the triangle at the end of the box on the bottom of the Save window labeled "Save as Type" and select the format you wish (see Figure 4-8). If you are working in Microsoft Word® 2007 and want to enable someone to open the file using Microsoft Word® 2003, you would select "Word 97-2003 Document (*.doc)." Then you would click Save.

For word processing files, there is also a universal format that can be opened by any Microsoft Windows®–compatible word processor. This format is abbreviated **rtf** and is known as a rich text format. Thus, one can save a Microsoft Word® 2007 file in this format, and it can be opened by Corel Word Perfect®. Many programs can also save a file in the format of a file from an application by a different vendor.

DISK ORGANIZATION

When the files are saved, they go to a **logical** (i.e., one visible to the user but which may have no relationship to the actual physical placement of the file) location on the disk. All internal hard disks are organized into folders that are similar to files in a filing cabinet except that the "folders" may have other folders nested within as well as files. Other disks can also be organized into folders. The ease with which one can find a file is directly proportional to the organization of the folders on the disk.

On the internal hard drive in a PC, the base folder where you store files may be called "My Documents" or, in Microsoft Vista®, "Documents." In an attempt to keep pictures separated from documents, another folder called "My Pictures" is seen in PCs (Pictures in

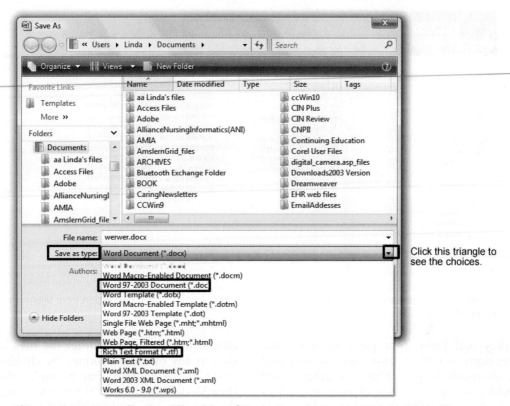

Click this triangle to see the choices.

Figure 4-8 • Saving a file as a different type (Microsoft product screen shot reprinted with permission from Microsoft Corporation).

Microsoft Vista®). Folders are organized in what looks like a hierarchical organizational chart with the top of the chart, or what could be called "the boss," being the base of the hard drive or the base of the external disk.

Personal style is reflected in how a filing cabinet is organized and how users name their files and folders. In some organizations, protocols for both file naming and folder organization are used by everyone to facilitate finding files that more than one person will use. Creating and using some type of organization will make backing up files to smaller disks a much easier process.

Figure 4-9 shows a view of folders and files in Microsoft Vista Windows Explore®[4]. On the

left are the folders, and on the right, the contents of the open folder. On the top of the screen, you see "▶ Linda ▶ Documents ▶ Nursing 401 ▶." This information tells you that this account belongs to Linda and that the folder Nursing 401, the open folder, is a folder in her Documents folder. The names on the right-hand side of the screen are the folders and files in her folder Nursing 401. Notice that in this folder she has both subfolders and files. For hard drives, consider the base folder, in this case Documents, to be the top of the organizational chart for files. There is no limit to the number of nested folders one can have, just be sure that there is some organizational principle behind the nesting.

This account holder has changed the default so that file extensions show. These extensions belong to files created by software applications from Microsoft Office® 2007.

[4] To open Windows Explore, *right* click on either the Start button (XP) or the Microsoft Logo (VISTA) in the lower left corner of the screen.

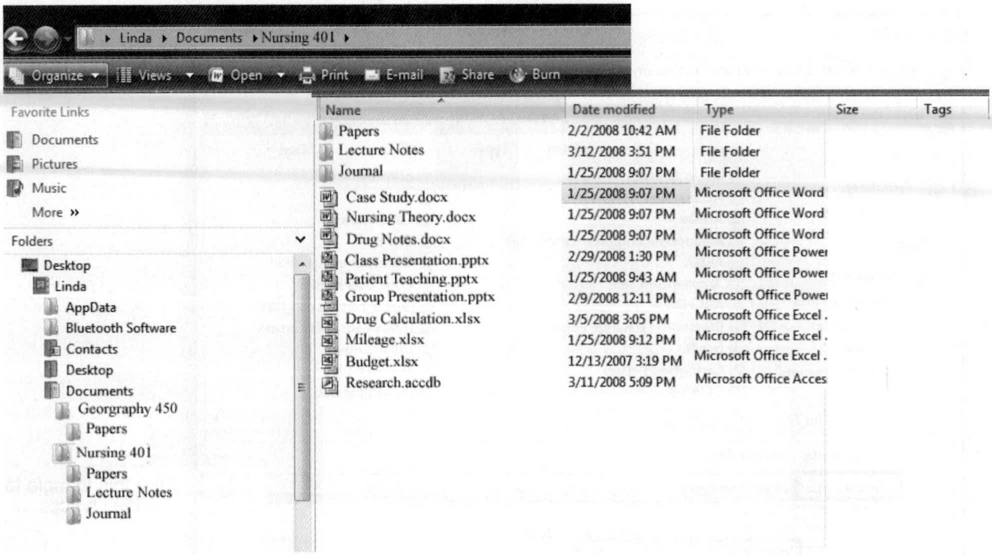

Figure 4-9 • Folders and files (Microsoft product screen shot reprinted with permission from Microsoft Corporation).

If they had been from prior versions, the extensions would be just three letters and the Microsoft Access® 2007 (a database) files would have an extension of mdb instead of accdb. To see the files in another folder, Linda would click the folder name in either the left or right side of the screen. To open any of these files, she would click the file name, which would open the program that has created the file as well as the file itself. Although the Microsoft Explore Windows® looks different in prior operating systems, the principles are identical, just as they are on other storage items such as flash drives.

VIEWING A FILE LIST

There are several options for viewing file lists either in Microsoft Explore Windows® or from the "Open File" choice in a program. The main choices for viewing the file names are lists, details, tiles, and different sizes of icons. Unless you are viewing pictures, the two most important views are the list and details views. Details view provides information about the file such as its size and the date on which it was created. The default listing of files in either view is alphabetical. You can reorder the files by the data in any of these columns by clicking the name of the column. For example, clicking Date Modified will order the files starting with the one that was modified first. Clicking Date Modified a second time will reverse the file order in the list, that is, placing the one modified last first. The list view shows only the file name with the icon of the program that created it and the extension if this is enabled. Figure 4-9 is a detailed view[5]. The order in which the files will appear in list view is determined by the last reordering of the files in the details view. In Figure 4-9 they are organized by file type.

TAGS

Although we organize our files in folders, sometimes making a distinction as to what folder a file belongs in is muddied because it may be useful in more than one circumstance. To permit this type of file management,

[5] In VISTA if the data that you wish to see is not an item under details, right click on a blank portion of that bar, click on More . . ., and select an item from that list.

Microsoft Office® 2007 added the ability to label a file using what is called a **tag**. For example, you are writing a paper for a course and want to file it under the course folder. However, you realize that next time you want information about this topic, you may not remember for which course you wrote it, so you tag it with a label that tells the topic of the paper. This feature, however, is only available for files created with Microsoft Word®, Microsoft Excel®, and pictures that have an extension of "jpg."

SAVING TO A SPECIFIC LOCATION

Understanding how files are organized on a disk makes it possible to save a file to the desired folder. When you click the Save icon (Figure 4-3) or the Logo button in Microsoft Office® 2007 applications and select "Save," the file list will look a lot like Figure 4-9. If there are many files and folders, there will be scroll bars, either horizontal or vertical, depending on how the files are viewed. Except for navigating to a folder lower in the hierarchy, which is done by clicking on the folder name, navigating to the desired folder is done a little differently, depending on which version of the operating system you are using and the vendor of the program. In versions of the Microsoft Windows® prior to the Microsoft Vista® operating systems, to move up folders in the hierarchy, at the end of the box with the open folder name, click the folder icon of an open folder that has a sideways "L" with an arrow pointing up. In Microsoft Vista® you can move up a folder by clicking on the folder name on the folder name bar of the folder that you wish to open or the folder name in the left column. To create a folder, use the Help function and search for "Create folder."

COPYING OR MOVING FILES

Copying or moving files or folders is a relatively simple procedure. It can be done by using the Cut or Copy options together with the Paste option from any Edit menu or by dragging the file in a Microsoft Windows Explore® window. Cut, Copy, and Paste work exactly as they do with any other object. In the file list, select the file and apply either Cut or Copy and Paste, depending on your need. To drag a file or folder, select it on the right panel, and holding down the left mouse button, drag it to its new location in the left panel. There is a basic principle that you need to understand when copying or dragging a file. When a file is dragged or copied to a new location, if the new location is a different folder on the same disk, the file will be moved (analogous to cut) so that it is only in one location on the disk. If the new location is a different disk, the file will be copied.

Universal Key Presses

When there are mouse-activated features that you use frequently, you may want to learn to use the alternate key presses for those features. With all programs, with the exception of Microsoft Office® 2007 applications, when a menu is opened by clicking, the key presses that will activate that feature are listed on the right side of the menu, as can be seen in Figure 4-10. The ones in this figure are universal to all versions of Microsoft Windows®–compatible applications. There are many others including Ctrl + Home that moves the insertion point to the beginning of a document and Ctrl + End to move it to the end. An excellent resource to discover universal key presses for both PCs and Macs is at http://www.computerhope.com/shortcut.htm

Multitasking

Living in today's world you no doubt multitask; for example, you talk on the phone and look for a patient record at the same time. Since the advent of the graphical user interface (GUI) you can **multitask** with your computer. In computer terminology this means having more than one program open at the same time and being able to quickly move between them. You can have as many programs open at one time as you wish, however, depending on the RAM and other facets of your computer; if you open too many at one time the computer may

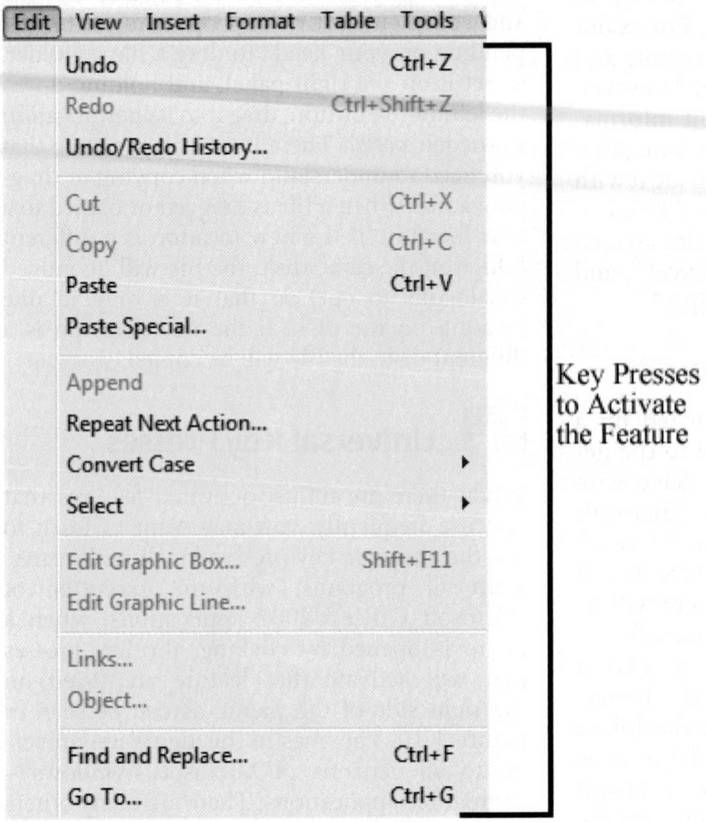

| Edit | View | Insert | Format | Table | Tools |

Undo   Ctrl+Z

Redo   Ctrl+Shift+Z

Undo/Redo History...

Cut   Ctrl+X

Copy   Ctrl+C

Paste   Ctrl+V

Paste Special...

Append

Repeat Next Action...

Convert Case   ▸

Select   ▸

Edit Graphic Box...   Shift+F11

Edit Graphic Line...

Links...

Object...

Find and Replace...   Ctrl+F

Go To...   Ctrl+G

Key Presses to Activate the Feature

Figure 4-10 • Key presses (Edit menu from Corel's WordPerfect® x3).

slow down. Most computers today will allow at least four or more programs to be open at the same time without losing efficiency. Thus, you can have your word processor and spreadsheet open while you are creating a presentation in another program. Each program that you open will leave its icon and name on the task bar; clicking the icon and name bar will switch the active window to that program. Using the clipboard you can easily copy objects from one program to another.

HAVING DIFFERENT FILES OPEN IN ONE PROGRAM

With most programs today, you can also have more than one file open at the same time in a program. There is a difference in how one accesses open files in the same program, depending on the application. In all Microsoft Office® applications, every open file in a program opens another item on the task bar. In most other programs, open files within the same program are accessed by clicking "Windows" in the menu bar of the application.

EMBEDDING AND LINKING

Any program that supports object **linking** and **embedding**, which includes all of the office applications, allows you to either embed a file from one program into another program or link to that file. For example, you may wish to have data from a spreadsheet in your word processing document. There is, however, a big difference in these processes. If you embed the file, you place

TABLE 4-1 ● *Linked and Embedded Files*	
Linked	**Embedded**
Changes made to either the spreadsheet while embedded in the document or the spreadsheet when open in the spreadsheet program will be reflected in both the document and the spreadsheet.	The spreadsheet will reflect the document at the time that it was embedded. Any changes made to the spreadsheet from within the word processing program will not be reflected in the actual spreadsheet, nor will changes made to the spreadsheet in the spreadsheet program be reflected in the document.

a copy of the worksheet as it is when you embed the file in your document. It is termed static because the document will not reflect further changes to the worksheet. If you click the embedded file, changes you make are only in that document, they do not affect the spreadsheet. When a spreadsheet is linked to a document, what is seen in the document will change if the linked spreadsheet changes. Clicking the linked object will open the spreadsheet and changes you make will be reflected in the word processing document after the spreadsheet is saved with the new changes (Table 4-1).

For example, let's say that you keep a record of the monthly expenses for supplies for a unit on a spreadsheet. You need to report these expenses every month along with a narrative explaining some of the expenses. Because each document reflects that month, you want the document to reflect the spreadsheet as it looks when you create the document. Then you embed the file and save the document for that month. If, instead, you need to do a report that is identical each time you report it, except for the data, you would link to the spreadsheet instead. Keep in mind that if you link, you will not have a record of any past documents. To learn how to do either, use the program's help feature.

SLEEP (STAND BY) OR HIBERNATE

Chapter 3 discussed closing programs and shutting down Microsoft Windows®, but not the options available to you when you close

Windows. If you are using Microsoft Vista®, you will see a list of these options when you activate the Close option by clicking the Start logo and clicking the tiny triangle on the lower right side of that window. In other versions of Microsoft Windows®, once you click the Start button and select Shut Down, it is necessary to open the drop-down box to see these options. Most of these options are fairly clear; the two that may be confusing are **Sleep**, known as Stand by on many computers, and **Hibernate**. They are both power-saving features, although turning off the monitor in PCs is also a big power saver.

The Sleep option saves all the information in all your open files plus information about which programs are open to RAM. This cuts power consumption to a minimum because the monitor is powered down and the disk drives are completely stopped. Hibernate, however, saves all this information to the hard drive and shuts the computer completely down, thus requiring no power. Of course when you again use the computer, it will recover very quickly from Sleep mode because RAM retrieval is faster than hard disk retrieval. The downside is that if the power goes off while the computer is in Sleep mode, all the information that was not saved is lost.

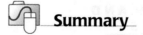 **Summary**

Computers are tools used to manage information. The task of learning to use a computer to manage information is facilitated when a user

understands some of the computer conventions such as how to use a mouse, edit text, find files, and use the "Help" function. Help is useful to both beginners who need direction on many things and more experienced users who need to learn a new feature or who infrequently use a feature. Many functions such as opening or saving a file, entering text, or printing follow the same principles in all application programs. Similarities also occur in the methods a computer uses with graphical objects, whether they are clip art, a drawing, an object that has been scanned, or the result of a screen capture. Understanding these principles makes transferring knowledge from one situation to another easier.

To make files easily retrievable, files are organized on a disk in a manner similar to a hierarchical organizational chart. Folders can contain nested folders and files. A well-organized disk facilitates making copies of files for backup purposes. All important files should be on at least two different disks such as the hard disk and a floppy diskette, and if very important, one copy, at least, should be stored in another geographical location.

Knowing shortcuts for computer tasks such as the universal key presses and becoming accustomed to multitasking are work- and time-savers. Work is further facilitated when you know how to use linking and embedding features. In this age when we are aware of global warming, using power-saving principles such as Sleep and Hibernate are ways of helping the environment.

When learning to use a computer, remember to give yourself permission to make mistakes—the computer could care less. It is you who becomes upset. Even experienced users make mistakes—there are very few from which it is not relatively easy to recover. Remember Ctrl+Z to undo!

APPLICATIONS AND COMPETENCIES

1. Examine a healthcare information system to see how many of the common features in this chapter are used. For example,

   a. Are there drop-down menus, dialog boxes, scroll bars, or tabs?
   b. Does F1 get help, or is there a question mark icon available?
   c. How is text edited?
   d. If text is selected and you type another character, does it replace that text?
   e. Is there context-sensitive help?
   f. Is there a taskbar and system tray on the screen?
   g. Will Ctrl + C copy an object? If it does, when should this *not* be used.
   h. Select something and tap the right mouse button. What happens? (Try this in an office suite program.)

2. You have selected a sentence and wish to move it to a new location in the paragraph. Which option would you use after selecting the sentence: Cut or Copy? Why?

3. Files, Folders, and Multitasking
   a. Open Microsoft Windows Explore® and navigate to the disk that you will use for backup copies (or originals if working in a lab).
   b. Using help create two new folders.
   c. Keeping Explore open, open a word processing program, create a simple file, and save it to one of the new folders using the word processing program.
   d. Using the task bar switch to Explore and move this file to the other folder by dragging it. Move it back to its original location using the universal key presses, Ctrl + C (Copy) and Ctrl + V (Paste).

4. You are working on an important paper that will take several sessions at the computer to complete. How will you preserve this?

5. Using Figure 4-9 draw an organizational file chart with Documents as the "boss."

6. Every month you need to do a report of the infections on your unit, which is kept in a spreadsheet along with a narrative that is in the word processor. This narrative will vary each month, but you wish to preserve each month's report. Will you embed the spreadsheet or link it, and why?

7. Make a chart of about 8–10 key presses that substitute for mouse actions for features that you use frequently.

8. You need to leave your computer for about 30 minutes. Which feature will you use, Sleep (Stand by) or Hibernate, and why?

CHAPTER 5

Computers and Networking

Learning Objectives

After studying this chapter you will be able to:

1. *Discuss the overall technology of computer networking.*

2. *Analyze the different methods of connecting to the Internet.*

3. *Differentiate between the Internet and the World Wide Web.*

4. *Identify uses of WWW technology for networking within an organization.*

5. *Protect a computer against computer malware.*

Key Terms

Active Server Pages (ASP)
Active X
Adware
Bandwidth
Bookmarks
Broadband
Case sensitive
Client/Server Architecture
Computer Malware
Computer Virus
Denial of Service
Digital Subscriber Line
Domain Name System
Download
Dynamic IP Address
Extensible Markup
  Language (XML)
Extranet
Favorites
Fiber Optic Cable
File Transfer Protocol (FTP)
Firewall
Graphical User Interface
  (GUI)
Hard Wired
Hoax
Home Page

HyperText Markup
  Language (HTML)
Internet
Internet Protocol (IP)
Intranet
IP address
Java
JavaScript
Local Area Network (LAN)
Markup Language
Megabits Per Second
Modem
Net Neutrality
Network
Nodes
Peer-to-Peer Network
Pharming
Phishing
Plain Old Telephone
  Service (POTS)
Plug-In
Rich Internet Application
Spyware
Static IP Address
Streaming
Telephony

Transmission Control
    Protocol (TCP)
Trojan Horse
Universal Resource
    Locator (URL)
Upload
Urban Legend
Virtual Private Network
    (VPN)

Web Browser
Web Cookies
Wide Area Network (WAN)
Wired Equivalent Privacy
    (WEP)
Wireless
World Wide Web
    (WWW/W3)
Worm

A nurse encounters a patient with an unfamiliar disease. From an email message, the nurse learns that a document on a computer in another country has information about caring for patients with this disease. Within 60 seconds of logging on to the Internet, the nurse prints out the document. This ability to exchange information on a global scale is changing the world. No longer do healthcare professionals have to wait for information to become available in a journal in the country in which they live. Nurses and other healthcare professionals can and do use computers to network with colleagues all over the world.

Healthcare depends on communication: communication between the nurse and the patient, communication between healthcare professionals, communication about organizational issues, and communication with the general public. As you can see from the previous paragraph, the methods used to communicate in healthcare are today being augmented with computer networking. Since the first computers talked to each other in the late 1960s, networking has progressed to the point where not only computers in an organization are connected to each other, but also institutions are connected to a worldwide network known as the **Internet.**

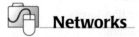 **Networks**

A **network** can range in size from a connection between a palmtop and a personal computer (PC) to the worldwide, multiuser computer connection – the **Internet**. Variation in network size or the number and location of connected computers is often seen in the name used to denote the network, such as a **local area network (LAN) or a wide area network (WAN)**. A LAN is a network in which the connected computers are physically close to one another, such as in the same department or building. A WAN is a network in which the connections are farther apart. Often, a WAN is an internetwork of LANs. WANs are sometimes referred to as enterprise networks because they connect all the computer networks throughout the entire organization or enterprise.

NETWORK ARCHITECTURE

There are many different variations in how networks are constructed, or what is referred to as their architecture, often depending on the purpose of the network. For a home network, a **peer-to-peer network** in which each connected computer is a workstation is a normal approach. In this scheme, each computer can have a shared folder that is accessible by the other computers. Often, the network is primarily for connecting to the Internet or for sharing hardware such as a printer.

Another type of architecture, often seen in healthcare agencies, is **client/server architecture**. The principles behind this model vary, but for most healthcare applications they are similar to the "dumb terminal" model. A client computer has software that allows it to request and receive information from the server. The

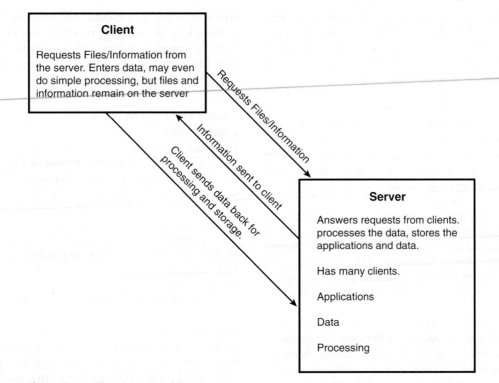

Figure 5-1 • Client/server architecture.

server has software that can accept these requests, find the appropriate information, and transmit it back to the client (Figure 5-1). The client views the information, enters data, and sends it back to the server for processing. Under this model, the client computer does no processing. Beyond making the initial request, rarely is any of this process visible to the user. Users sometimes have the misperception that the software and data reside on the computer/terminal that they are using, instead of the server.

There are other variations for networks. A computer in a healthcare facility may function as a client for the patient care information system, but may have application software that allows users to do things like word processing, in which case it acts like a regular computer. This computer may also be networked to another server that stores the files created by the networked computer, or the files may be stored on the computer that was used to create them. This computer may even be connected to the Internet through another server. Printers are usually connected to a network so that more than one computer/client can use them. Managing networks is an ongoing maintenance task performed by the network administrator.

CONNECTIONS

Networks are connected physically with a variety of materials such as twisted-wire cables, phone lines, fiber optic lines, or radio waves. Computers that are wired together are said to be **hard wired**. When you see the term "hard" with another item, this means that the item is permanent, or that it physically exists. Most healthcare agency networks, even those that use **wireless**, are hard wired to some extent.

Wireless transmissions are limited in distance, so they do not compete with other radio traffic. When a wireless system is installed, **nodes** are placed at strategic locations throughout the institution, locations that are determined after a thorough assessment of the building. A node in a wireless connection is a single point on the network that consists of a tiny router with a few wireless cards and antennas. These nodes pick up the signals sent by a user and transmit them to the central server, or even to another node for rebroadcast, and transmit signals back to the user's computer. Successful wireless communication depends on an adequate number of nodes or hardware that send or rebroadcast the signal and on their placement. The distance of a device from the node will affect both the speed of transmission and whether one can use the network.

Wireless transmission is less secure than hard-wired transmission because the signal is available for use for anyone in range. Security depends on the network administrators who follow procedures to secure the transmission. Many wireless networks, including those at home, use **wired equivalent privacy (WEP)**, the goal of which is to prevent disclosure or modifications of messages in transit. When this is employed, to connect to a network, a user must have the WEP key to enter before being allowed to use the network. In many cases, once a WEP key is entered on a computer, the computer remembers it and will automatically find the network any time a user is in range. Another newer, more secure form of protection is WPA (Wi-Fi Protected Access) (Webopedia, 2007). It features improved data encryption and better user authentication.

PROTOCOLS

For networks to function correctly, it is necessary that there be agreements known as **protocols**, which prescribe how data will be exchanged between participating computers. These protocols include standards for tasks such as how the system will check for transmission errors, whether to use data compression, and if so how, how the sending machine will indicate that the message it has sent is complete, and how the receiving machine will indicate that it has received the message.

Internet Protocol and Transmission Control Protocol

To ensure interoperable data transmission on the Internet, the **Internet Protocol (IP)** and the **Transmission Control Protocol (TCP)**, sometimes referred to as TCP/IP, were introduced in 1974 and are still in use, although consideration is being given to moving beyond the capabilities of these two protocols. The IP enables computers to find each other, and the TCP controls the tasks associated with data transmission.

Although invisible to the user, messages sent on the Internet are not sent as a whole. Instead they are broken up into what are called packets. Each packet may even take a different route to its destination. For each packet, a device called a router scans the routes available to the final destination, selects what is the shortest and the least congested route at that moment, and then sends the packet to another router that again makes a decision about the best route at that moment. This process continues for each packet until all the packets in a message reach their final destination. Under this process, it is not uncommon for packets in a message to take different routes to their destination.

File Transfer Protocol

Another process used on the Internet is the **file transfer protocol (FTP)**. This is the method used to download files (as opposed to retrieving a page from the Web) from another computer. Until the early 1990s, this was a manual process and users had to learn commands to do it. Today, **Web browsers** have automated this process for files that are retrieved from the **World Wide Web (WWW/W3)**. People who create pages for the WWW on their own computers use an FTP program to place their files on the server.

Internet: A Network of Networks

The **Internet** is, as its last three letters indicate, a network. Granted, it is a worldwide, amorphous network of interconnected computers, but it still is a network (see Figure 5-2). Nothing in the world before has become so quickly assimilated into daily use. In the early 1990s, the Internet was relatively unknown by all but a few academics. By the summer of 1994, the popular culture took note of this phenomenon, as evidenced by a cartoon in the *New Yorker* showing two dogs at a computer, with one remarking to the other, "On the Internet no one knows you are a dog." Since then the Internet has started to change how and with whom we communicate. It crosses national boundaries disregarding long-established international protocols and has created a situation in which laws designed for national entities are inadequate.

THE BEGINNINGS OF THE INTERNET

One of the positive legacies of the Cold War, the Internet was devised as a means of communication that would survive a nuclear war and provide the most economical use from then scarce, large computer resources. The journey from ARPANET (Advanced Research Projects Agency NETwork), which was established in 1969 to connect four nodes – the University of California, Los Angeles; Stanford Research Institute; the University of California, Santa Barbara; and the University of Utah (Howe, 2007) – to today's Internet has been amazing. It is "one of the most successful examples of the benefits of sustained investment and commitment to research and development of information infrastructure" (Leiner et al., 2003).

The underlying technical feature of the Internet is open architecture networking (Leiner et al., 2003). That is, the choice of how connected networks were set up, or their network architecture, was immaterial as long as

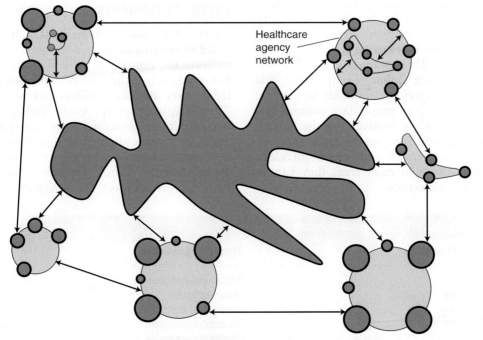

The Internet is millions of connected computer networks that span the globe.

Figure 5-2 • The Internet is billions of connected computer networks that span the globe.

they could work with other networks using a metalevel "Internetworking Architecture." The government, industry, and academia have been, and continue to be, partners in evolving and implementing the Internet. The free and open access to basic documents, especially protocol specifications, has been a key to the rapid growth of the Internet.

INTERNET SERVICE PROVIDER

An **Internet service provider** (ISP) is any organization that provides access to the Internet. It can be an educational institution, an employer, a hotel, or a coffee shop. For home or business use, a private ISP provides this service. If you are using a dial-up Internet connection, the ISP can be any service; however, common sense says that the dial-up number should be a local number. For **broadband** connections, you are limited in your selection of ISPs to whoever provides telephone or cable service to your location. A typical ISP offers email with one or more addresses per account. The cost varies; for dial-up it can be as low as $10 a month, while for broadband it may be bundled with either phone or cable service.

There are two types of ISPs: basic ISPs and online services. Three of the largest online services are America Online, CompuServe, and MSN. These services offer not only an Internet connection, but also proprietary content and features that are not available on the general Internet. However, access to these services, unless you are using dial-up, may be an added expense, because in most areas they cannot offer home connections.

IP ADDRESSES

To make it possible for each computer on the Internet to be electronically located, each has what is called an **IP address**, even the one you use to connect to the Internet at home. Because numbers are difficult for most people to remember, and because they may change, each computer is also assigned a name. Each time a message is sent, the Internet **Domain Name System** translates the computer name into its IP address. Using this system, only the **domain name system** must be updated when an IP numerical address change is required.

IP addresses can be static or dynamic. A **static IP address** will be the same each time the computer is logged on to the Internet. A **dynamic IP address** changes each time a user connects to the Internet. To facilitate each online computer having its own IP address, each ISP is assigned a given number of IP addresses, which they then assign to online computers, in either a static or a dynamic format.

INTERNET DOMAINS

As part of the **domain name system**, it was decided to assign a suffix to a computer name to indicate the domain to which the computer belonged. When the Internet was first established, six domain suffixes, as shown in Table 5-1, were set up. As the Web grew, the need for more domain names also grew. In 2000, two years after its designation by the U.S. government as the authority for overseeing Internet naming policies, the International Corporation for Assigning Names

TABLE 5-1 ● *Original Domain Suffixes*	
Characters	**Type of Organization**
edu	Educational institution
mil	Military computer
gov	Government source
org	Nonprofit organization
com	Commercial enterprise
net	Network, often an ISP provider

and Numbers (ICAHN – http://www.icann.org/) approved seven new domain suffixes.

Originally, one could tell the type of organization sponsoring the Web page by the domain suffix. This practice is still generally followed, but no organization monitors it. One should pay attention to the domain suffix in a Web address (URL) because people intent on deceiving others will take the name of the computer of a respected organization and obtain an Internet address with that name but with a different domain suffix. If you wonder whether this has been done, in the address bar of a browser, enter the same computer name, but use a different domain suffix.

CONNECTIONS TO THE INTERNET

The last mile of connection to the Internet is determined by the user. When institutional networked computers are connected to the Internet, the connection is generally provided at the network level and is invisible to the user. For home computers, the user has several choices.

TYPES OF CONNECTION

There are different ways to connect to the Internet, many of which are determined by your ISP. They fall generally into two broad categories: **plain old telephone service (POTS)** and broadband. These choices, somewhat limited by geographical location and available ISPs, determine the speed of the connection; that is, how quickly information will be transmitted. This speed is referred to as **bandwidth**. The higher the bandwidth, the faster the speed. Bandwidth varies throughout the Internet.

Telephone Modems

The original method of connecting computers to the Internet was through telephone lines. This system, still used especially in rural areas, requires a **modem**, or a device that will translate computer output (digital format) to electronic impulses that can be transmitted over telephone lines (analog format). Telephone modems are connected to the computer through a serial port and to the Internet through a telephone line. The speed with which information can be sent over a telephone line has increased dramatically from the original 25 characters per second (which was measured in baud) to 56,600 kilobits per second. Data transmission, however, often does not live up to its full capacity. To attain full speed, the phone line must be clear of noise or interference. More noise on the line, which is common in older lines, slows the connection. Picking up a phone extension while the line is being used for a computer connection and call waiting produce enough noise to interrupt a regular telephone connection to the Internet. This type of connection, which is known as dial-up or POTS, has probably already reached its top speed.

Broadband Connections

Broadband refers to telecommunication in which one wire transmits a wide band of frequencies. This allows more information to be transmitted, just as a six-lane highway will permit more cars to travel at the same time. POTS allows only a single frequency to be transmitted at one time; hence a broadband connection offers more speed. There are different broadband connections available for using the Internet, such as **digital subscriber lines** (DSL), cable, and satellite.

Fiber Optic Cable. **Fiber optic cable** is a popular connection for LANs. This cable consists of very thin, pure glass, which allows more fibers to be bundled in the size of a copper wire (What is fiber optic cable and why would I want it for my business?). Data travel over this cable in the form of light and is capable of speeds up to 186,000 miles per second; however, the technology to use all this speed has not yet been developed. The light signal in one fiber does not interfere with signals in other fibers, so it provides both faster data transfers and clearer phone conversations. Besides these advantages, the fiber does not corrode and has no known distance limitations. Its main disadvantage is that it is more fragile than wire, difficult to splice, and more expensive to install (Fiber optics, 2006). Despite this, fiber connections to the home are becoming more common because at this time they can offer speeds of 1,000 **megabits per second** (What is fiber optic cable and why would I want it for my business?), a speed that will continue to increase.

Digital Subscriber Lines Connections. DSL, one form of broadband, offers much faster speeds than POTS, although it still uses a basic copper phone line. Various types of DSL are available, and you will sometimes see it referred to as xDSL, meaning all the varieties. Asymmetric digital subscriber lines (ADSL), which provide a faster connection than the original DSL, are an improvement to DSL; most DSL connections today in North America are of the ADSL type. Another type of DSL, symmetric digital subscriber line (SDSL), is more common in Europe (Beal, 2005). The name symmetric is used because the data transmission rate is identical for upstream and downstream.

All types of DSL are able to use regular phone lines by employing a sophisticated scheme that packs digital data onto the existing phone lines, avoiding the translation of data to the analog format. A special modem is required for DSL service, along with what is called a splitter, on all the phone lines with the same number. Because DSL transmission uses parts of the telephone line not used in voice communication, unlike POTS service, DSL users can talk on the phone at the same time they are accessing the Internet.

With ADSL, **download** speed, that is, receiving information from the Internet, is usually set to be faster than the **upload** speed in the belief that most users download much more than they upload (Marples, 2004). Although ADSL is faster than POTS, the distance from the central office of the telephone company is still a factor. As you get farther away, the signal becomes weaker and the connection speed slows. The limit for ADSL service is now about 20,000 feet (6,096 meters). Speeds also vary with the type of DSL, but it is always at least 100 times faster than POTS.

TV Cable Connections. The last mile can also be provided by the cable used to transmit television. Like DSL, which uses unused portions of the telephone line, cable connections use unused bandwidth on a cable television network. A cable connection can attain speeds from 320 kilobytes per second to 10 megabits per second (International Engineering Consortium, 2007). Subscriber needs can be met by configuring the upstream and downstream rates. The transmission of television signals is not interrupted by the use of the Internet. Cable connections, like the varieties of DSL, can make use of **telephony**, that is, the use of the Internet as a telephone by subscribing to a third party such as Skype® (Wikipedia, 2008).

Cable or DSL?

Whether cable or DSL is faster has been debated since the move from POTS, and as of yet there is no clear winner. Although cable modem download speeds are typically two times faster than DSL, because this technology is based on shared bandwidth, many factors influence this speed (Wikipedia, 2008). With the varieties of DSL, the connection is only yours; with cable it is shared with other users. Hence the speed varies with the number of users on the network. Cable providers seldom publish the speed of the connection. For uploading information, the speed is usually about the same. There are many Web sites that you can access to test the speed of your connection; search by using the type of connection and speed.

Satellite. Satellite Internet connections offer broadband connections to rural areas that cannot receive either DSL or cable. The speed of approximately 1,500 kilobits per second download and from 128 to 256 kilobits per second upload is slower than either DSL or cable, but faster than POTS. The cost is higher than DSL or cable for the setup, but the monthly cost is not much higher than other broadband services (Web Hosting Geeks). The connection requires an antenna, transmit-and-receive electronics, and a satellite dish (High Speed Internet Access). The satellite dish needs a clear view of the skies, and heavy rainstorms or other severe weather are likely to cause outages. Also, because of the distance that the Internet signal has to travel, there is a built-in delay of about a quarter of a second (Kawamoto, 2005). Although this does not affect viewing Web pages, it makes telephony operate in a walkie-talkie manner that may require saying "over" at the end of a transmission (Web Hosting Geeks). Like cable connections, subscribers compete with one another for bandwidth. A satellite connection may, however, be an answer for underdeveloped countries because it can be powered by a generator or battery power that is able to support a desktop computer system (Gardena, 2008).

NETWORK NEUTRALITY

Today, with the use of the Internet for everything from its original purpose of open access for academic information to downloading full movies, the traffic on the Internet has grown to the point where there are traffic jams. This has raised several questions. Should payment for the privilege of being on the Internet be a flat fee for everyone, or should it be based on the amount of usage, much like cell phone service is billed? Another question involves the right of those who provide Internet service to prevent users from accessing some sites, or prevent them from using any device from a nonsponsored vendor to connect to the Internet.

These have all become an object of concern in what has been named **net neutrality**. The definitions of this term vary, but the main meaning is that the Internet be free of restrictions on use or equipment used to access the Internet, or the type of use, regardless of the service that is providing connectivity to the Internet (Network neutrality, 2007). Several bills concerning net neutrality were introduced into the first session of the 110th Congress, none of which advanced beyond the committee stage. In the second session of the 110th Congress, a new bill addressing this issue was introduced, the Internet Freedom Preservation Act of 2008 (HR5353), which died in committee. This act "proposed adding a new section to the Communications Act of 1934, which regulates the telecommunications and media industries and which was amended with the Telecom Act of 1996, to regulate broadband Internet communications" (Morgan, 2008). Expect to see this issue addressed again in the new Congress.

Some ISPs are already altering service in an attempt to control bandwidth usage. One ISP has been slowing the transmission speed of those using some high-bandwidth applications and even discontinuing service to individuals who use as much bandwidth as some business customers (Spring, 2008). Other ISPs are experimenting with a tiered pricing that raises prices for those who have a high-bandwidth usage. Where and how this will end is still up in the air; expect strong lobbying by both sides. The underlying fact is that the infrastructure required to keep the Internet working has to be paid for, and with the increase in traffic it will need updating.

RICH INTERNET APPLICATIONS

A **Rich Internet Application** (RIA) is a Web application that has the features and functionality of a regular desktop application, with the processing done on the user's computer, but the data and program stored on the application server (Rich Internet application, 2008). It is called "rich" because it offers more user-interface functions than traditional Internet offerings. Some of the benefits are that there is usually no need for software installations, any updates are automatic and done on the applications server, the application and data can be used from any Internet-connected computer, they are generally less apt to be infected by a virus, and there is a reduced need for external data backup.

The World Wide Web

The WWW or W3, although the term is often used interchangeably with the term Internet, is a part of the Internet, but it is far from being the entire Internet. It began as a networked information project in 1989 at the European

Organization for Nuclear Research (CERN). Its originator, Tim Berners-Lee, devised the system to enable the sharing of research materials and collaboration between physicists at many different locations. It first became operational in 1990. From that beginning, in less than 20 years it has become a large factor in the economy and lives of many in the world. Since Gutenberg's invention of movable type, there has not been an innovation that has so changed the speed with which new information could be made available and the methods we use to access this information.

The WWW can be regarded as a huge, worldwide library. By using it, one can find valuable information, such as the latest in cancer treatments, the full wording of bills pending before Congress, and any information that someone who has a point to make and access to a Web site wants to publish. Like its container, the Internet, the WWW is based on a set of protocols and conventions. Files are created using a markup language known as the **HyperText Markup Language (HTML)**. Although the Web is a wonderful contribution to the spread of knowledge, the fact that anyone can obtain a Web site and post anything on it means that users must carefully evaluate the information they find on the Web, a topic addressed in both Chapters 12 and 15.

WEB BROWSERS

The tool that enables users to retrieve and display files from the Web is called a Web browser, or just a browser. Using the client/server model of networking, to retrieve a Web document, the browser on the client computer requests a file using a transmission protocol known as the hypertext transfer protocol (HTTP). With this same protocol, the server, using special server software, receives that message, finds the file, and sends it off to the requesting computer. If you use a PC, you are familiar with Microsoft Internet Explorer® (IE). Other well-known browsers are Mozilla Firefox®, Apple Safari®, Opera Software Opera®, and AOL Netscape®, all of which are free to download.

MARKUP LANGUAGES

One of the protocols used by the Web is a **markup language**. Markup languages create computer files that combine data and extra information that provides more information about the data. It was derived from the term used in publishing, to mark up the margins of a manuscript with symbols for the printer (Markup language, 2008). Today there are several markup languages; the first standardized of these was the standardized generalized markup language (SGML). Using syntax from SGML, Sir Time Berners-Lee developed the markup language most used on the Web, HTML. The **extensible markup language (XML)** finds a user in healthcare to extract information from electronic messages and documents.

HyperText Markup Language

HTML is, as the term "markup" implies, a system of marking up a document. HTML adds tags to objects such as text or images that define the manner in which they should be displayed. The tags provide a browser with information about the color, font, attributes, and size to be used to display the text. The tags also provide instructions for hypertext links to other Web pages and instructions for displaying any image files that the document contains. Figure 5-3 shows some of the tags that are used to markup a Web document and how it is displayed by the browser. Between the two title tags is the name that would be displayed at the very top of the browser; the body tag starts the document and the p tag tells the browser to display all the text within this tag as a paragraph. Notice that tags exist in pairs. What symbol is used to tell the browser that this is the end of that type of formatting?[1] To see some live examples of html, on your browser's View tab click "Page Source" or simply "Source."

Extensible Markup Language

Another markup language, XML, is starting to be used in healthcare. It is also a system of

---

[1] The backslash in the tag, for example, </title>.

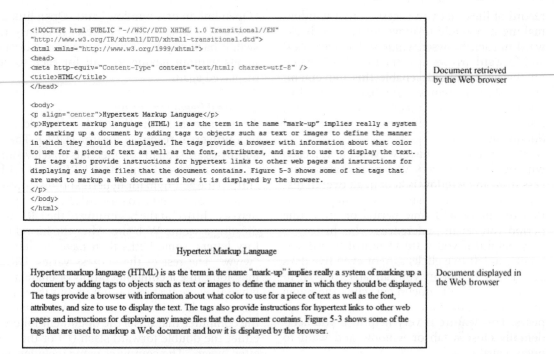

```
<!DOCTYPE html PUBLIC "-//W3C//DTD XHTML 1.0 Transitional//EN"
"http://www.w3.org/TR/xhtml1/DTD/xhtml1-transitional.dtd">
<html xmlns="http://www.w3.org/1999/xhtml">
<head>
<meta http-equiv="Content-Type" content="text/html; charset=utf-8" />
<title>HTML</title>
</head>

<body>
<p align="center">Hypertext Markup Language</p>
<p>Hypertext markup language (HTML) is as the term in the name "mark-up" implies really a system
 of marking up a document by adding tags to objects such as text or images to define the manner
in which they should be displayed. The tags provide a browser with information about what color
to use for a piece of text as well as the font, attributes, and size to use to display the text.
 The tags also provide instructions for hypertext links to other web pages and instructions for
displaying any image files that the document contains. Figure 5-3 shows some of the tags that
are used to markup a Web document and how it is displayed by the browser.
</p>
</body>
</html>
```

Document retrieved
by the Web browser

Hypertext Markup Language

Hypertext markup language (HTML) is as the term in the name "mark-up" implies really a system of marking up a document by adding tags to objects such as text or images to define the manner in which they should be displayed. The tags provide a browser with information about what color to use for a piece of text as well as the font, attributes, and size to use to display the text. The tags also provide instructions for hypertext links to other web pages and instructions for displaying any image files that the document contains. Figure 5-3 shows some of the tags that are used to markup a Web document and how it is displayed by the browser.

Document displayed in
the Web browser

Figure 5-3 • Web documents and HTML formatting tags.

tags, but the purpose of these tags is to define the meaning of the data, thereby making it easier to find information within a document, database, or Web site. Much healthcare information is in a free text or narrative format that lacks any structure (Schweiger, Hoelzer, Altmann, & Dudeck, 2002). Trying to reduce this to a computerized format often results in important information being omitted. XML enables tags to be used to identify items such as diagnosis, patient name, gender, and birth date in free text. XML is useful for both exchanging data between incompatible systems and extracting information from free text. Like information in a database, information tagged with XML tags can be displayed in many different ways, including on the Web (J. Quiggle, personal communication, 2008).

WEB NAVIGATION

Navigating within a Web document is identical to most applications in a **graphical user interface (GUI)** operating system. The four arrow keys will move in the document just as they will in any computer document, and the action of the vertical and horizontal scroll bars is also identical. Navigating from document to document (called pages) on the Web is done using hyperlinks. Clicking a hyperlink, which is also known as a hot area, will retrieve the document whose Web address is specified by that link. On most pages, hyperlinks are identified in text by the color blue and an underline.[2] Images can also be a hot area. A sure indicator that you are over a hot area is that the mouse pointer changes to a hand with the index finger pointing up.

Although the screens vary among the various browsers, they all have some things in common. For each open window they keep a

[2] Some Web designers whose desire to demonstrate that their design capabilities exceed their desire to make a site user friendly will use different attributes to designate a hyperlink.

record of files that you access in that window, making it possible to move forward or backward in each browser window. The backward and forward arrows near the top of the screen on the left-hand side enable this movement. Hence, if in one window you have opened five documents, you will need to click the back arrow five times to return to the original document.

Not only is this history available for each window, but also every Web page that you access from any window is kept in an overall history. How long this history is kept depends either on the default time period or on a time period you set in preferences. This history is very helpful if you want to return to a document you left five clicks ago, or even five days ago. To see the history you can tap Ctrl + H. To return to a specific document, click the name of the desired document on the menu that appears. This feature is very helpful if you accidentally close a tab or window and want to open it again.

Sometimes when a link is clicked, a document opens in a new window, often smaller than the original, instead of in the current browser window. In this case, the back arrow on the menu line is grayed out. To return to your original document, you must close this window. Although sometimes opening another window is beyond your choice, you can always choose to have a link open in either a new window, or, in most browsers today, a tab in that window. To see these choices, right click a hot area. Two of these choices will be "Open link in new window" and "Open link in new tab." Using either of these, it is easy to switch back and forth between various documents without having to wait for each to be displayed again.

Universal Resource Locators

All documents on the WWW have an address, or a **universal resource locator (URL)**. These addresses are seen in commercials on television or in print advertising. Most URLs start with "http" (the acronym for hypertext transfer protocol), a colon, and two forward slashes, or you may see "https" at the beginning of the URL, indicating a secure Web site. After the introductory letters, some URLs then have the letters "www." The rest of the address varies. URLs may look like a conglomeration of characters when they are first encountered, but there is a pattern to them (see Figure 5-4). The name of the computer that hosts the document follows either the double forward slash (//) or the dot after "www." The computer name includes the domain suffix, which is the letters following the last dot in the name before the leftmost single forward slash (/). The letters after the name of the computer are the name of the folder or folders on the host computer where the document is stored.

Some URLs have more than one directory name in them. For example, in the URL http://dlthede.net/Informatics/Chap05Computer Communications/Chap05.html, there are two directory names between the name of the computer (dlthede.net), "Informatics" and

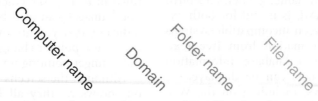

To find the home page for a site, delete all the characters back to the domain name, in this case "com."

Figure 5-4 • Anatomy of a URL.

"Chap05ComputerCommunications" and the file name. Just as on a storage disk, directories are organized hierarchically. A forward slash (/) separates each folder from the one above it. The last part of the URL may or may not end with a file name. File names end in a dot and usually the letters "htm," "html," "pdf," or "asp."

Given the myriad features now offered on the Web, marked by some very complicated disk organization, it is not surprising that many URLs are very long and have many characters in them, such as some cited in this book. These elements are all integral parts of an address and must not be omitted. One thing that all Web addresses have in common, however, is that they contain no spaces and all slashes are forward slashes. Additionally, the characters in a URL after the domain name are often **case sensitive**; that is, if the letter in an URL is uppercase, it needs to be entered in uppercase; if in lowercase, it must be entered in lowercase. Because URLs can become very complicated, whenever you need to enter a complex URL, which is not a hyperlink, but is in an electronic document, select it, copy it to the clipboard, and paste it in the address bar of the browser. For this reason, all the URLs in this book will be on the Web page for the book, so you can just click to access them (see http://dlthede.net/Informatics/Informatics.html).

Home Page

A concept that came with the WWW is the idea of a **home page**. On a browser this refers to the page that opens when the browser is first opened. On Web sites, however, the home page is the primary point of the site, or the top page from which all others are linked. If you are accessing a page and want to know more about the originator of that page, in the address bar delete the names of all the folders back to the domain suffix and tap the Enter key.

OTHER WEB PAGE TOOLS

Active Server Page

You may have noticed that not all Web addresses end in "htm" or "html." The Web has grown to where it needs interactive pages. One of the most popular ways to create these is

to combine HTML for the text part, and use **Active Server Pages (ASP)** to create interaction (ASP101). ASP is server based, so independent of which browser a user has. It allows Web pages to dynamically access databases to present real-time data.

Java and JavaScript

Java and **JavaScript**, both useful on the Web, are two different items. Java is a programming language developed by Sun Microsystems® that is used to create small applications called applets that can be downloaded from the Web. JavaScript is a scripting language written by Brendan Eich (Wilton-Jones) that allows Web designers to create interactive pages. A scripting language is enabled when it is run while a programming language like Java is precompiled (already converted into machine language; thus starts quickly). JavaScript is an open language that can be used without purchasing a license.

Active X and Active X Control

Active X is a set of programming technologies and tools for the Web, created by Microsoft®, used to create a self-sufficient program that can be run in Windows and Macintosh operating systems. An Active X control is a program similar to a Java applet. However, unlike Java applets, Active X controls have full access to the operating system, and they work only with IE. To protect you from unauthorized access to your operating system, when Active X is working on a Web site, the newer versions of IE will place an Information Bar near the top of your screen and warn you that a program wants to install something on your computer. Be certain of the legitimacy of a site before you agree to this.

FAVORITES (BOOKMARKS)

Entering URLs from a keyboard can become very tiresome as well as prone to transcription error. For this reason, browsers provide a way for users to easily record the URLs of sites that are frequently accessed. To access a site that has been recorded, click **Favorites** (IE) or

Bookmarks (Netscape and Firefox), and click the site name on the list. To add a site to these lists, with the document displayed, click Favorites (Bookmarks) and select Add. These Bookmarks (Favorites) can be organized into folders.

SECURE WEB PAGES

Many Web users shop online, giving out their credit card numbers. A level of security is provided by Web browsers by placing a locked lock icon on the screen when the site is a secure site. The placement of the lock varies; it is generally near one of the four corners of the screen. Some browsers will also change the color of the address bar; for example, in IE the line becomes gray.

WEB COOKIES

A great deal of fear and misinformation are linked to **Web cookies**. Web cookies are a collection of data that are sent to your computer by some Web sites and generally make the use of the Web more convenient. The browser stores the information in a cookie file on your computer. They may be used when a user fills out a form on the Web that has more than one page, so the information can be remembered between pages. Some cookies, known as session cookies, expire when the user leaves the site. Persistent cookies exist for a given time (Beal, 2007a).

Cookies do not normally act maliciously on computer systems (Beal, 2007a). However, a trend toward using cookies that store and track your activity online exists. This information is used to build a profile that is sold to advertisers who use the information to target you for specific advertising. Cookies cannot be used to spread viruses, and they cannot access or read your hard drive. Cookies stored on your computer can be read by users, but the information is gibberish to most of us. Protections are, however, available against cookies. Today's browsers allow you to set a default to delete any cookies when you exit the browser. Additionally, many antivirus

programs today will flag suspicious spyware or adware cookies when scanning your system for viruses. To learn more about managing cookies, check the Help section of your browser.

PLUG-INS/HELPERS

A **plug-in** is a helper program for a browser. Browsers alone are capable only of interpreting html. The Internet, however, is capable of transmitting other types of files, such as those created by multimedia-authoring languages. Before one can use these files, his or her computer must have a program that can interpret the file and show it either in the browser or on a separate screen. Plug-ins perform this function.

One of the most common plug-ins is the Adobe Acrobat Reader®, which is used to read files that are in the portable document format (PDF). Unlike regular Web pages that print according to the dictates of the printer used to output them, PDF files are designed to print in a specified way. This type of file is useful for things like forms that are intended for printing. PDF files, however, are difficult to read online and take longer to download. Most plug-ins intended to display files from the Web, such as Adobe Acrobat Reader, Real Player, Apple QuickTime, or Shockwave, may be downloaded for free.

STREAMING

Streaming is a method of delivering information, usually either audio or video on the Internet. It allows the user to start seeing or hearing the file before the entire file has downloaded. This technique is becoming important because of the increase in the number of large files, such as multimedia applications, that users want to download. Its ability to work depends on the receiving computer's ability to collect the data and deliver it in a steady stream, despite the unsteady rate at which data are transmitted on the Internet. Audio files and video clips are sometimes sent in this manner.

Other Uses of WWW Technology

INTRANET

An **intranet**[3] is a private network, usually within a corporation that uses html-formatted documents and the TCP/IP. They provide a cost-effective way to share information within agencies. Anyone in an organization who has struggled either to find the latest version of a procedure or to see that all who need updated information have it in their possession can appreciate an intranet. Intranets can be extremely useful for storing documents that need frequent updating, such as procedures, clinical pathways, policies, and drug information. Because there is only one official copy of these items, all that is required to make current information accessible is to update the one document on the intranet.

An intranet may or may not be connected to the Internet. If it is connected, the contents of the intranet will be protected from the outside world. Those within the institution can access both the intranet and the Internet, but outsiders cannot access the information on the intranet. Intranets can also provide some of the same kinds of features provided on the Internet, such as email, mailing lists, or news groups, although unless they are connected to the Internet, these features will be limited only to those on the intranet.

Like information on the Internet, information on an intranet is also not limited to text. Graphics and multimedia files can also be made available through the intranet. Digital video cameras can be used to record a procedure, and the file placed on the intranet, giving users the ability to play it in slow motion, or to stop and start as necessary. This makes the intranet an ideal way to offer in-service continuing education programs and access to proce-

dures. Preparing these documents does not need to be difficult. Although they often comprise a very large file, or one not really suited to the full Internet, all the major application programs (word processors, databases, spreadsheets, and presentation programs) convert documents to Web documents with a few mouse clicks. When preparing material for the intranet, thought should be given to adapting the material to take full advantage of browser capabilities, especially hyperlinking.[4]

EXTRANET

An **extranet** is an extension of an intranet with added security features. Like an intranet, it uses HTTP and TCP/IP. It provides accessibility to the intranet to a specific group of outsiders, often business partners. To access the extranet, a valid username and password are needed. An extranet can be viewed as part of a company's intranet that is extended to users outside the company.

VIRTUAL PRIVATE NETWORK

A **virtual private network** (VPN) is a private network that uses a public network, usually the Internet, to connect the nodes (Beal, 2007b). The information that the VPN transmits uses an encrypted tunnel and cannot be read by anyone else. It can be described as an extranet with an added layer of security. It can be used to provide access to current patient data from patient monitors to authorized healthcare professionals who are not physically present in the hospital.

Online Security

One does not have to be Web familiar to have heard about Web security problems. Most of these can be prevented by a savvy user. Before

---

[3] Internet, because it is a formal name, is always capitalized; intranet is not a formal name, thus should not be capitalized.

[4] Chapter 15 provides more information on creating a Web page, and Chapter 23 includes educational principles to follow for online learning.

becoming overly paranoid about this, know that most of the problems occur if one is lax about Internet security. Anyone connecting to the Internet with any type of broadband connection needs to protect their computer systems against invaders or viruses. POTS users, although less vulnerable, also need to take precautions.

COMPUTER MALWARE

Computer malware is a term given to all forms of computer software designed specifically to damage or disrupt a computer system. Several types of such programs exist, all of which operate differently, but they all damage a computer.

Phishing and Pharming

Phishing and **pharming** are forms of Web scams, and both try to get an individual to reveal personal information such as a bank account number or a social security number. In phishing, the victim is sent an email message with a Web address hyperlink in it, with instructions to go to this Web site to confirm an account or perform some other task that will involve revealing personal information. Although the hyperlink text in the message looks authentic, clicking it will take a user to a Web site that is not the one seen in the URL in

the message, although it may be a mirror image of the real one. One can protect oneself against this type of fraud by placing the mouse pointer over the hyperlinked Web address and looking at the lower left corner of the screen. In that area you will see the real address to which you will be taken if you click this link (see Figure 5-5). Pharming, on the contrary, results when an attacker infiltrates a Domain Name Server and changes the routing for addresses. Thus, when users of that Domain Name Server enter an URL for a pharmed site, they are pharmed to the evil site. It results from inadequate security for the Domain Name Server server. Protection against this type of attack rests with those who maintain the Domain Name Server servers.

Computer Viruses

A type of malware that you hear about most often is a **computer virus**. These are small software programs that are designed to execute and replicate themselves without your knowledge. Before the widespread use of the Internet, they usually were introduced by a disk inserted into the computer's drive. Today, they usually arrive from the Internet, with an email attachment, a greeting card, or an audio or video file. They can corrupt or delete data on your computer or use your email program

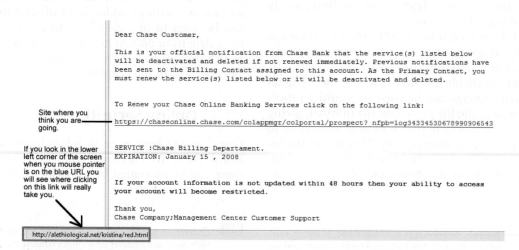

Figure 5-5 • Email scam.

to send themselves to everyone in your address book, or even erase your hard drive.

Like the human variety, computer viruses cause varying degrees of harm. Some can damage hardware; others only cause annoying effects. Although a virus may exist on a computer, it cannot infect the computer until the program to which it is attached is run. After their initial introduction, viruses are usually spread unknowingly by sharing infected files or sending emails with an infected attachment.

Email Virus.   This type of virus can be attached to an email message. One type, not too common anymore because of increased security, replicates itself by accessing the victim's address book and mailing itself to those in the list. More common is a virus that is attached to a file created by a legitimate program such as a word processor or a spreadsheet. To prevent this type of virus, most antivirus programs thoroughly vet each email message.

Worm.   A **worm** is a small piece of malware that uses security holes and computer networks to replicate itself. It is not completely a virus in that it does not require a human to run a program to become active; rather it is considered a subclass of virus because it replicates itself. To accomplish replication, the worm scans the network for another machine with the same security hole, and using this, copies itself to the new machine, which in turn repeats this action creating an ever-growing mass of infection. Unlike a plain virus, worms do not need to attach themselves to an existing program. They always cause harm to a network, even if only by consuming bandwidth.

Trojan Horse.   A **Trojan horse** is not technically a virus because it does not replicate itself. Like the historical Trojan horse, it masquerades as something it is not. For example, a Trojan horse may appear to be a program that performs a useful action, or is fun, such as a game, but in reality when the program is run, it damages your computer. Trojan horses may also create what is called a backdoor to the computer, which provides malicious users access to the computer. Trojan horses do not infect other files or self-replicate.

A keylogger trojan is malicious software that monitors keystrokes, placing them in a file and sending it to the remote attacker (Landesman, 2008a). Some keyloggers record all keystrokes; others are sophisticated enough to only log keys when you open a specific site such as a bank account. This type of software is also sold to parents to monitor their children's online activities. Some sites prevent keylogging by having a user use the mouse to point to a visual cue instead of using the keyboard.

Adware and Spyware

Adware and **spyware** are neither a virus nor spam. Most adware is legitimate, but some software that functions as adware is actually spyware, which at the very least is a nuisance, or it may actually invade your privacy by tracking your Internet travels or installing malicious code (Beal, 2004).

Adware.   Adware is a software that is often a legitimate revenue source for companies that offer free software. Software programs, games, or utilities that are designed and distributed as freeware, such as the email program Eudora, often provide their software in what is called a sponsored mode (Beal, 2004). In this mode, depending on the vendor, most or all of the features will be enabled, but pop-up advertisements will be seen when you use the program. Paying to register the software will remove the advertisements. This software is not malicious, but just paid advertisements that are randomly displayed when the program is used. It does not track your habits or provide personal information to a third party, but is a legitimate source of income to those who provide free software.

Spyware.   Spyware, in contrast to adware, tracks your Web surfing to tailor advertisements for you. Some adware unfortunately is spyware (Beal, 2004). This has given legitimate adware a bad name. Spyware can be compared to a Trojan horse because it comes aboard masquerading as what it is not. Downloading and installing peer-to-peer file swapping products, such as those allowing users to swap music files, is a common way to become infected. Although spyware appears to operate like legitimate adware, it is usually a separate program that can monitor keystrokes including passwords and credit card numbers and transmit this information to a third party. It can also scan your hard drive, read cookies, and change default home pages on Web browsers. Sometimes a licensing agreement, which few of us read before clicking Accept, informs users that spyware will be installed with the program, although this information is usually in obtuse, hard-to-read legalese, or misleading double-edged statements.

PROTECTION AGAINST MALWARE

Whether malware is a type of virus, spyware, or Trojan horse is not important. What is important is that a computer be protected against them, or that if a computer is infected they be promptly removed. The first line of protection is to be careful of sites whose reputation is unknown. Downloading a file that you find in an open Web search is always problematic. If you really must download it, scan the file with your antivirus program before installing or executing it. In fact, this is a good standard procedure with *any* file that is downloaded, no matter what the source.

Firewalls

A **firewall** for computers is like a firewall in a building; it acts to block destructive forces. On a computer it is a program or hardware device that works closely with a router program to filter the traffic both coming into and, for many firewalls, going out of a network or a private computer. The difficulty comes with deciding what should be let through, that is, what level of security to set. For networks such as those in healthcare agencies, the network administrator sets the limits. For a private computer, the best method is to accept the defaults. Most routers for home use come with a built-in hardware firewall, but given that new methods of attack as well as new viruses come on the scene almost daily, installing a software firewall and keeping it up-to-date is a good idea.

Antivirus Software

Although not having antivirus software is not a realistic option today if one is ever on the Internet, keeping copies of all important files and, if they are really important, storing them in another geographical location, is the first step toward protecting one's data. There are many different vendors of antivirus software, including free versions, some of which are of high quality (Landesman, 2008b). Details may differ between vendors, but antivirus software operates by scanning files or your computer's memory or both, looking for patterns based on the signatures or definitions of known viruses that may indicate an infection. Because virus authors are continually creating new viruses, antivirus software must be continually updated. In fact, once installed on your computer, most antivirus software immediately go to the Internet and download updates. Most antivirus software allow you to make continual updating automatic, for example, every Tuesday at noon. If the computer is not online at that time, or if you do not set automatic updates, you need to access the software and manually update it.

Once antivirus software is fully installed and updated, you should run a complete scan of the entire computer. After that, depending on the software and your choice, you may be able to configure the software to automatically scan specific files or folders at intervals that you set (McDowell & Householder, 2004). Scanning the entire computer is often a lengthy process; it may even take two to four hours. This process uses much of the processing ability and usually slows down any work that you may wish to do. Therefore, you may want to set the scan for times when you are normally not using the computer, but it is on.

Antivirus software can also scan individual files, which is usually a quick process. Scanning any email attachments of Web downloads is an excellent way to protect your system from malware.

The response when an antivirus program finds a virus varies with the software and whether the virus is found during an automatic or a manual scan. Some software packages will present you with a dialog box asking you if you would like the virus removed, and others will remove the virus without asking you.

Today, most antivirus software is combined with software to detect and remove both viruses and spyware as well as to have firewall-type protection. Once installed, this software operates in the background and checks all the incoming and outgoing data for malicious operations. If it is not regularly updated, however, it cannot offer much protection.

HOAXES

The world has never known a shortage of practical jokers, or those who enjoy sending sensational news to friends. Unfortunately, email lends itself beautifully to these misguided individuals.

Virus Hoaxes
Emails that warn of viruses are a **hoax** 99% of the time. Although, with few exceptions, these hoaxes are not harmful; they are a waste of time and clutter up the Internet and internal networks with useless messages. Hoaxes sound very credible, frequently citing sources such as an official from Microsoft® or Symantec®. The message contains the information that this virus will destroy a hard drive or perform other dire computer damage. They always tell the recipient to forward this message to anyone she or he knows. Despite containing the statement that "This is not a hoax," such messages are a hoax. Discard these messages and do not forward them. When there is a real virus, you are most likely to hear about it in the regular mass media, especially if the virus is new and your antivirus program does not have any protection

against it. There are several Web sites where a virus warning can be checked to see if it is a hoax. One such site is (http://www.trendmicro.com/vinfo/hoaxes/default.asp) About.com at http://urbanlegends.about.com/cs/nethoaxes/ht/emailhoax.htm provides excellent information on how to spot an email hoax.

Urban Legends
Urban legends often are stories thought to be factual by those who pass them on. They may be cautionary or moralistic tales passed on by those who believe them. They are not necessarily untrue, but are generally sensationalist, distorted, or exaggerated. They can even be found in a news story, but today these are mostly passed via email. The sender alleges that the incident happened to someone they or their friends know. Before passing on such information, check with a site that reports on urban legends such as Snopes (http://www.snopes.com/).

Damaging Hoaxes
There is another type of hoax that is not exactly a hoax, but a malicious practical joke that is also spread by email. A user receives a message saying that if a file named "such and such" is on the recipient's computer, the recipient should delete it immediately because it is a logical virus that will execute in so many days and damage the computer, files, and so on. Included are elaborate instructions for how to determine whether the file is on the computer, and equally elaborate instructions for deleting it. When a user searches for this file, it is found on the computer. Believing the message, the user deletes it. Unfortunately, it is often a file that is part of the operating system, or other application program on the computer. Deleting the file causes a problem when the system or application program needs that file. Repairing the damage is often a lengthy chore.

If a recipient has any doubt that a message such as the one discussed in the previous paragraph is a malicious practical joke, after finding the file, he or she should maximize the Find Screen and look at the date that the file was created (use the details view). The recipient will probably find that the date the file was created shows that the time period mentioned in the warning has exceeded long ago; hence the file is not malicious. If the file is part of the operating system, the date will be the date that Windows was installed on that computer or that a patch was applied. As a rule of thumb, except for deleting files that were user created with an application program, proceed very cautiously in deleting any file. Know exactly what the file that is to be deleted does, and be 100% certain that it is not an important file. A good way to discover what a file does is to enter the name into a Web search tool.

Characteristics of This Type of Joke

Email warnings should arise suspicions if any of the following characteristics are present (McDowell & Householder, 2007):

▼ The message says that tragic consequences will occur if you do not perform a given action.
▼ It is mentioned that you will receive money or a gift certificate for performing an action.
▼ Instructions or attachments claim to protect you from a virus that is undetectable by antivirus software.
▼ The email says that it is not a hoax.
▼ The logic is contradictory.
▼ There are multiple spelling or grammatical errors.
▼ You are asked to forward the message.
▼ The message has already been forwarded multiple times, which is evidenced by a trail of email headers in the body of the message.

SECURITY PITFALLS

Believing that antivirus software and firewalls once installed are 100% effective is a guaranteed step toward problems. Although combining these technologies with good security habits reduces risk, if protective software is not updated frequently, you are at risk

(McDowell, 2006). If you do not protect your computer, believing that there is nothing important on it, it becomes a fertile field for use by attackers who, unbeknownst to you, plant software that is used to attack other people in what are called **denial of service** attacks. Some operating systems will not install a program without informing you, but it is only a matter of time until attackers learn to bypass this. Slowing down of your computer may be a sign that there are other processes or programs running in the background without your permission, usually to yours or the Internet's detriment. Ignoring patches for either the operating system or the software is another risk situation.

Summary

The time since the first two computers "talked" to each other to today's Internet has been short, but it has been a long journey. Never before in history have the methods of communication been as rapidly changed. The worldwide reach of the Internet and its features, such as the WWW and email, provides the tools that are creating a truly international community.

Ways of connecting to the Internet have speeded up connections from the original 300 baud (slow enough to read the text as it was sent to your computer) to 56 kilobytes per second for POTS and up to 1,000 megabits per second for fiber, with the potential to keep increasing. Building on the use of protocols that join the Internet, the WWW has introduced a new level of knowledge dissemination. From the original HTML language have come variations such as Java and ASP, which have added new features to the Web.

Organizations, understanding the benefits of Internet connections, have created network connections such as LANs and WANs. Unfortunately, people intent on doing damage to others have also been active in creating viruses, Trojan horses, and other methods of spying on Web users. Fortunately, methods of protecting against these threats have kept up, and with common sense, it is possible to protect oneself against damages. Computer networking is here to stay and will continue to expand the ways that it can be used, limited not by technology, but by imagination and the willingness to adopt new methods.

APPLICATIONS AND COMPETENCIES

1. How do you see the rapid communication and availability of knowledge via the Internet affecting society in general? Healthcare?
2. Visit a Web site with many directory names. Parse the URL by working your way backwards until you read the domain name. What did you learn about the sponsor of the site?
3. Add two sites to Favorites (if using IE) or Bookmarks (if using Netscape or Firefox).
4. Learn how your browser manages cookies. Does it erase them when you close the browser, when you leave the site, or are they kept for a given number of days?
5. View the page source for a Web page. Identify a tag for a paragraph.
6. Compare and contrast two Internet security products using a site that reviews these products. Which one would you select and why?

REFERENCES

ASP101. *What is ASP?* Retrieved November 17, 2008, from http://www.asp101.com/wrox/asp2samp/ 2459ch01.asp

Beal, V. (2004, November 11). *The difference between adware & spyware.* Retrieved November 17, 2008, from http://www.webopedia.com/DidYouKnow/Internet/2004/spyware.asp

Beal, V. (2005, June 3). *Cable vs. DSL.* Retrieved November 17, 2008, from http://www.webopedia.com/DidYouKnow/Internet/2005/cable_vs_dsl.asp

Beal, V. (2007a, May 18). *What you need to know about cookies.* Retrieved November 17, 2008, from http://www.webopedia.com/DidYouKnow/Internet/2007/all_about_cookies.asp

Beal, V. (2007b, June 1). *What makes a virtual private network private?* Retrieved November 17, 2008, from http://www.webopedia.com/DidYouKnow/Internet/2007/virtual_private_network_VPN.asp

Fiber optics. (2006, July 13). Retrieved November 17, 2008, from http://webopedia.com/TERM/F/fiber_ optics.html

Gardena, E. (2008, January 23). *Satellite Internet.* Retrieved November 18, 2008, from http://ezinearticles.com/?Satellite-Internet&id=944996

High Speed Internet Access. *Satellite Internet service.* Retrieved November 17, 2008, from http://www.high-speed-internet-access-guide.com/satellite/

Howe, W. (2007, January 16). *A brief history of the Internet.* Retrieved November 17, 2008, from http://www.walthowe.com/navnet/history.html

International Engineering Consortium. (2007). *Cable modems.* Retrieved November 17, 2008, from http://www.iec.org/online/tutorials/cable_mod/topic01.html

Kawamoto, W. (2005, February 1). *Web management satellite equals broadband lite.* Retrieved November 17, 2008, from http://www.smallbusinesscomputing.com/webmaster/article.php/ 3466881

Landesman, M. (2008a) *What is a keylogger trojan?* Retrieved November 17, 2008, from http://antivirus.about.com/od/whatisavirus/a/keylogger.htm

Landesman, M. (2008b). *Review: Free antivirus software.* Retrieved November 17, 2008, from http://antivirus.about.com/od/antivirussoftwarereviews/a/freeav.htm

Leiner, B. M., Cerf, V. G., Clark, D. D., Kahn, R. E., Kleinrock, L., Lynch, D. C., et al. (2003, December 10). *A brief history of the Internet.* Retrieved November 17, 2008, from http://www.isoc.org/internet/history/brief.shtml

Markup language. (2008, November 15). Retrieved November 17, 2008, from http://en.wikipedia.org/wiki/Markup_language

Marples, G. (2004). *How DSL Internet access works.* Retrieved November 17, 2008, from http://www.howitworks.net/how-dsl-internet-access-works.html

McDowell, M. (2006). *National cyber alert system, Cyber security tip ST06-002: Debunking some common myths.* Retrieved November 17, 2008, from http://www.us-cert.gov/cas/tips/ST06-002.html

McDowell, M., & Householder, A. (2004). *National cyber alert system cyber security tip ST04-005: Understanding anti-virus software.* Retrieved November 17, 2008, from http://www.us-cert.gov/ cas/tips/ST04-005.html

McDowell, M., & Householder, A. (2007, May 3). *National cyber alert system cyber security tip ST04-009: Identifying hoaxes and urban legends.* Retrieved November 17, 2008, from http://www.us-cert.gov/cas/tips/ST04-009.html

Morgan, T. P. (2008, February 19). Net neutrality comes around on the ferris wheel again. Retrieved November 18, 2008, from http://www.itjungle.com/tlb/tlb021908-story06.html

Network neutrality. (2007, September). Retrieved November 17, 2008, from http://en.wikipedia.org/wiki/Network_neutrality

New domain names coming next year? (2007, May 11). Retrieved November 17, 2008, from http://www.msnbc.msn.com/id/18608110/

Rich Internet application. (2008, November 13). Retrieved February 19, 2008, from http://en.wikipedia.org/wiki/Rich_Internet_application

Schweiger, R., Hoelzer, S., Altmann, U., & Dudeck, J. R. J. (2002). Plug-and-play XML. *Journal of the American Medical Informatics Association, 9*(1), 37–62.

Spring, T. (2008, February 18). *Get ready for a crackdown on broadband use.* Retrieved November 17, 2008, from http://www.macworld.com/article/132144/2008/02/broadband.html

Web Hosting Geeks. *Ka band -affordable satellite Internet on the way!* Retrieved February 19, 2008, from http://webhostinggeeks.com/articles/broadband-internet/7643.php

Webopedia. (2007, June 15). *The differences between WEP and WPA.* Retrieved November 17, 2008, from http://www.webopedia.com/DidYouKnow/Computer_Science/2007/WEP_WPA_wireless_security.asp#5571765847448233914

What is fiber optic cable and why would I want it for my business? Retrieved November 17, 2008, from http://www.cpifiber.com/AboutCPIFiberOptics.html

Wikipedia. (2008, October 13). *Cable modem.* Retrieved November 17, 2008, from http://en.wikipedia.org/wiki/Cable_modem

Wilton-Jones, M. *The early Internet and the first generation browsers.* Retrieved November 17, 2008, from http://www.howtocreate.co.uk/jshistory.html

UNIT II

Computers and Your Professional Career

CHAPTER 6   Professional Networking
CHAPTER 7   Word Processing
CHAPTER 8   Presentation Software: Looking Professional in the Spotlight
CHAPTER 9   Spreadsheets: Making Numbers Talk
CHAPTER 10 Databases: Creating Information From Data

SOME of you have grown up in the world of computers and look at the world before them as the dark ages. But there are also some of you who are being thrown into the world of computers feeling very much a foreigner. No matter into which category, or where on the continuum between them, you find yourself, the use of the computer as a tool in writing, calculating, analyzing data, and presenting, are a necessary instrument for your professional and personal life.

The unit opens with professional networking, or using computer networking personally, and professionally. Collective intelligence tools such as wikis, blogs, and mashups are explained as is the full world of email including the use of email discussion lists. Chapter 7 addresses using a word processor beyond its use as an electronic typewriter. This includes features that even some "digital natives" (those born to computers) do not use such as automatic headers and page numbering, outlining, footnotes, and mail merge; features that when ignored robs one of time. Presentations are the topic of Chapter 8. This chapter looks at both the pluses and minuses of using slide presentation programs and offers help to make their usage truly informational. Chapter 9 examines spreadsheets, software that can assist in managing numbers. The mathematical priority in formulas, tips to better spreadsheets, the use of graphs, and other spreadsheet features such as protecting data are investigated. Chapter 10, the last chapter in this unit, introduces databases, which are the key ingredient of all information systems. Starting with searching databases, the chapter examines other uses in nursing, such as for analyzing data pertinent to a unit, database structures, and the, "one piece of data, many views" concept and concludes with the use of data mining.

Professional Networking

Learning Objectives
After studying this chapter you will be able to:

1. *Discuss Web 2.0 features.*

2. *Use email effectively.*

3. *Manage email accounts.*

4. *Be a responsible member of a discussion list.*

Key Terms

Backwardly Compatible
Bcc
Blog
Cc
Collective Intelligence
Email
Emoticon
Flame
Flame War
Folksonomy
Grass Roots Media
Hypertext Markup
    Language (HTML)
Instant Messaging
Internet Mail Access
    Protocol (IMAP)
Internet Service
    Provider (ISP)
Listserv
Login Name
Mashup
Pharming
Phishing
Podcast

Post Office Protocol
    (POP)3
Rich Text File (RTF)
Real Simple Syndication or
    Rich Site Summary Feed
Semantic Web
Simple Mail Transfer
    Protocol (SMTP)
Spam
Telephony
Threaded Messages
User Id
Vodcast
Voice over the Internet
    Protocol (VoIP)
Web 3.0
Web Conferencing
Web 2.0
Webcast
Webinar
Wiki
Wikipedia®
Zipped File

Christina is a nurse in the quality improvement department of a rural county hospital. Kerrie is a nurse in a critical care step-down unit. Both Christina and Kerrie (not their real names) are working on nursing degrees and have become dependent on electronic communication, but both have had to devise "work-arounds" to get access to the Internet. Christina has access to the email and the Internet from her hospital but not at home. In the evenings and on weekends, she takes her laptop and textbooks and drives to the local library or coffee or sandwich shop to check email and complete online course assignments. Kerrie doesn't have email or Internet access at work, so to stay in touch with her instructors and fellow students during breaks, she checks email using her smartphone.

Like the two nurses above, online communication has become so important to daily life that when it is not easily available, people go out of their way to become connected. Free Wi-Fi™ (wireless fidelity)[1] connections to the Internet have become a selling point for coffee shops and hotels. Never before in history have new communication methods like those provided by the Internet and its by-products made such quick inroads into society. The Internet has given us inexpensive asynchronous discussions, synchronous instant communication, email, electronic mailing lists, and the library known as the World Wide Web (WWW). Creative users, not content to have the WWW as just a repository of information, have given us social networking, interactive sites, instant news, and personal opinions not regulated by traditional media.

The networking thus provided allows us to communicate with colleagues worldwide and to stay abreast of standards of care and practice. History has taught us through recent devastating disasters that electronic networking can provide a means for organizing and

delivering healthcare provider volunteer assistance, pharmaceuticals and medical supplies, as well as a way to provide care to those in need. Nurses trapped within the disasters have been able to connect to the Internet and chronicle events using email and online blogs.

Synchronous Internet Communication

Synchronous Internet Communication refers to communication that is done in real time, just like a telephone or face-to-face conversation. There are several different types: text-based instant messaging, telephony, and Web conferencing.

TEXT-BASED INSTANT MESSAGING

Instant messaging (IM) is becoming a transparent part of email and an optional feature in most course learning management systems (LMSs). You can see "who else is online" and then send them a text message. IM has been controversial in the classroom because students instant message each other in class similar to the days when some of us passed paper notes. Text messaging (short message service [SMS]) and multimedia messaging (MMS) are similar features that are standard on mobile phones.

Chat is interactive email that has been around for a long time, but it has morphed into newer types of instant communication. Chat is an optional feature that is available in course LMSs. In this milieu, the computer screen shows a list of the participants as they enter the chat room. Chat users use their real names or a "handle or alias," type their conversation, and tap the Enter key to send the message. Others in the chat room respond with their replies.

TELEPHONY

Telephony refers to computer software and hardware that can perform functions usually

---

[1] The Wi-Fi Alliance is a trade group that owns WiFi™, which is the trademark to Wi-Fi.

associated with a telephone. Telephony products are often referred to as **voice over the Internet protocol (VoIP)**. VoIP provides a means to make a telephone call anywhere in the world with voice and video using the Internet, thereby bypassing the phone company. The free versions provide phone communication from computer to computer. All you need is a microphone, speakers, and a sound card. If you have a video camera, you can have video calls. Some VoIP software include conference and video calls. The connection, computer processor, and software determine the number of people and quality of the connection. For a small fee, you can choose to call telephone numbers on mobile phones and landlines using the Internet.

TELECONFERENCING VIA THE INTERNET

Conference calls using the telephone have become a way of life for those belonging to committees whose members live in different geographical locations. In **Web conferencing**, videos such as slideshows and other visuals can be added to the meeting. Some Web conferencing software feature the ability of participants to mark up documents or images, as well as "chat" using a keyboard. Web conferencing is similar to an open telephone call, but with the added element of video. A **Webcast** is generally a one-way presentation, usually with video, to an audience who may be present either in a room or in a different geographical location. Methods for the distant audience to ask questions are usually provided (Molay, 2007). A **Webinar**, on the other hand, is more like a live seminar. Although there is a speaker, the audience can ask questions, and the speaker can ask for feedback as the information is delivered.

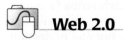 **Web 2.0**

In the quest to make the Web function in a more personal manner, a concept called **Web 2.0** was born. It does not have strict boundaries from the original Web but is about people interacting, sharing, and collaborating. The term "Web 2.0" was first coined by O'Reilly and others to describe what online companies/services that survived the dot.com bubble burst in 2000 had in common (O'Reilly, 2005). Web 2.0 is more of a philosophy than a technology and has many interpretations. It is based on a common vision of its user community. The objective of all Web 2.0 services is to mutually maximize the collective intelligence of the participants and add value for each participant by formalized and dynamic information sharing and creation (Högg, Meckel, Stanoevska-Slabeva, & Martignoni, 2006).

Web 2.0 services are an interactive development process (Högg et al., 2006). Information sharing can be video, data, text, or metadata such as annotations of history. The format is determined by the provider, with the basic idea being that information is created and shared among many users maximizing the collective intelligence. The results can be commonly accepted content or opinion. This type of intelligence requires some type of regulating, often from users of the site. User recommendations on eBay are one example as are reviews of various travel facilities by those who have used them.

Web 2.0 provides a rich medium to nurses and other healthcare professionals for interactive networking. A professional networking Web site is like a visit to one's colleague's office or home where one can see personal pictures and other decor that reflect his or her ideas and personality.

COLLECTIVE INTELLIGENCE TOOLS

Collective intelligence is defined as knowledge and understanding that emerges from large groups of people (The Horizon Report, 2008). Analysis of data that is collected over time will allow new patterns to emerge and in turn will result in new knowledge. The notion of collective intelligence has implications for changes in the educational process and the nursing profession. Use of collective intelligence applications in nursing education provides opportunities for grassroots problem solving and knowledge construction by students worldwide.

Wikis

A **Wiki** is one example of a collective intelligence application. A "Wiki" is a piece of server software that allows users to freely create and edit a Web page's content using any Web browser. Wiki supports hyperlinks and has a simple text syntax for creating new pages and cross-links between internal pages on the fly (What is Wiki, 2002). Wikis are Web sites designed for sharing and collaborative work on documents. They are used for committee work, clubs, classrooms, and knowledge management. Wikis can be private or public, for example, a Wiki designed for committee work would be private. The Wiki administrator identifies the membership using email addresses, and the Wiki automatically emails members with information on how to register for the Wikispace. Wikispaces provides a video tutorial on creating a Wiki at http://www.wikispaces.com/site/tour#introduction. Free Wikispace will have advertisements, but you can pay a small fee for an advertisement-free space.

The culture of the group is a factor that affects the effectiveness of collaboration (Watson & Harper, 2008). Users must be willing to share knowledge and exchange ideas. They must be open-minded and willing to seek new knowledge. When Wikis are used as an updatable knowledge management repository, users must have the technical skills to upload and edit documents.

Wikipedia® is an example of a public Wiki. It is a popular, free, online encyclopedia, which began in 2001. Within the first six months of development, users had contributed 6000 articles (Neus, 2001); as of November 2008, there were over two and a half million articles written in English (Wikipedia, 2008). Wikipedia articles are collaboratively created and improved by users. To make any changes to Wikipedia articles, users must register and then log in to the site. Tabs at the top of the article provide a means for collaborative discussion on the topic, editing the topic, or viewing the history of changes (an audit trail). All changes are recorded and can always be undone. The strength of Wikipedia is that it provides information on an ever-expanding number of topics. Critics are quick to point out that the quality of the articles is inconsistent. For technical information, it is often one of the most up-to-date and best source.

Web 2.0 Office Suites

With Web 2.0 have come many tools that allow groups of users to work together virtually. Many of the tools are free and very easy to use. The only requirement is the use of a computer with an Internet connection. Two examples of online office suites that allow group collaboration are Google Docs™ and Zoho Office. Google Docs (http://www.wikispaces.com/site/tour#introduction) includes word processing, spreadsheet, and presentation software. The documents are usually created off-site and then uploaded where they can be shared and edited by others. The documents can also be downloaded and saved. Zoho® at http://zoho.com provides collaborative access to word processing, spreadsheets, presentation tools, an online notebook, an online planner, a Wiki, Web conferencing, Web application creation, and chat. The Web site allows users to import files from other office applications. Joining either of these is free; all one has to do is create an account.

Sharing Media

The Sketchcast (http://sketchcast.com/) tool allows a registered user to draw and narrate an idea and then share it via a Web page or blog. Slideshare (http://www.slideshare.net/) allows users to embed a slideshow into a Web site or a blog, synch audio to slides, and join groups who share the same interests. Presentations can be downloaded to the user's computer or shared with others. The search terms "nursing" and "nursing research" at this site will find slideshows pertinent to the nursing profession. "Slide" at http://www.slide.com/ also allows you to create online slideshows including music videos as well as create a guest book for your site on which friends can share their pictures.

Evolving Collective Intelligence Applications

New collective intelligence applications are on the horizon. Freebase at http://www.freebase.com is an open shared knowledge database. The Web site provides an introductory video designed to guide new users to efficiently search the database. To contribute you must register and receive a login and password. The Google Image Labeler at http://images.google.com/imagelabeler/ uses a gaming strategy to improve the quality of Google images search term results. Users are randomly paired with an online partner. The players are shown a set of images over a two-minute period and asked to describe the image with as many labels as possible. When the two players agree on a label, the players receive points.

Folksonomies

Folksonomy, or management by people, is a method of classifying material (Anissimov) that is another form of collective intelligence. Tagging Web sites by group consensus for easy retrieval is one form. The social bookmarking site Delicious (http://delicious.com/), where people share and tag their favorite Web sites, is an example. At this site you can add your favorite Web sites to a label and see those of others with the same label. Another example is Technorati (http://technorati.com/), which tracks the links and comments of bloggers in their blogs.

BLOGS

A **blog** is an online Web log or discussion. Although blogs can be collaborative, more often, they are started by one person known as a blogger, and although comments are usually allowed, they generally revolve around the blogger's posts. Blog has many definitions, but basically, it is a Web site on which the blogger, or bloggers, share ideas and thoughts, often about a given topic, with posts in reverse chronological order. It is, or should be, updated regularly. Their quality and content vary, from personal musings to those that are more serious and informative.

There are many different ways to use blogs in both education and healthcare (Kawamoto, 2004). Because blogs are a Web site, nursing educators can easily incorporate their use into online course content. Family blogs that share experiences about care for a loved one with medical problems could be used as case studies for nursing students and provide insights into those affected by the illnesses. The teaching/learning effectiveness of patient-centered blogs is enhanced when readers are encouraged to participate in the conversation and to post personal reflections (Sandars, 2007).

Blogs can also be used to share information about a particular health topic. One example of this type of blog is the *Scoliosis News*, where news reports about scoliosis are posted. Health blogs have varying authors including healthcare professionals, patients, and someone interested in a topic who reads widely on a subject and wants to share his or her knowledge. Nurses in both hospital and education settings use blogs to share learning. For example, the nurses at Saint Joseph Hospital (Orange, California) have created a nursing research blog (http://evidencebasednursing.blogspot.com/search/label/ResearchatSt.JosephHospital0Orange) in which they communicate the research activities of their staff as well as the results of group discussions about research articles.

A blog is relatively easy to create using free tools such as Google's (http://www.blogger.com/start), Live Journal (http://www.livejournal.com/), and Xanga (http://www.xanga.com/). Some of these tools also allow readers to post comments to the postings. Authoring a blog is not something to be taken on lightly; they are time consuming and need to be constantly updated if others are to find them interesting. Like all Web sources, information from a blog needs to be carefully evaluated (Kawamoto, 2004).[2]

RSS FEEDS

Because blogs are updated, but generally not on a fixed schedule, you can subscribe to an

---

[2] Evaluating Web sites is discussed in Chapter 12.

Figure 6-1 • The RSS icon.

RSS feed, which will notify you when there is new information on a blog. RSS feed is an acronym for both **Real Simple Syndication** and **Rich Site Summary** (your choice). RSS feeds are not confined to blogs. You can have RSS feeds of new items from Web sites including electronic library searches, news, and blogs sent to your personalized Web browser home Web page, such as iGoogle or MyYahoo. The signal that a Web site is amenable to being subscribed to is the orange icon on the page itself, or in the location bar (see Figure 6-1). Since December 2005, this icon has become the industry standard denoting RSS feed availability. Using the Help menu in your Web browser or email application you can easily create an RSS feed for any site where you see the icon.

MASHUPS

A **mashup** is a Web application that takes data from more than one source and combines it into a single, integrated tool (Merrill, 2006). There are several varieties of mashups. One type involves mapping, in which data is overlaid on a map. This type of mashup was given a push with the advent of Google Maps, which, developers discovered, could be overlaid with current data from various sources. This type of mashup could be used in healthcare to place cases of infectious diseases on a geographical area. In a smaller example, overlaying data about infections on a unit over a blueprint of rooms would provide more information than the data alone.

Another type of mashup involves associating videos or photos with the metadata about the picture such as who took the picture and the location where it was taken. There are also search and shopping mashups such as the comparative shopping tools that draw data from various sources. News mashups are another variety in which news from various sources is synthesized into personalized news.

GOOGLE® GROUPS

Google Groups™ discussion forums, similar to Wikispaces, allow for sharing of documents as well as a group discussion. Unlike Wikispaces, all Google Group users must have a Gmail address. Google Groups can be private or public, or serve as an electronic bulletin board. Private Google Groups has a feature that alerts all the members when there is a change to the workspace. Google Groups are also used for collaborative work such as committee work, classrooms, and clubs. Yahoo also provides the same service.

GRASS ROOTS MEDIA

The ability to share photographs and videos is a rapidly growing trend! The term **Grass Roots Media** refers to the widespread creation and posting to the Web of media such as videos, slides, and blogs by nonprofessionals. There are multiple ways to create digital photos or videos that can be posted to the Web. Many cell phones include both the ability to take photos and videos. Inexpensive but "good-enough" digital camcorders are also available. One inexpensive digital video camera is even small enough to fit inside a pocket (Pure Digital Technologies, n.d.). There are also disposable camcorders that take up to 20 minutes of audio and video (Money.com., 2005).

Online Photos

Web sites such as Flickr™ (http://flickr.com/) and Shutterfly (http://www.shutterfly.com/) are specifically designed for photo sharing. They both allow photos to be shared privately and publically. Shared photos is an excellent way of sharing experiences from professional meetings and conferences.

Online Personal Videos

Video-on-demand Web sites, such as YouTube (http://www.youtube.com/), allow users to upload, view, and broadcast videos to a worldwide audience at no charge. To find and view a video from YouTube, enter a search term in the search box. To upload a video, register for an account, complete a short form where you indicate your account type, contact information, gender, and age, and agree to the Web site terms of use. Although free online videos vary in quality and length, users are guided to useful resources such as the ratings of other users. Faculty and healthcare professionals are using the video-on-demand sites to deliver lecture material. When uploading video on healthcare topics, users must adhere to all privacy guidelines to protect patient confidentiality.

Podcasts and Vodcasts

Podcasts, or audio messages available online, and **vodcasts**, video and audio online, allow anyone with the appropriate hardware and software to create and publish audio and video contents on the Web. Some developers publish these as a theme series on a specific subject that are available as an RSS feed. They can be identified by the orange icon with the word "POD." There are three ways through which you can listen to a podcast: using an MP3 player, listening on a computer with special software such as the Windows Media Player®, and with VoIP by dialing a number (Little, 2007). Free podcatching software (the name given to software that allows users to play podcasts on their computer) is also available from iTunes (http://www.apple.com/itunes/download/) and Juice (http://juicereceiver.sourceforge.net/). There are also many excellent resources for podcasts at these sites.

Although podcasts and vodcasts are often referred to with only the term "podcast," they are in different file formats. Many MP3 players play both. Podcasts, like blogs, are available at just about every news Web site. Educators are taking advantage of podcasting by recording their lectures and then uploading them as a podcast to the iTunes store or other places. To subscribe to a podcast, open the command to subscribe in podcatching software and then copy and paste the URL for the podcast.

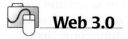

Web 3.0

It's hard to believe, but the Web is now thought of in context of generations. Web 1.0 provided information. Web 2.0, which was discussed in the last section, is characterized by Web sites that promote sharing and collaboration, and is still a work in progress. How **Web 3.0** will eventually look is not yet known, but the goal is to make it more of a guide and less of a catalog. To accomplish this, Web scientists are trying to provide a level of Web artificial intelligence that would think instead of just following commands, a task that has eluded researchers for more than half a century (Markoff, 2006). Some call this the Semantic Web (Metz, 2007), but others think that it is just a precursor to the real Semantic Web (Iskold, 2007).

In the **Semantic Web**, the data in documents will be processed, transformed, assembled, and even acted on, instead of requiring reading, interpretation, and action by humans (What is the Semantic Web?, 2007). Under this scheme, let's say that you have a patient who needs self-care information about a rare disease. It is one with which you are not familiar, so you search for this disease using your favorite search engine. The results, however, are not satisfactory. You receive a list of 1,500 items, some of which are advertisements for questionable products, others are from non-English-speaking countries, and there are many long, involved, articles. After looking at a few, you realize that they are mostly concerned with the etiology and prevention and are not appropriate for self-care. The prospect of looking at each link to find what you need is daunting. In a Semantic Web–enabled environment, you would be able to search using your specifications that this not be a commercial for a product, and that the information be research based and about self-care for a person with this condition. Your results would be greatly reduced, but would be more relevant to your needs.

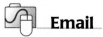

Email

Sending and receiving **email** on the computer is one of the primary uses of the Internet. Email offers many advantages to nurses and other healthcare professionals. Before 1995,

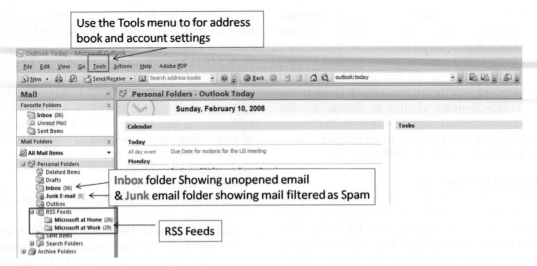

Figure 6-2 • Microsoft Outlook illustration.

only those who shared the same network connection could exchange email. For instance, those using CompuServe as their **Internet service provider (ISP)** could only email others who also used CompuServe. Today, with most computer networks being part of the Internet, the exchange of email is possible with anyone in the world who has an Internet email address. Being knowledgeable about how to use and manage email makes you a more efficient professional communicator.

As seen in the introductory scenario, email enhances communication with speed and convenience. Most messages arrive at their destination only a few moments after they have been sent, even if the destination is halfway around the globe. Email offers a way to avoid "telephone tag" and to create a written message that the receiver can read several times, convert into voice with special software, or save. To use email, you need email software (called an email client) and an email account.

EMAIL SOFTWARE

An email client is software used to access email from an email server so it can be viewed and read. An email server is simply a computer that uses server software to receive and make email

available for those who have an account on that server. Operating systems come with email software such as Windows Mail® (formerly, Outlook Express®). Other free email clients usable by both personal computers (PCs) and Macs can be found at Eudora (http://www.eudora.com/), or Mozilla's Thumberbird (http://www.mozilla.com/en-US/thunderbird/). There are similarities in the menus for all of the email clients. Figure 6-2 shows an example of the Microsoft Outlook 2007 window.

Email software can keep a copy of all messages that are sent and received, however the default is to delete these messages when the email software is closed. Many people like to be able to search and view these messages after more than one session. To accommodate this, the default is easily set to keep the messages. Because these folders can become huge, if the default is reset to keep the messages, one needs to open and delete the messages on a regular schedule, perhaps every month. Email software also provides a way to create folders so that incoming mail can be saved into a specific folder for future reference. Email is ideal for communicating across time zones, particularly those where night and day are opposite, not only because the sender and receiver can respond at times that are most convenient for them, but also because it saves postage and telephone expenses.

EMAIL ACCOUNTS

Access to the Internet is through an ISP, either a private one at home or through a college, work, or establishment that offers free Wi-fi. There are many ways to create an email account and get an email address. ISPs provide email accounts, usually two to five per account, for their customers. Colleges also provide email accounts for their students, and many healthcare agencies create email accounts for their employees. It is also possible to get a free email account at Google, Microsoft, or Yahoo by visiting their home page and opening an account.

Email Addresses

Like postal mail, email requires sender and receiver addresses. At first glance, an email address may look forbidding, but a closer look at the address will reveal the formatting rules. An email address has two parts separated by the @ sign. The first part, or the letters before the @ sign, is called the user name (sometimes called the login name) and identifies the sender. The part after the @ is the name of the email server where the email is received. The characters after the last dot in an email address constitute the suffix that identifies the domain or main subdivision of the Internet to which the computer belongs (see Figure 6-3).

User Name

The computer name and domain suffix are dependent on which email server you are using; these are assigned by the ISP that hosts the email account. Most institutions assign a **login name (user id)**, which includes at least part of the user's name. If you create an account for yourself, remember that the user name reflects on you. Email messages can be forwarded anywhere, and the email address of the person who created it, as well as anyone who receives it, is also forwarded. For this reason, healthcare providers should always select a user name that conveys their profession appropriately; cutesy names are never appropriate.

Configuring an Email Client

To configure an email client that is on your PC to send and receive email, you need just five pieces of information: the email account type, the name of the incoming server, the name of the outgoing server, your login user name, and your logon password. The account type and name of the incoming and outgoing server are assigned by the ISP where you have your account. The type of email account is usually **POP3 (Post Office Protocol)**, but may also be **IMAP (Internet Mail Access Protocol)**. Outgoing servers use **SMTP (Simple Mail Transfer Protocol)**. In private accounts such as one from your own PC or one created with one of the free email clients, you select your own login or user name and password when you open an account. The logon user name and password allow you to retrieve your email from your account. To simplify this process, Outlook® 2007 automatically configures the email accounts using the email address and email server password.

PLANNING EMAIL ACCOUNTS

Email users should consider having several email accounts, each with a different purpose. One email account should be used for official communication with coworkers and colleagues. Students should use an account dedicated to

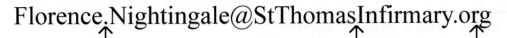

Florence.Nightingale@StThomasInfirmary.org

Userid (Login)   Computer Name   Domain Suffix

Figure 6-3 • An email address.

official school communication with other students and faculty. A third email account, using free online email software or a home ISP, should be used for personal communication. In addition, a fourth email account might be used for online shopping to trap potential resulting spam.

If you have more than one email address, you may want to configure your email client to download from more than one server. For example, if you create a free email account at Google® or Yahoo®, you can set your email client to download mail from there by using the account settings. Unless you are an expert, use only one outgoing server.

CREATING AND SENDING EMAIL

When you activate the Write feature of your email client, your address will already be on the "From" line. Your first step is to enter the address(es) of the receiver(s) on the "To" line. If you have put the recipient's name in your email client's address book, when you start to enter the beginning of the name, the address book will automatically finish it for you. After entering the recipient's name, enter a brief word or phrase about the message on the subject line. Emails with no subject line may be classified as junk mail by the user's email server and not be received by the recipient. Finally, create your message and add a signature that clearly identifies you.

There may be times when you want to send the same message to more than one person. This is simple if the message is a reply to a message that was also addressed to others to whom you wish the reply to be sent; select "Reply All" to start your message instead of "Reply." If you routinely send email to the same group of people, such as to members of a committee that you are on, you can use the address book to create a group. With a group, you then place the name of the group on the "To" line, instead of each name. Use Help to learn how to create a group of recipients. When sending a duplicate of a message to others, you have the option of using "**Cc**" or "**Bcc**." The acronym "**Cc**" is derived from

earlier days of the typewriter carbon copy. The "Bcc" indicates a blind copy where the receiver is unaware that others have also received a copy of the message. Blind carbon copies should be used judiciously; the sender must consider the ethics of secrecy when using the function.

Sometimes you want to forward a message that you have received to someone else. Before forwarding a message, give thoughtful consideration to the sender and receiver. In consideration to the sender, send a copy of the email to the original sender when forwarding the email to others. When forwarding a message, edit the message to remove the email addresses of prior recipients. Avoid passing on chain letters; most people do not want them, and many agencies will terminate your account if you do this. Messages warning about viruses or other dire things that will happen to your computer if you don't do something are generally hoaxes.[3]

EMAIL SIGNATURE

Email written by professionals should always include a signature with the sender's name, title, company name, and geographical location. A signature is similar to the return address on a postal letter; however, personal information such as street addresses and home phone numbers should be avoided. Most signatures are one to five lines; a signature may be personalized by including a favorite quotation. Instructions for creating a signature for Windows Outlook®, Windows Mail®, Netscape®, or Mozilla Thunderbird® go to the Web page for Chapter 6 the book at http://dlthede.net/Informatics/Informatics.html. In Gmail, the signature can be created from the Settings window. In some email packages, a user creates the signature as a "txt" file with a program like Notepad® and then, using account settings, tells the email client where to find it.

---

[3] See Chapter 5 for more information about viruses and hoaxes.

EMAIL FILE FORMATTING

There are three main file formats for creating and sending messages: plain text (TXT), **rich text file (RTF), and hypertext markup language (HTML)**. TXT files have no formatting, which makes them ideal for electronic mailing lists because any email client can read them. RTF files allow for some formatting, but not the robust features of a word processor. HTML files use HTML tags to display formatting of text. Not all email software can read HTML messages, especially in less developed nations. For file formats that are either rtf or html, you can use the formatting functions, such as bold, italics, and bullets in your email client.

THE DO'S AND DO NOTS OF EMAIL CONTENT

As convenient as email is, it must be used appropriately. Care must be taken in deciding what is included in a message that is sent via email; contents of email must always adhere to common decency. Email should never be used to give bad news, such as a poor evaluation, work layoff, or pay decrease. A rule of thumb is not to include anything in an email message that you wouldn't want to read on the front page of the newspaper since it is very easy for a recipient to either accidentally or purposely forward your message to someone else. All messages carry headers that can be traced to the original sender. Even if the sender uses a remailer, a service that strips the identifying header so that email can be sent anonymously, sender information can be traced by contacting the remailer service (Freeman, 2007).

EMAIL PRIVACY ISSUES

There is no guarantee that email that is sent using an educational facility or employer email server or email provider service will be private. A growing trend is for institutions to monitor email to avoid potential litigation and investigations from government agencies (AMA/ePolicy Institute, 2008; Clearinghouse, 2006). There is still no definitive case law on whether students or employees have the right to privacy in email. This includes situations in which the institution has said that your email is private because if the message can be construed as damaging to the institution, privacy promises may be legally invalidated. There are several court cases that have set precedence and ruled in favor of the employer (Bourke v. Nissan Motor Corporation in the United States, 1993; Smyth v. The Pillsbury Company, 1996 Sykes, 2000).

EMAIL ETIQUETTE

Email etiquette, like regular mail letter etiquette, is essential for professional communication (Jones, 2006). The rules for creating email are important. First of all, always include a short pertinent subject line. When replying to email, make sure to include appropriate information from the prior message in the reply. Email is a special form of communication, not as interactive as the telephone, but more interactive than written communication. Because it often seems very personal and quick, there is a tendency to regard it as a verbal conversation and forget that the recipient may have been involved in many complicated matters since he or she last sent you a message. For this reason, mailers provide an option to include the prior message with the original when you reply. To prevent messages that rapidly become too large and uncommunicative, edit the prior message so that only the parts pertinent to your reply are included. In general, email should be short and to the point, but not too short. A message that is too short may be misinterpreted by the recipient, who may feel that the sender was being abrupt or curt.

Use the appropriate font and case when writing email. According to email etiquette, use of all uppercase letters (all caps) indicates that the user is shouting, so all caps should never be used for sentence construction. Use font colors thoughtfully. Depending on the message, a red-colored font may be interpreted as swearing (Cleary & Freeman, 2005). Finally, email should always be signed. Professional email should include a signature,

---

Box 6-1 • Email Recommendations

- Managing Accounts
  - Be familiar with your employer's policy on the use of official email
  - Use employer email only for official business
  - Use several email accounts – one for official email, one for school email, and the others for personal activities
- Sending Email
  - Always check your email for spelling, grammar, and punctuation before sending
  - Include a signature with contact information (title, organization, address)
  - Be aware that all email, even if it is deleted, is potentially discoverable

- Be sure that your email does not violate common decency laws
- Never open attachments that you do not expect to receive
- Never send confidential information in email
- Use email appropriately – never use it to avoid face-to-face communication
- Managing Email
  - Create email filters to avoid spam and other unwanted email
  - Never respond to spam
  - Organize your email using folders and alerts
  - Try to respond to email within 24 hours

---

title, and contact information, such as a mailing address of the agency, phone number, and home page URL. (see Box 6-1).

There are some major differences between email and letters sent by postal mail. Postal mail letters generally have the reader's full, undivided attention. In contrast, because of the sheer volume of email, the reader may not read the message thoroughly, causing misunderstandings resulting in problems in relationships. If there is a chance for disagreement, or email messages seem to be causing disagreements, use email to set up a time for either a person-to-person meeting or a telephone conversation.

ACRONYMS AND EMOTICONS

Email is devoid of the nonverbal commands of face-to-face communication. Thus, expressions of subtle meaning and tone are easily lost. With the informality of much email and the limited typing skills of many who send email messages, it is only natural that common acronyms and icons have developed. They are only valuable when the recipients understand them. Acronyms use the first letter of words or word parts to communicate a common phrase (see Table 6-1). They are commonly used in informal email and instant messaging. Acronyms are not appropriate for professional communication.

To provide the appropriate body language tone, telecommunicators have devised icons called **emoticons** (emotional icons), sometimes called smileys, which can be created on the keyboard. For example, one that is frequently used is :-). When tilting your head to the left, which is the position for "reading" keyboard character emoticons, you can see a smiling face (see Table 6-2). Some email clients include graphic emoticons. A classic graphic emoticon is a round, yellow button with two dots for eyes and half circle for a smile. Use emoticons sparingly, if at all, in professional business communication. (See http://www.windweaver.com/emoticon.htm for more examples of emoticons.)

TABLE 6-1 ● *Common Email Acronyms*

Acronym	Meaning
BTW	By the way
FAQ	Frequently asked questions
f2f	Face-to-face
FWIW	For what it is worth
<g>	Grin
IMO or IMHO	In my opinion or in my humble opinion
OTOH	On the other hand

TABLE 6-2 ● *Common Email Emoticons*

Emoticon	Meaning
☺ or :)	Smiley
☹ or :(	Frown
:O	Shock or disappointment
:[	Serious or sad
;)	Wink
> :(or > :O	Upset or angry

ATTACHMENTS

Many people use email to send files created with other software, such as a word processor or spreadsheet. When including attachments in your email, use the following guidelines. First, always alert the receiver before sending an attachment and verify that the receiver has the software that can view the attachment. For example, if a file is created and saved with Publisher® with the Publisher file extension ".pub," the recipient will not be able to view the file unless he or she has Publisher on their computer. Be sure that the recipient has the appropriate version of the software that you are using; many file formats from the same vendor's program are not **backwardly compatible**. If you need to save the file in a different format before sending, see Chapter 4.

Attaching files to email messages increases the size of the message, which in turn increases the time required to both send and receive it. If the attached file is large, consider "**zipping**" it. Zipping a file involves using a piece of software that compresses the file to make it smaller. In general, text files can be compressed much more than graphics files. Files may be zipped separately or as a group (archived). Before zipping a file, make sure that the recipient has unzip software in his or her computer and that the person's email server allows for zipped attachments (some email servers remove attachments with certain file formats, such as a zipped file, to prevent the spread of potentially harmful viruses). Most of today's operating systems include some type of zip/unzip software. Use the Help feature to learn to use it.

An alternative for attaching a large file or zipped file is to use file transfer Internet Web sites. Examples include YouSendIt (http://www.yousendit.com/), SendThisFile (http://www.sendthisfile.com/), and LogMein (http://secure.logmein.com). The file transfer Web sites provide free as well as fee-based services; both require the user to register to receive a login and password. To send a file, go to the Web site, log in, enter the recipient's email address and an email subject, browse (find in your folders) to the file, select it, click open on that window, and click Send It. The recipient receives an email with a Web address (URL) to download the file. If you are in the habit of exchanging large files with someone whose email account is limited in sending or receiving large files or if you are limited in this respect, one or both of you may want to get a free email account where the size of attachments is not as limited.

MANAGING EMAIL

Taking a few minutes to organize and manage email can save you much time and energy later (see Table 6-3). Whether you use a stand-alone or Web-based client, the email management processes are similar. All email clients have Help menus to guide you through the process of organizing email. You can use email alerts to assist in prioritizing email. Alerts include flags, stars, and font colors. Use email filters to automatically file incoming email into designated folders and send you personal alerts for email from certain senders. You can also use filters to filter unwanted mail such as spam (unsolicited commercial email) to the deleted items folder.

OUT-OF-OFFICE REPLIES

There are times when you will not be answering email, such as when out of town. This, however, does not stop your email. When you do not answer, your correspondents may become upset. To show consideration for them, it is smart to have an automatic response sent to them informing them that you are unable to read and

TABLE 6-3 ● *Managing Email: Tools May Vary According to the Email Agent*

Tools	Function	How to Use
Folders and labels	Provide a way to categorize email.	Drag and drop email into the folders or create a filter to automatically move the email to the folder. Examples of categories are committees, school, and work.
		If using a filter to move email into a folder, consider providing yourself an alert that the email has arrived.
Flags or stars	Used to give a visual alert for importance and/or follow-up.	After you have read the email, you can click a flag or star to indicate importance and follow-up.
Colors	Provide a visual cue to help organize email.	Create rules to use color to categorize email.
Sound	Provides an auditory alert for the arrival of email.	Use sound alerts to check email as it arrives into the mailbox.
Filters	Provide rules to the software to perform actions on email.	Use filters to delete spam that escapes your Internet Mail Provider spam filter. Filters can be used to apply rules to automatically perform an action on email with identified senders, receivers, subject, and/or message words.

respond to their message and letting them know when you will be able to do so. Most ISPs provide this service; to activate it go to your account on their server and use Help to learn how to do this. If you are using Gmail, look for "Vacation Responder" in the Settings menu.

SPAM

Spam (junk email) is not only a nuisance, it is potentially harmful. As annoying as junk email can be, it is important to recognize it to proactively limit or eliminate it. A first clue of junk is the sender's email address. If you don't know the sender, the email is probably junk. To proactively limit or eliminate junk mail, learn how to develop email filters and rules. In Windows Mail® 2007, using the junk email options on the Tools menu can be used to filter spam to the junk folder to decide what to do with mail determined to be junk. In Gmail the "Filters" window can be used to discard spam. Some online email clients allow the user to report spam with the click of a button.

Spam is the electronic version of junk postal mail, except that it shifts the costs of advertising to the receiver; it exists because it is a cheap way to advertise. It also fills the Internet with unwanted messages. Usually, spam originates from a false address, so replying is a waste of time. If, however, you receive a spam message and you know from the email address that the ISP exists, such as one of the online services, you can forward it to postmaster@online.service (substitute the name of the service for online.service). Most services and ISPs take a very dim view of spamming and terminate the account of anyone who sends junk email, or if someone's identity has been illegally assumed, the ISP will look for ways to prevent this from happening again.

All email users must be knowledgeable about spamming practices and malware, such as **phishing** and **pharming**.[4] One of the best ways to avoid spam is to not give out an email

---

[4] See Chapter 5 for a discussion on phishing and pharming.

address to any Web site. An alternative is to acquire a free mailbox site and use that email address when completing online forms, for example, when shopping online. Records of online shopping are then emailed to the free designated account along with any advertisements that they might send. When visiting the free email account, legitimate email can be forwarded to another address and spam can be deleted. Users should never open a known spam message! Finally, users should never purchase a product or service advertised from unsolicited email (Project, 2007).

RETRIEVING EMAIL FROM A REMOTE EMAIL ACCOUNT

Perhaps you normally use a stand-alone email client such as Outlook®, Windows Mail®, or Mozilla Thunderbird® to retrieve email, but you want to check your email when you are not at the computer that you usually use. Many ISPs will allow you to retrieve your mail directly from the server. Or, you can configure a Web-based client such as Gmail, Hotmail, or Yahoo to retrieve the email from your server when asked. Web-based email clients may also offer software designed for mobile devices. Mobile email clients allow users to retrieve and download remote email to handheld devices such as personal digital assistants (PDAs) and smartphones.

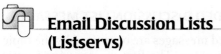

Email Discussion Lists (Listservs)

An email discussion list, sometimes referred to as a **listserv** (no "e" at the end) from the first software that was used to create one, is made up of a group of subscribers with a common interest. The software allows subscribers to receive discussion postings via email. Subscribing, or joining, a list is generally free. Instructions for subscribing are specific to a list and are generally found on the Web site for the list or as a click at a place where you find information about the list. Once subscribed to

a group, copies of any message posted to the group are sent to all members mailboxes (see Figure 6-4). Members can reply to any of the messages or send an entirely new message to the group. The tasks of keeping track of subscribers and sending copies of messages are accomplished by a software program. Other kinds of email list software include Majordomo®, Mailbase®, and Listproc®.

Once subscribed to a group, copies of any message posted to the group are sent to all members mailboxes. Members can reply to any of the messages or send an entirely new message to the group. Most lists are automated, that is, the software immediately sends out any messages posted to the group's posting address; some groups are moderated, that is, the message is first vetted by the list owner before posting.

Most mailing list software offer many options for subscribers beyond just sending messages. For this reason, there are two addresses for each group: one that manages the list, performing such tasks as subscribing a new member or evoking the available options such as temporarily suspending mail from the group; and another address that is used *only* when one posts a message to the group. This information is included in the information that is sent to all new subscribers. It is important to save this message because it not only provides you with the administrative address but also tells you how to unsubscribe, find the names of other participants, digest your mail (so that you receive one message per day with all of that day's postings), and temporarily stop your mail from the list (*very* important if you are not able to check your mail for a while). The instructions for use of email lists vary. When replying to a list message pay particular attention to whether you need to use Reply or Reply All. With some lists, the Reply feature will permit you to reply to all list participants; with other lists, you need to use "Reply All" to send the reply to more than the person who wrote the last message. Make sure that you sign the email posted to mailing lists with a standard "signature" that includes at least your name and email address. Some lists "strip" the email address of the participants in the header.

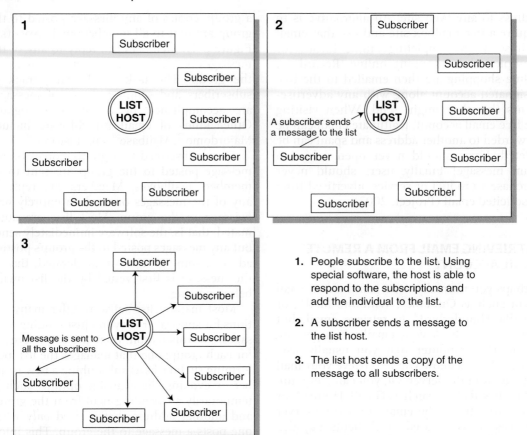

Figure 6-4 • Listserv topography.

1. People subscribe to the list. Using special software, the host is able to respond to the subscriptions and add the individual to the list.

2. A subscriber sends a message to the list host.

3. The list host sends a copy of the message to all subscribers.

FINDING A NURSING DISCUSSION LIST

There are electronic mailing lists for just about every nursing and other healthcare specialty imaginable; finding the right one is not always easy. Although you can search the Web using the term "nursing discussion lists" or "nursing listserv," staying up-to-date on what mailing lists are active is almost impossible. Check the Book Web page for current places where information about nursing mailing lists can be found. Examples of popular nursing discussion lists are as follows:

▼ Student nurse listserv at http://listserv .buffalo.edu/archives/snurse-l.html
▼ Nursing informatics listserv at http:// mailman.amia.org/mailman/listinfo/nrsing-l

▼ Nursing educator listserv at https://lists .uvic.ca/mailman/listinfo/nrsinged

THREADED DISCUSSION LIST MESSAGES

Threaded messages are organized by the topic of the message. The first message for a topic starts the thread followed by the other messages about the topic. Often the number of other messages on the topic is noted in parentheses after the topic of the group. If you receive list mail in the digest format, the messages are often threaded. You can also organize your personal email by topic to have threaded messages.

Regular listserv messages are not threaded, but if the group has an archives page, the messages are usually threaded on that page. The threading concept works only when posters preserve the original subject, either by using the Reply or Reply All function or by copying and pasting the original subject on the subject line prefaced by "Re:". It breaks down when posters use the Reply function to start a new topic without changing the subject line. In online courses, messages are also threaded, so learning to use threaded messages is an important skill.[5]

DISCUSSION LIST ETIQUETTE

Listserv etiquette is similar to that used for standard email. It is extremely important to be respectful of the other group members. Discussion list members represent an invisible number of individuals with a variety of experiences who may live anywhere in the world. Thus, messages need to be understandable to all. In messages avoid acronyms, which are often not understood even by people in your own area. Keep messages on the topic of the list; information about the allowable topics is provided in the welcoming message.

Lists are maintained or "owned" by the person who is responsible for the list. It is a thankless task for which there is no payment. For this reason, as well as consideration of the other members, you should consider being a member of a list, a privilege that conveys responsibilities. Send nothing except messages to be posted to the group to the email address that is used to send you group messages. For all other requests, like unsubscribing, use the administrative address or Web page of the group; information about how to implement these features is in the welcoming message. If you are going to be away for a while, either unsubscribe from the list or set the mail to no-mail (called noack in some list software). This is important to prevent a "full mailbox error," which is not happily received by the list owner who must then take the time to manually unsubscribe you. If you want to receive

only one message from a list a day, you can use the Web page or administrative address to set the mail to digest. If you receive messages in the digest mode and use the reply function of your email to reply to a message, delete the subject that is automatically on the subject line and copy and paste the subject of the message to which you wish to reply on that line prefaced by "Re:".

New list users may think that a list is a way to avoid doing a needed literature search. Don't expect other list members to do this for you. If you want information about a topic, when asking for help indicate the sources you have found. When a member indicates that he or she has done homework and is willing to share, other members are very happy to provide more help. Do remember to sign your email and use a contact signature, which includes your email address and the name and address of your affiliating organization.

FLAME WARS

Messages sent to an electronic mailing list go to many people whom the sender does not know. The messages will be read under a variety of conditions, by people in different moods. Given these circumstances, it is not surprising that occasionally a member takes umbrage at what another says and posts an overheated message. A message of this sort, called a **flame**, can easily deteriorate into a **flame war** when others respond derogatorily with other positions on the disputed topic. In most groups, this ends on a conciliatory note when cooler heads prevail. Flame wars can happen in any group, but tend to be more common in groups with controversial topics.

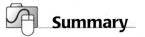 **Summary**

The WWW provides many opportunities for professional networking. As the Web has matured, many new features have been added such as the interaction permitted by Web 2.0. From the sharing of documents to discussion groups, these features make possible a collective

---

[5] Online education is discussed in Chapter 22.

intelligence as many people from all geographical areas and walks of life contribute their knowledge in such formats as Wikis and blogs. Grass Roots Media has become a possibility with blogs and media-sharing facilities such as YouTube®, all of which can be useful in healthcare for providing both continuing education and patient education. Email has become a way of life, necessitating learning a new way of communicating that is between voice mail and letter writing. Email has also provided a method of networking through email discussion groups often known as listservs. When healthcare professionals effectively use these new tools, they improve healthcare, both in the practice of the professional and for the patient.

APPLICATIONS AND COMPETENCIES

1. Examine the technology use policies and procedures for your educational or healthcare provider workplace facility for
   a. procedure to set up an email account,
   b. policies and procedures for use of the institution's email server,
   c. a privacy policy for user email,
   d. policies and procedures for approved email attachment file types, and
   e. policies and procedures for email communication with patients and families (healthcare provider).
2. Discuss how the policies and procedures benefit email users. Discuss any limitations that you noted. Compare your findings with those of your classmates.
3. Add three names and email addresses to an email address book and create a group for those three individuals.
4. Join a discussion list that relates to your nursing interest.
   a. Identify the address to be used to post a message to the group.
   b. Access the list's administrative Web site and experiment with the various options.
   c. Discuss advantages and limitations of the discussion list.
   d. Resign from the list using the Web site when you no longer want to be a member or your

email address is going to be terminated such as when you leave a place of employment, graduate from school, or change ISPs.
5. Explore one or more of Web 2.0 social networking features that could be beneficial to you as a student/healthcare professional. Explain the benefits and compare your experiences with other students or nursing colleagues.
6. Open iTunes (or download the software at http://www.apple.com/itunes/) and then search for free nursing resources in the iTunes store. Discuss the pros and cons for two of the resources.

REFERENCES

AMA/ePolicy Institute. (2008, February 28). *2007 electronic monitoring & surveillance survey.* Retrieved November 17, 2008, from http://press.amanet.org/press-releases/177/2007-electronic-monitoring-surveillance-survey/

Anissimov, M. *What is a folksonomy?* Retrieved November 17, 2008, from http://www.wisegeek.com/what-is-a-folksonomy.htm

Bonita P. Bourke et al. v. Nissan Motor Corporation in U.S.A., No. B068705 (Cal. Ct. App. 1993). Retrieved November 23, 2008, from http://www.loundy.com/CASES/Bourke_v_Nissan.html

Clearinghouse, P. R. (2006, February). *Employee monitoring: Is there privacy in the workplace?* Retrieved November 17, 2008, from http://www.privacyrights.org/fs/fs7-work.htm

Cleary, M., & Freeman, A. (2005). Email etiquette: guidelines for mental health nurses. *International Journal of Mental Health Nursing,* 14(1), 62–65.

Freeman, E. H. (2007). Email privacy and the wiretap act: U.S. v. councilman [Electronic version at http://epic.org/privacy/councilman/]. *Information Systems Security,* 16(3), 182–185.

Högg, R., Meckel, M., Stanoevska-Slabeva, K., & Martignoni, R. (2006). *Overview of business models for Web 2.0 communities* [Electronic version at http://www.alexandria.unisg.ch/EXPORT/DL/31412.pdf]. Paper presented at the GeNeMe 2006, Dresden, Germany. Retrieved November 23, 2008.

The Horizon Report. (2008). The new media consortium and educause learning initiative [Electronic version from http://www.nmc.org/pdf/2008-Horizon-Report.pdf].

Iskold, A. (2007, March 19). *Web 3.0: When Web sites become Web services.* Retrieved November 17, 2008, from http://www.readwriteweb.com/archives/web_30_when_web_sites_become_web_services.php

Jones, J. R. (2006). Sending the right message. *Nursing Standard,* 20(4), 72.

Kawamoto, K. (2004). Health related blogs [Electronic version at http://bcis.pacificu.edu/journal/2004/01/kawamoto.php]. *Interface: The Journal of Education, Community and Values,* 4(1).

Little, J. K. (2007, June). *Podcasting: A teaching with technology white paper. Educause.* Retrieved November 17, 2008, from http://connect.educause.edu/blog/jklittle/podcastingateachingw/44653?time=1184094157

Markoff, J. (2006). *Entrepreneurs see a web guided by common sense. Business.* Retrieved November 17, 2008, from http://www.nytimes.com/2006/11/12/business/12web.html?ex=1320987600&en=254d697964cedc62&ei=5088

Merrill, D. (2006, October 16). *Mashups: The new breed of Web app.* Retrieved November 17, 2008, from http://www.ibm.com/developerworks/xml/library/x-mashups.html

Metz, C. (2007, March 14). *Web 3.0. PC Magazine.* Retrieved November 17, 2008, from http://www.pcmag.com/article2/0,1759,2102852,00.asp

Michael A. Smyth v. The Pillsbury Company, C.A. NO. 95-5712 (Pa. District Court 1996). Retrieved November 17, 2008, from http://www.loundy.com/CASES/Smyth_v_Pillsbury.html

Molay, K. (2007, March 1). *Webinar or webcast – what's the difference?* Retrieved November 17, 2008, from http://wsuccess.typepad.com/webinarblog/2007/03/webinar_or_webc.html

CNNMoney.com (2005, June 5). *Disposable video camera: $29.99.* Retrieved November 17, 2008, from http://money.cnn.com/2005/06/06/technology/personaltech/cvs_camera/

Neus, A. (2001). *Managing information quality in virtual communities of practice.* Paper presented at the Proceedings of the 6th International Conference on Information Quality at MIT. Retrieved November 17, 2008, from http://opensource.mit.edu/papers/neus.pdf

O'Reilly, T. (2005, September 30). *What is Web 2.0.* Retrieved November 17, 2008, from http://www.oreillynet.com/pub/a/oreilly/tim/news/2005/09/30/what-is-web-20.html

Project, P. I. A. L. (2007, May). *The volume of spam is growing in Americans' personal and workplace email accounts, but email users are less bothered by it.* Retrieved March 1, 2008, from Pew Internet & American Life Project. Retrieved November 17, 2008, from http://www.pewinternet.org/PPF/r/214/report_display.asp

Pure Digital Technologies. (n.d.). *Introducing the Flip video ultra series.* Retrieved November 17, 2008, from http://www.theflip.com/

Sandars, J. (2007). The potential of blogs and wikis in health-care education. *Education for Primary Care,* 18(1), 16–21.

Sykes, C. Big brother in the workplace [Electronic version at http://www.hoover.org/publications/digest/3491686.html]. *Hoover Digest: Research and Opinion on Public Policy,* 2000(3).

Watson, K., & Harper, C. (2008). Supporting knowledge creation: Using Wikis for group collaboration [Electronic version]. *EDUCAUSE Center for Applied Research: Research Bulletin,* (3), 1–13.

What is the semantic web? (2007). Retrieved November 17, 2008, from http://www.altova.com/semantic_web.html

What is Wiki. (2002, June 27). Retrieved November 17, 2008, from http://www.wiki.org/wiki.cgi

Wikipedia. (2008, January 15). *Wikipedia: Size comparisons.* Retrieved November 17, 2008, from http://en.wikipedia.org/wiki/Wikipedia:Size_comparisons

Word Processing

Learning Objectives
After studying this chapter you will be able to:

1. *Apply many common word processing features.*

2. *List word processing features that are applicable in other application programs.*

3. *Be able to increase your word processing skills.*

Key Terms

Attribute	Mail Merge
Endnote	Object
Font	Overtype
Footer	Page Break
Footnote	Page Orientation
Header	Typeover
Justification	Word Processor
Macro	

Software programs designed to help a user manipulate text, edit, rearrange, and retype documents on a personal computer are called **word processors**. The popularity of word processing attests to the fact that written communication, whether in the printed or electronic format, is still the primary means of spreading information and knowledge. Effective usage of a word processor is part of computer fluency and is necessary to advance in nursing. One of the benefits of mastering basic word processing skills is the transferability of these skills to other application programs, most of which use the basic editing features of word processors when any text editing is required.

Word processing software packages vary in some of the features they offer, but all packages, even the text-editing software that comes with an operating system, offer the ability to insert, delete, cut, and paste text; search and replace words; and store and retrieve documents.

With the exception of the Microsoft Windows™ Accessory program, Notepad, all others also offer word wrap (the automatic insertion of line breaks when text exceeds the width of the page). Even email software offers many of these features. Full-featured word processors such as Corel WordPerfect®, Lotus WordPro®, and Microsoft Word®, however, offer the writer many more features.

The Document

Open a word processor and a blank document appears, in some ways resembling a blank piece of paper. The top of the screen has menus or tabs and icons that provide access to the features of the word processor. The bottom of the screen usually has what is called a status line, or a line that provides information about the document, such as the number of the current page, the distance of the insertion point from the left margin, the number of words in the document, and whether the Caps Lock is on or off. In the blank section of the screen, the user types a document, which often will be printed when finished. Although typing skills are a great help in entering text, it is the only resemblance that a word processor has to a typewriter. In fact, thinking in terms of the printed page, as one does with a typewriter, interferes with maximizing word processing features. In word processing, a user should separate the tasks of writing from those of formatting the page. Concentrate first on writing and format later is a good rule for word processing.

The available views of a document that a user can access support separation of formatting from writing. The draft or normal view shows just the text and is ideal for writing. In this view, when a new page becomes necessary, a solid or dotted single line appears to indicate a page break. The top and bottom page margins are not visible and do not interfere with one's thinking, nor is one tempted to paginate (create artificial page breaks) before editing is completed. In print view (page view in some word processors), one sees items that will appear on the printed page, such as footnotes or page numbers. Some word processors also have a Web view, and most can be used to create Web pages. When used for this purpose, they may create files that are very large or have hypertext codes that are not compatible with all Web browsers.

Text Characteristics

The flexibility of entering and manipulating text in a word processor makes writing and editing very easy. Some basic word processing features that are common to many other programs such as word wrap, erasing text, undo and redo, navigating a document, and default mode are discussed in Chapter 4 and will not be discussed here.

TEXT-ENTERING MODES

Two modes are available for entering (inputting) text in a word processing program: Insert and **Overtype**. In many programs, users can toggle between these two modes by tapping the Insert key.[1] The Default mode is the insert setting. In this mode, when the user enters new characters, the original text automatically makes room for it. In **Typeover** (may be called Overtype or Strikeover) mode, any new characters will replace those already in the document. Because the Insert key can be accidentally tapped, if you find that keys you type are overwriting text, tap the Insert key. If in doubt about which mode a user currently is in, the status line (except in Microsoft Word® 2007) usually provides this information. There are times when one wishes to use overtype, such as when

---

[1] In Microsoft Word® 2007 search help using the word "overtype" to find out how to implement this feature.

TABLE 7-1 ● *Font and Point Size*		
Different Fonts and Sizes		
8 point	*12 point*	*20 point*
Arial	Arial	Arial
Courier	Courier	Courier
Times New Roman	Times New Roman	Times New Roman

entering text into an electronic word processing form (not on the Web).

CHANGING THE APPEARANCE OF THE TEXT

The appearance of text can be changed in many ways. Changing the appearance of something is known as changing the attribute. An **attribute** is a characteristic that changes the appearance of an **object** (remember, an object is anything that can be manipulated). Attributes that can be applied to characters in most word processors include boldface, italics, color, and various types of underlines. Attributes can be turned on before or after characters are typed. To change an attribute before typing, choose the appropriate symbol from the toolbar, or click Format > Font (Page Layout tab in Microsoft Word® 2007). To make the change after typing, select the text and apply the attribute in the same manner.

FONTS (TYPEFACES) AND FONT SIZE (IN POINTS)

A **font** is the name given to the typeface style that is used for the characters in the document. The font and its size can be changed for the entire document or for just a small section. Like other attributes, changes can be made before or after text is entered. A drop-down box for both fonts and size is generally found on the toolbox near the top of the screen, or they are available in the Font menu under Format on the menu line (Home menu in Microsoft Word® 2007.). Some programs use the term "point size" to refer to the size of the print. Font sizes, however, vary with the font and attributes (see Table 7-1).

CUTTING, MOVING, AND PASTING TEXT

With word processing, as in all application programs, the user has the ability to copy and/or move sentences, paragraphs, pages, and the entire document. The same principles of cut (removing from one location) and copy (making a copy) as discussed in Chapter 4 apply in word processing. The text to be moved or copied must first be selected, then placed on the clipboard, and then pasted. These options are on the toolbar or in the Edit menu (Home tab in Microsoft Word® 2007).

Saving and Retrieving Files

As with all computer applications, it is a good idea to save frequently when creating a document in a word processor. Review principles of saving in Chapter 4. Files saved by a word processor are in a proprietary format, or one that is specific to the brand of the word processor that created it. Sometimes it is necessary to give a file to someone who uses a different type of word processor. To do this, you can save the file in an RTF format that usually maintains all the font attributes when transferred from one application to another (see Figure 4-8 in Chapter 4).

To retrieve a document, the user needs to know the location and name of the file. If a file was saved to a flash disk, to retrieve it, you can use the File Open feature and navigate to the appropriate disk. See Figure 4-3 for the icons that also invoke retrieving a file. Or, you can open My Computer (Computer in Microsoft Vista®) and click the appropriate disk. Then navigate to the appropriate file and click it. This will open both the program and the file.

Paragraphs

JUSTIFICATION

Justification, or text alignment, refers to how the left and right margins of the paragraph appear. Different justification can be applied to a paragraph, paragraphs, a page, or an entire document. Text can be justified in four ways (Box 7-1). Unless a very good printer and font are available, the easiest documents to read are those in which the text is aligned left, creating a straight left margin and even spacing between words.

PARAGRAPH FORMATTING

The default formatting for a paragraph is often indenting the first line a half inch to the right. Paragraphs, however, may also be formatted as outdented or hanging paragraphs, as required by fifth edition of the American Psychological Association's (APA) format for references (Box 7-2). All these styles are easily created by a word processor by placing the insertion point anywhere in the paragraph, right clicking and selecting paragraph, or under the Format menu. If you indent one paragraph, some word processors will assume that all subsequent ones should be similarly indented. If you want a following paragraph formatted differently, you must manually change the style as above.

Box 7-1 • Justification (Alignment) Examples

Left Justification (Left Margin Straight)

Learning to use a word processor is not so much a factor of learning the commands, but of knowing what is possible. Once you know what is possible and can ask, "How do you do x?" instead of being oblivious to the fact that it is possible to do x, you are 75% of the way to using a function effectively.

Right Justification (Right Margin Straight)

Few writers, even professionals, get it right the first time. Rewriting is as germane to writing as breathing is to staying alive. A word processor makes rewriting relatively painless, thus allowing a writer to appear at his/her best. Editing, however, leads to unintended results when one formats manually.

Center Justification (Text Centered Horizontally)

When an individual first moves from a typewriter to a word processor, and before one has learned to think "let the computer do it," some features in word processing can cause confusion, and yes, frustration! Much of the frustration new word processor users experience comes from ideas ingrained by the use of typewriters and a fixed page.

Full Justification (Both Margins Straight)

Those reared in the printed page world sometimes find it very anti-intuitive that they do not have to, indeed should not, use the enter key to paginate. This results in unintended results when the document is edited. New pages created using the Enter key are fluid and change their location as text above is added or deleted. The result is that the text that was supposed to start a "new page" is in the middle of a page with blank spaces above.

Page Properties

The printed page is the ultimate focus of a word-processed document. A page has many properties that can be used to change its

---

Box 7-2 • Examples of Paragraph Formatting

....

Hanging Paragraph

Manually creating a hanging paragraph instead of using this feature not only wastes time but also creates problems when one needs to edit the text.

Indenting of Both Margins

Create page breaks only when it is imperative that the new text be on a fresh page and then use the forced page break (Ctrl + Enter). If it is necessary for all of a given set of text to always be on the same page, use the "Keep text together" feature found under Format (Paragraph in some word processors).

---

printed appearance. Most are accessible from the Page Setup menu, which is usually found under File on the menu line (Page Layout tab in Microsoft Word® 2007). Like all programs that offer printing, including Web browsers, pages can be printed in either portrait or landscape mode in word processors.[2]

CENTERING A PAGE VERTICALLY

Sometimes it is desirable to center the text on a page not only left to right but also vertically, or top to bottom. This can be useful in creating a title page. In many word processors this feature is found on the File menu under the Layout tab in Page Setup. (In Microsoft Word® 2007 click the drop-down arrow on the Page Layout command box, then Layout, then change Vertical alignment to Center.)

MARGINS

Both changing the **page orientation** and centering a page vertically must be applied to an entire page. Left and right margin changes,

---

[2] Page orientation is discussed in Chapter 4 (see Figure 4-7).

---

however, can be applied to one paragraph, to a page, or to the entire document. The usual margin is 1 inch on all four sides. This may or may not be the default setting for the word processor. If this is not the case, the left and right margins should be changed to 1 inch for formal papers. When page margins are changed, you can make 1 inch margins the default for any future documents. Top and bottom margins and defaults may also be changed. These settings are found under Page Setup in the File menu. (In Microsoft Word 2007 look on the Page Layout Tab in the Page Setup commands.)

Printing

In Windows-compliant programs, tapping Ctrl + P automatically starts the printing process. The File menu also contains a Print function (Microsoft Office button in Microsoft Word® 2007). Using this option, a block of text, one page, a range of pages, or the entire document can be selected for printing. Although many features that improve the appearance of a printed page, such as a header or page numbering, can be applied anytime, others, such as entering page breaks to improve the cohesiveness of the pages, should not be introduced until all editing is finished and the document is ready to be printed.

PAGE BREAKS AND KEEPING TEXT TOGETHER

Page breaks work the same way as word wrap; the computer starts a new page when it finds that it is needed. Like a line break caused by word wrap, this page break is fluid and will change as needed when the document is edited. If you want a hard page, that is one that will always start at a given location, tap the Ctrl + Enter at that location in the text. Do *not* attempt to paginate, that is determine where a new page will start, as you write unless you know that subsequent text must start on a new page, such as after a title page, or when creating the first page in the Reference section. Using a

Header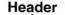

New Page   1

Use a hard page break when you want to force a new page, for example, after the title page, or to start a reference page. If you want certain text to always be on the same page, instead of a page break use the "keep lines together" feature. Never force a new page by tapping the enter key.

If a file was saved to a flash disk, to retrieve the file you will need to navigate to the appropriate disk. This can be done using the "open file" option, or by opening My Computer and double clicking on the disk name. Then select the appropriate file and click on it to open both the file and the program that created the file.

Retrieve File   1

Footer

Figure 7-1 • Headers and footers.

hard page break will ensure that no matter how much text is added or removed above it, the text on that page will always start on a fresh page. Under no circumstances use a soft page break or force a new page by using the Enter key. When a page break is forced by tapping the Enter key, editing by adding or removing text will cause it to move accordingly, because the computer regards tapping the Enter key as just creating a new line, not a new page.

Sometimes, although one does not necessarily need a new page, one wants to be sure that a given block of text when printed will always be on the same page. This can be done by using the "keep paragraph (text) together" feature. Use the Help feature to learn how this is done. You may find this information under "Insert a page break."

HEADERS, FOOTERS, AND PAGE NUMBERS

A **header** is text that is printed on the top of each page, and a **footer** is that printed on the

bottom of every page (Figure 7-1). Some formal documents require headers on all pages. On others, the user may want to use a header as clarification for the reader. Manually entering headers and footers results in their moving to a location other than the top of a page when there is any editing of the document that either adds or deletes a line. For this reason, headers and footers should be inserted using the word processor Header/Footer function. Headers and footers may have any attributes that can be applied to text, and can be left, center, or right justified. Some word processors print a header above the margin, thus creating a smaller top margin. This can be reset. A header or footer can include page numbers, or page numbers may be inserted without using headers or footers. If both are needed, include the page number as part of the header. The page number will then not try to print in the same location as the header. Check the application's Help option to learn the use of the functions, Header, Footer, or Page Numbers.

Some Common Word Processor Features

Most people use only a very small portion of their word processor's capability, ignoring features that can make a document more professional looking as well as saving time.

SPELL CHECK

Many misconceptions exist about how spell check works. A computer does not think; it only makes comparisons (Box 7-3). When spell check is used, the computer compares each set of characters between spaces with the words that are in its dictionary. If it finds a set of matching letters, it assumes that the word is spelled correctly.

Most word processors use a wavy red line at the point of entry to underline any words that are considered misspelled. When this line appears, to find out how the word processor thinks the word should be spelled, place the mouse pointer over the word and right click. A list of suggestions will appear. If one of those words is the correct one, click it, and the spelling checker will replace the misspelled word. If No Suggestions appears, and the user knows the word is spelled correctly, the user can add that word to the dictionary. If one is engaged in writing for a specialty field for which many of the words are not part of the default dictionary, additional dictionaries, such as a medical dictionary, can be added.

One function related to the spelling checker is the ability of word processors to automatically change what is seen as a misspelled – or more usually mistyped – word to what it considers the correct format. This function is often referred to as Auto Correct or Quick Correct. To provide for this function, the word processor stores a list of common misspellings together with the correctly spelled word. If a word is typed in a way that matches the misspelling, the correct word is automatically substituted for the misspelled one. New words can be added to this function, and those that may not be a misspelling in a certain context can be deleted, such as ADN, which the speller insists should be "AND."

THESAURUS

Although not as large, the Thesaurus is set up much like a printed one and is much quicker to use. Like spell check, the Thesaurus is located in the Tools (sometimes under Language) menu (Review tab in Microsoft Word® 2007). To use the Thesaurus, place the insertion point on the word for which a substitute is desired and click it. A window pops up that lists some possible synonyms. Some word processors also provide antonyms. Select the proper word and click the box that tells the computer to replace it.

GRAMMAR CHECKERS

Perfect functionality has not yet been reached with grammar checkers. Still, using one will not hurt anything. They are excellent at picking up syntactical errors such as subject–verb disagreement and run-on sentences. In this day of using a word processor, there is no excuse for either in a document. Grammar checkers may also be located under Tools (Review tab in Microsoft Word® 2007). Grammar problems are often underlined with a green wavy line in the text. With your insertion point on that section, right click to find options.

Box 7-3 • Speller Peccadilloes

I have a spelling checker
I disk covered for my personal computer (PC).
It plane lee marks for my revue
Mistakes I cannot see.

Eye ran this poem threw it.
Your sure real glad to know.
It very polished in its weigh,
My checker told me sew.

LINE SPACING

Single, double, one and a half, and triple spacing – the choice of spacing is yours. When submitting a paper, the preferred choice is usually double spacing. This does not mean that you have to write the paper double spaced; just that before you print it, or submit it electronically, you change the spacing so that the lines are double spaced. To change spacing, select the portion of text you wish to change (tapping Ctrl + A will select the entire document) and then proceed. In some word processors, right clicking a portion of the selected text will present a menu from which you can choose Paragraph and then submit the change under Line spacing. For others, this feature will be found in Format. Use the Help feature if you have difficulty finding it.

Some word processors assume that you are writing a business letter and will automatically set the spacing to one and a half lines. They may also add extra space before or after a paragraph. You may need to change these defaults for a formal paper. They can be changed the same way as for changing spacing.

FIND AND REPLACE

Find and Replace is another very useful tool. Find will locate every instance of a set of characters, which is usually a word or phrase. This feature is available in most application programs, including Web browsers and email packages. The Find and Replace feature can replace one set of characters with another. Suppose a user types the word "nurse" when he or she really wants to write "Registered Nurse." By accessing Find and Replace on the Edit menu (on the Home ribbon in Microsoft Word 2007), the word processor can be told to find every instance of "nurse" and replace it with "Registered Nurse." The replacement can be automatic, or the user can decide which occurrences to replace.

FOOTNOTES AND ENDNOTES

Footnotes and **Endnotes** are different features, but each is accessed and entered the same way. A footnote is a piece of text printed at the bottom of a page. It is usually additional information that may add to a reader's knowledge. An endnote is a piece of text that is printed at the end of a document, for instance, a list of references. Word processors automatically place these notes in the proper position and number them accordingly. The drop-down box to access this feature is found on the Insert menu.

GRAPHICS

Graphical objects, any object other than a table or text, can be inserted into a document using File > Insert, or by Copy and Paste. They can also be dragged from a Web page opened with Microsoft Internet Explorer® into any program that accepts graphics. Once in a document, you can resize them just as you would any graphical object by dragging the edge.[3]

You may need to move the object in the word processor. In some word processors, you can easily accomplish this by dragging the graphic where you wish it placed, or selecting it and using the arrow keys to move it. In others you will need to right click the object, select Format Picture, then Layout from the next menu, and change to a square or tight format. (In Microsoft Word 2007, right click and select Text Wrapping to place text either to one or either side of the graphic.)

COLUMNS

Column creation is accessed from the Format menu (Page Layout ribbon in Microsoft Word® 2007). Users are then asked to designate the number of columns and can either accept the default spacing between the columns or change it. Using a forced page break (Ctrl + Enter) in a column forces the text to the top of the next column.

TABLES

Tables can be created by clicking the Table icon on the toolbar (Insert ribbon in Microsoft Word® 2007) and dragging to create the

---

[3] Chapter 8 discusses resizing a graphic in more detail.

desired number of rows and columns. Extra columns can be added or deleted at any time. If the default column size does not match a need, columns can be resized by placing the mouse pointer on the grid line between columns until it changes shape to an east–west arrow,[4] depressing the left mouse button and dragging the line. To enter text into a table, simply type. The rectangle, or cell, will enlarge as needed.

Many options for formatting a table are available. Although some word processors have more detailed features, all provide the following functions:

▼ Adding a row to the bottom of the table by placing the insertion point in the rightmost cell on the bottom row and tapping the Tab key.

▼ Navigating in the table by tapping the Tab key to go to the cell on the right, Shift + Tab to go the cell on the left, or using the arrow keys to move the insertion point up or down a row.

▼ Changing the appearance or style of a table. This includes removing all the borders, or changing their attributes. Several readymade formats are part of each word processor package. Table attributes can be accessed either by right clicking the table or by clicking the Table icon on the menu line.

▼ Calculating using elementary formulas.

▼ Changing cell sizes, either by a menu or dragging row or column borders.

▼ Joining and splitting cells either vertically or horizontally.

Selecting cells you wish to change and right clicking will produce a menu of options.

SORTING

When typing a list of names, it is not always convenient to enter them in alphabetical order. The Sort function, however, can automatically alphabetize them based on the word

(e.g., first, second) in the line that the user designates. Sort can be applied to a list, a table column, or paragraphs. The sorting function is useful in organizing references for a paper. Use the Help function to learn how to sort.

MAIL MERGE

Mail merge takes a set of data and places the different pieces into the desired place in a letter. To use names and addresses in a form letter, the user first creates a set of data that includes fields such as title, first name, middle name, last name, address, and so forth. The data for the letter can be in a spreadsheet, a database, a table, or in some word processors created as a separate document. After the data is entered, a letter, or form, is then planned in which these items are placed appropriately (Figure 7-2).

AUTOMATIC NUMBERING AND BULLETS

If you need to outline something, or want a numbered or bulleted list, word processors will easily do this. Like most word processor features, you can select this one before you enter the text, or afterward. To start a bulleted list in Microsoft Word® 2003 or earlier versions select Format (Home ribbon in Microsoft Word® 2007). Some word processors have this function under the Insert menu.

If you enter the number one (1), a period, and a space and then enter text, some older word processors automatically assume that this should be a numbered list and will enter a number 2, a period, and space when you tap the Enter key. The maneuver to stop the numbering varies with the word processor, but tapping the Enter key twice will delete the unwanted number. The advantage to automatic numbering is that it saves the effort of entering the numbers when a list is wanted; but even more valuable is that if the items in the list are reordered, the numbers change automatically so they remain in sequence. That is, if item 4 is moved to the line after item 1, the number 4 automatically becomes 2, and the former number 2 becomes 3, and so on.

The automatic numbering feature is not an outline feature because the default generally

---

[4] An east–west arrow is a horizontal line with an arrow at each end (↔). A north–south arrow is a vertical line with arrows at each end (↕). A north–south–east–west arrow is horizontal and vertical lines crossed in the middle with arrows at all four ends.

(Title)Ms.
(First Name)Lucy
(Middle Name)X.
(Last Name)Caro
(Address)25 East Southwick Drive
(City)Anywhere
(State)Any State
(Zip)42424-1001

Sample of one record in a data set

(Title) (First Name) (Middle Name) (Last Name)
(Address)
(City), (State) (Zip)

Dear (Title) (Last Name):

   You have been selected from many people to enjoy a special vacation at our new resort at the beautiful seashore. (First Name), we know that you will not object to paying a small fee of $2000 for this privilege. You need to contact us by Friday at the latest to take part in this great opportunity. Call us at 1-800-BELIEVE.

Sincerely,

Joe Barnum
A sucker is born every minute

Sample of a form letter

Ms. Lucy X. Caro
25 East Southwick Drive
Anywhere, Any State 42424-1001

Dear Ms. Caro:

   You have been selected from many people to enjoy a special vacation at our new resort at the beautiful seashore. Lucy, we know that you will not object to paying a small fee of $2000 for this privilege. You need to contact us by Friday at the latest to take part in this great opportunity. Call us at 1-800-BELIEVE.

Sincerely,

Joe Barnum
A sucker is born every minute

Form letter after it has been merged

Figure 7-2 • Dataset, form letter, and result of merge.

has only one level. To create a multilevel list, it is necessary to change the format of the numbering feature. This can be done either before one enters any numbers and text or afterward. This feature is on the Insert menu in some word processors and the Format menu in others (Home ribbon in Microsoft Word® 2007). This function is very useful for creating an outline for a paper or a multiple-choice test.

   When the outline or bullet function is on, tap the Enter key to create the next numbered item. To move to the next lower level, tap the

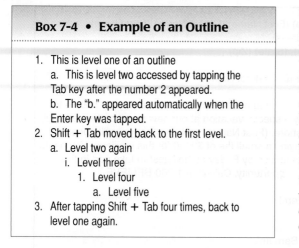

> ## Box 7-4 • Example of an Outline
>
> 1. This is level one of an outline
>   a. This is level two accessed by tapping the Tab key after the number 2 appeared.
>   b. The "b." appeared automatically when the Enter key was tapped.
> 2. Shift + Tab moved back to the first level.
>   a. Level two again
>   i. Level three
>   1. Level four
>   a. Level five
> 3. After tapping Shift + Tab four times, back to level one again.

Tab key. To change to a level above, tap Shift + Tab keys. Box 7-4 illustrates an outline format. The user can change the labels for each level (e.g., number 1, a.). A regular outline format with Roman numerals as the top level and uppercase letters for the second level can be selected, or the user can select or create any desired style.

CROSS-REFERENCING

With the popularity of the Web, publishers of word processing software have added the ability to insert a Web link into a document. Clicking the link, if the user is online, will retrieve the page in the link just as it does in a regular Web page. Links within the document, known as cross-referencing, are also possible (e.g., "see page X-23"). The page number then is "generated" before printing to ensure its accuracy. It is also possible to use referencing or to mark items to be included in a table of contents.

MACRO

A **macro** is a small program that automates a function. If the same functions are continually accessed, such as creating a superscript, a macro can be created to perform this function automat-ically. Although complex macros are pro-grammed, it is also possible to create a macro by recording keystrokes as a function is performed. After creating a macro, it can be placed on the toolbar or assigned a key. To place a macro on the toolbar, place the mouse pointer on the toolbar and click the right mouse button, and then follow the directions. To record keystrokes to create a macro, click "Tools/Macro/Record" (View ribbon in Microsoft Word® 2007), enter a name for the macro, implement the keystrokes, and stop the recording by clicking the square on the small window that is present when a macro is being created. In Microsoft Word® 2007 macros can only be placed on the "Quick Access toolbar."

Increasing One's Skills in Word Processing

Using only a small fraction of the features that their word processors offer limits output and results in time wasted. Manually entering things like headers and page numbers renders it impossible to easily edit a document. The ability to edit is what makes a word processor superior to a typewriter. Few documents exist that cannot benefit from heavy editing. Learn to make your word processor work for you, not the other way around. Online help gets better with every version of the office software suites and is a great source of assistance in increasing one's word processing skills. Classes can help too, but they only open a door to the intricacies of the program; one must enter that door and try the features not only in class but in all settings. Becoming aware of what a word processor can do, then learning the features in a "just-in-time" manner, can keep the learning to a manageable level.

Before experimenting with a new feature, save the document. By doing so, if the result is unacceptable, you can always close the document without saving and retrieve the original document. The undo feature is also often a ticket back to square one. When learning new features, expect some frustration, but remember that you will be rewarded by saving time the next time this feature is needed.

Box 7-5 • Automatic Translations

....

English

The ocean shows signs of being windy, but we are sailing anyway.

Translated to Spanish

El océano demuestra muestras de ser ventoso, pero estamos navegando de todos modos.

Translated Back to English

The ocean demonstrates samples of being windy, but we are sailing anyway.

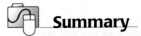

Language Translation

Given the global culture of today, there will be times when you want to translate something into another language. The Web has programs that will do this to some extent, but they are far from perfect. Translating the occasional phrase is one thing, but translating an entire document is fraught with misunderstanding and misinterpretation. One example of a free translation program is AltaVista's BabelFish (http://babelfish .altavista.com/). Play with it, but go easy on using it except in very informal situations unless you have a native speaker of the foreign language who also understands your language and can rewrite the document for you (see Box 7-5).

Word processors, however, do make it possible to write characters in another language, such as the *e* or an *a* with an accent (é á) or adding an umlaut to a *u* (ü). If you need to constantly write in a language other than the default on your computer, use the Help feature to learn how.

Summary

Word processors have become very popular. The basic editing skills pioneered in word processors are used in most application programs, including email programs. Once text is entered into a word processor it can be altered in many ways. Attributes can be added; the

font or font (point) size can be changed; and text can be deleted, copied, or moved. Learning to let the word processor perform such functions as line breaks and page breaks involves reconceptualizing the idea of a document from a fixed-page entity to a document that easily changes while it is being edited. Time spent learning to let the computer perform features such as centering a page vertically, formatting a paragraph, and entering headers and footers plus learning to cope with automatic numbering is returned many times over in creating future documents. Word processors have many other features that not only make tasks easier but also make them economically feasible, such as sorting, mail merge for personalizing notes, and cross-referencing to make it easier for a reader to locate information on another page of a document.

APPLICATIONS AND COMPETENCIES

1. Download the document "Multitasking.rtf" from Chapter 7 on the Web page http://dlthede.net/ Informatics/Informatics.html and open it in your word processor and do as follows:

   a. Select a paragraph and change the font and font (point) size.

   (If using Microsoft Word® 2007, before doing the next exercise click the Microsoft Office button, and on the drop-down menu in the lower right corner of the window click Word Options and then Advanced. If the box before "Use the insert key to control the overtype mode" is blank, place a check in it and click ok. If you will never use overtype mode, you may want to go back and uncheck that after you do the following exercise.)

   b. Place the insertion point at the beginning of the first word in the second paragraph, tap the Insert key, and enter the letters "abc" and see what happens.

   c. Click the Undo icon (or tap Ctrl + Z) to undo this change.

   d. Tap the Insert key again to stop this mode of entering text.

   e. Boldface any one sentence.

   f. Create a hard page before the word References at the end of the document.

g. Center the word References

h. Make the reference a hanging paragraph (may be under Indent paragraphs in Help).

i. Italicize the words and number "Nursing Assist 23."

2. Start a fresh page by making a hard page and experiment with automatic numbering. If using Microsoft Word 2007, before starting this exercise, on the Home ribbon, in the Paragraph commands, click the icon whose tip reads "numbering" when you rest the mouse pointer over it.

a. Enter the number 1, a period, and tap the Tab key, and then enter the word "house."

b. Tap the Enter key.

c. What happened? (If you do not see the number 2, use the Insert or Format tab [word processor dependent] and select Outline/Bullets and Numbering.)

d. Enter the word "car" after the "2," and tap the Enter key.

e. Type the word "boat," and tap the Enter key.

f. Stop the automatic numbering.

3. Experiment with multilevel numbering.

a. Find Bullets and Numbering on either the Insert or Format menu, and select outline numbered. (For Microsoft Word® 2007 select the Multilevel list icon from the Paragraph command on the Home ribbon.)

b. Select any of the multilevel formats.

c. After the 1 that appears on the screen:

   i. Enter the word "house," and tap Enter.

   ii. Tap the Tab key.

   iii. Enter the word "kitchen," and tap Enter.

   iv. Enter the words "family room," and tap Enter.

   v. Tap Shift + Tab.

   vi. Enter the word CAR, and tap Enter.

   vii. Turn off the outline feature the same way the automatic numbering was turned off.

4. Copy the entire document to another document:

a. Tap Ctrl + A to select the entire document. There are three ways to place the selected text on the clipboard so it can be copied. Select one and perform the activity.

b. Tap Ctrl + C

Or

c. On the toolbar click the Copy icon. (Home ribbon in Microsoft Word® 2007.)

Or

d. On the menu line click Edit > Copy. (Home ribbon in Microsoft Word® 2007.)

5. Create a new document by tapping Ctrl + N, and paste the text into the new document by either:

a. Tap Shift + Insert.

Or

b. Tap Ctrl + V.

Or

c. Click the Paste icon on the toolbar (Home ribbon in Microsoft Word® 2007.) in all word processors except Microsoft Word 2007.

d. On the menu line click Edit > Paste.

e. Return to the original document by clicking its icon on the bottom of the screen. (If a line of icons is not seen there, place the mouse pointer there until one appears.

f. On the Page Setup screen (On the menu line click File > Page Setup or Page Layout ribbon.):

   i. Change the page orientation to Landscape.

   ii. Change the margins to 0.75 inches (7 cm).

6. Insert a header that will automatically appear on each page that is right justified and contains a left justified running head, five spaces, and a page number. Use the Help feature to discover how to do this. You may have to experiment a little. (For Microsoft Word® 2007 see the instructions on Chapter 7 of the Web page http://dlthede.net/Informatics/Informatics.html)

7. Change the view of the document from the Print Layout to Normal (Draft) mode or the other way around if you are already looking at the document in the Normal (Draft) mode. (In the View menu in earlier Microsoft Word, in the Document View command group on the View ribbon in Microsoft Word 2007.) What happens to the header?

8. Create a table of three columns and two rows. Enter the following words:

a. In the first cell in the first row enter DATE.

b. Tap the Tab key.

c. Enter the word TIME and tap Tab.

d. Enter the word PROJECT and tap Tab.

e. In the Date column enter today's date and tap Tab.

f. Enter the present time and tap Tab.

g. Enter "Creating a table" and tap Tab. What happened?

h. Create a header row in the table. First, select the top row in the table, leave your insertion point there, and ask help how to make this a header row. To search help, for some word processors enter "header row: in the search bar, for others "format table" and scroll down.

Presentation Software: Looking Professional in the Spotlight

Learning Objectives

After studying this chapter you will be able to:

1. *Differentiate between information that can accurately be communicated with computer slides and that which needs a narrative.*

2. *Compare the differences in design between a slide presentation that is used as an aid to a live presentation and one used as a stand-alone message.*

3. *Apply principles of good slide design in creating a slide presentation.*

4. *Employ appropriate principles in creating handouts*

Key Terms

Attribute

Crop

Gradient Background

Lecture Replacement Model

Lecture Support Model

Progressive Disclosure

Storyboard

Y ou skipped today's lecture because you could get the PowerPoint® slides from the course Web site. Now you are looking at these slides and wondering how the pieces of information fit together – should you memorize all these bullet points? But how will you apply them? How can you make this information meaningful?

This is a dilemma that many face when they look at class slides, handouts from presentations, or PowerPoint® slide shows online. Most of us find ourselves frustrated in using information only from slides, or only from handouts of slides, even if we took notes along the sides of the slides. PowerPoint® may help us as presenters to outline our talk, but when they stand alone, do they help those on the receiving end understand the information that we are trying to communicate?

Nurses and students give many presentations, sometimes informally to one another, but often before a group. Feeling confident in this endeavor is something that comes with practice. Today the expectation of speakers is that they will use computerized slides. Not only knowing how to create these visuals, but also giving consideration to what the audience will take away from these slides is the key to developing useful visuals. Visuals can be distracting if not created and used appropriately.

It is doubtful whether today there is anyone who has not been subjected to computer-projected visuals that either detracted from the speaker or upstaged her or him. The computer slide show is your partner. It should not upstage you or detract from what you say or be expected to communicate a message alone.

Using Computer-Projected Visuals

A question that has been asked about the February 1, 2003, explosion of the space shuttle *Columbia* was "Did PowerPoint® make the space shuttle crash?" Evidence proves that it was a contributing factor. It seems that the National Aeronautics and Space Administration (NASA) had become too reliant on using PowerPoint® to present complex information instead of narrative technical reports. The nesting and subnesting of complex points caused those who had to make decisions about the safety of *Columbia* to not understand the true picture (New York Times, 2003; Tufte, 2003). One then must ask, "Could depending on PowerPoint® slides to communicate information create a healthcare mistake?"

A good slide design, as shown in Table 8-1, requires that one use only about 40 words per slide. This is about eight seconds worth of silent reading (Tufte, 2003). Kruchten (2004) believes that in many organizations, bullet points on slides have been substituted for real discourse, devastating our ability to completely and accurately communicate. Presenters need to be aware that slides should only be used to help an audience keep track of ideas and occasionally illustrate a point, and not be used as the basis of understanding. Audiences also need to realize that slides alone are only an outline of a talk.

Computer slides have two main uses: one as a guide for an oral presentation and another as a stand-alone information source such as for an online course. Common sense says that the design of each should be different (Springfield, 2007). The **lecture support model** can be effective to guide audiences to follow your

TABLE 8-1 ● Basic Rules for Creating and Using Visuals	
Creating and Using Visuals	
Text	Limit to 6–7 words in a line and 6 lines on a slide
Fonts	Choose a sans serif font for projected visuals. Limit the number of different fonts, to no more than three. Match font to reactions desired from the audience.
Font Size	Transparencies ≥ 18 points Slides ≥ 24 points
Colors	
Background	Match to lighting of room where presentation will be given. Light for light rooms, dark for dark rooms.
Text and Background	Contrasting – opposite sides of color wheel
For Emphasis	Be consistent
Number Used	Total of no more than 5–6.
Using Visuals	
Time on Screen	At least 10 seconds and never more than 100; break up a slide if needed, use progressive disclosure, or blank out screen.
Coordinate	Keep the talk focused on the slide in view.
Audience Reading	If the audience need to read an entire slide, give them time!
Blank Screen	To digress from the slides, tap the letter "w" to produce a white screen, or "b" for a black screen.

presentation, while the **lecture replacement model** needs more than just bullet points.

LECTURE SUPPORT MODEL

These slides should be used to communicate information that needs a visual backup such as body systems, or physiology (Springfield, 2007). During your lecture, on a slide place a question that is not easily answered with one or two words and get the audience involved in a discussion. If this is a question that involves more than one point of view, help the audience to bring out all views. Questions with right answers can be explored with the audience in a way that gets them to think. Presenters do not have to tell the audience everything; letting the group figure out something for themselves will result in greater retention, and perhaps bring out points that you alone would never have considered.

Trying to include too much information on your slides will lead the audience to read the slide and not hear what you are saying. Follow the guidelines in Table 8-1. If you want to use a quote, place it on the slide and give the audience time to read it; do not hurry them. When images are included on a slide, make them convey information that would otherwise be difficult to communicate, not just fulfill an obligation to have X number of images or add interest that may upstage you.

LECTURE REPLACEMENT MODEL

The first question to ask in this instance is, "Should I use slides, create a narrative with illustrations, or use the Notes section of PowerPoint® to expand on the points on the slides?" Start by thinking about the nature of the information that needs to be communicated. Can it be made meaningful with just bullet points? Information that is 100% memorization can perhaps be communicated in this fashion, but it is doubtful if learning beyond Bloom's first level of learning can be accommodated with bullet points alone.

Creating a narrative with illustrations for learning at the level of analysis or evaluation is the best approach. When on the Web, this information can be linked to other sources that are integrated into the narrative with discussion or questions. Or if the information to be communicated is at a low level, using the Notes section of PowerPoint® allows a designer to provide more information than just bullet points. Probably, the best method is to look at each objective and match the method to the objective. If the objective depends on learning from animation in PowerPoint® slides, there is a free download that can convert

Microsoft PowerPoint® slides to *Flash* files, or those with an "swf" extension that are smaller than a PowerPoint® file. (See PowerPoint Lite at http://www.authorgen.com/authorpoint-lite-free/powerpoint-to-flash-converter.aspx.) The resulting file can then be posted on the Web, complete with all video and audio (Perry, 2007).

Basics of Slide Creation

With the understanding that slides, when properly designed and used, can be a useful aid in communications, we will look at some of the basics of slide creation. Each brand of presentation software, as well as specific versions within that brand, varies in how features are implemented, but all packages have more similarities than dissimilarities. They all have different views of the slides from the show view to handouts view. Additionally, they all operate with layers that are like pieces of transparent paper that are overlaid on each other, starting with the background layer, then the layout, and finally the content layer. And they all treat images very similarly.

VIEWS OF THE SLIDES

Slide show creation programs allow users to look at their slides in many different ways. The view that audiences see is the Slide Show view. The default creation mode is what is called the Normal mode. In this view the left-hand side of the screen has a column with tabs that allow either a thumbnail view of several slides or, under the Outline tab, a view of the text on the screen. The top right has a view of the slide under construction, and at the bottom of the screen, a Notes section that can be enlarged to enter notes. There is also a Notes view in which the slide image takes up the top half of the screen and the Notes section the bottom. All of these except the Slide Show view allow the user to enter information on a slide or in the Notes section.

The Slide Sorter view is useful for viewing many slides at once. The number of slides in the view can be changed using the Zoom feature.

This view is especially useful for rearranging slides, or for copying slides from one presentation to another. When slides are copied, the slides placed in the new environment will take on the style of the new environment. Slides can be selected either one by one by clicking with the Ctrl key held down or as a contiguous group by selecting either the first or last slide and holding down the Shift key while left clicking the slide at the other end. These principles of selecting objects either one by one or as a group is a Windows® principle that can be applied to objects on a graphical screen or while dragging files in Windows Explorer®.

THE BACKGROUND LAYER

One of the first choices a user makes when creating a slide show is the background. This layer is often referred to as the master layer. Presentation programs all come with various background choices that the user can either accept as they are or modify. More background designs are often available on the Web site of the vendor of the slide program, or you can create your own.

This layer is important because it keeps all the slides in the presentation consistent in looks. The background layer has place keepers for the title and subtitle for the title page, and for bullet points, graphics, and other items for subsequent pages. Because the place keepers are located in different places in different backgrounds (called Themes in PowerPoint® 2007), if you change the background layer after you have designed the slides, you need to check to be sure that all your slides are still intact.

When selecting a background it is helpful to know the kind of lighting that will be used at the venue of the presentation. Borrowing from the days of 35 mm slides, when rooms were dark, many people still choose a dark background that is very appropriate with a dark room, but which allows content to get lost in a room that is lighted. Contrast is important, and having the background match the lighting in the room is a good principle to follow: light for light rooms and dark for dark rooms (Prost; Communicating Effectively with an Audience).

THE LAYOUT LAYER

The layout layer builds on the background layer in the number and types of placeholders it has for different types of slides. Opening up a document to create a new presentation will present you with a title page layout. When you add a new slide, it is assumed that you want to make bullet points. If bullet points are an appropriate communication method, use the Tab key to create a nested bullet point and the Shift + Tab to move back to a higher level just as in the outline feature of a word processor.

Explore some of the layouts beyond bullet points; they may very well be a better choice to communicate your information. For example, there is a layout that has only a title on which you can place any object that you need to communicate your message; there are also blank pages and those that will allow placement of a graphic on one side and text on the other. Keep in mind that any graphics on your background layer will show through any of these layouts. To change either the layout of a slide or to remove the background graphic for one slide, start by right clicking on a blank spot on the slide. To change the layout, select Layout from the drop-down menu and make the appropriate choice. To omit the background from one slide, from the drop-down menu select Background (Format Background in 2007) then check Omit Background Graphics from the Master (In PowerPoint® 2007 Hide Background Graphics.) then click Apply (Close in PowerPoint® 2007).

THE CONTENT LAYER

Entering text or other objects is done on the top, or on the content layer. The layouts have boxes visible only in the Normal view that guide the user in placing text. All word processing principles apply to the content layer, including the use of the spell checker!

TEXT

A facet of presentation packages that can be both an advantage and a disadvantage is the number of fonts available, many of which are unsuitable for text in a projected visual. Even though one is always tempted to select a "jazzy" font in the hope that it will enliven a presentation, too often this choice creates readability problems. When making a selection, remember that fonts can elicit an emotional response from the audience; thus, choose one that not only is visually appealing but also elicits the desired emotional response (see Figure 8-1).

The background templates for presentation programs have preselected fonts that are generally suitable for a presentation. These font styles can be changed either for an individual slide or for the entire presentation. However, changing a font after the completion of a presentation may disturb the layout on some slides because of the difference in size of the text in different fonts. For example, the font size in Figure 8-1 is the same, yet you can see that the text is not all of the same size. The measurement unit for text size is points. Point size, as you can see, is not always an accurate guide. Some fonts at 12 points, despite being one sixth of an inch in height, are very difficult to read. This is because of what is called the x factor, or the height of lowercase letters. The smallest easily readable text size for computer slides is 24 points.

Some fonts (e.g., Garamond, and to a lesser degree, Times Roman) have projections from the type body called serifs that are fine strokes across the ends of the main strokes of a character. Serifs create softer edges to the characters, which adds to readability on paper. When they are projected, however, they may have a tendency to look fuzzy. For projected visuals, use a sans serif (i.e., without serifs) font such as Arial (Figure 8-2). This font follows the basic

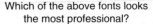
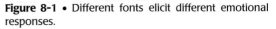

Which of the above fonts looks
the most professional?

Figure 8-1 • Different fonts elicit different emotional responses.

rule in choosing a display font – that the letters appear crisp and clean.

Identical to word processing, the appearance of text can be altered with **attributes** other than the type of font. Making a text boldface is one way to emphasize a point, as are underlining and italicizing. Italicizing, however, tends to make text more difficult to read; if it is used, give the audience more time to read the slide, a feature that can be used to advantage for a point that you wish the audience to read more slowly. If a point or points are emphasized with any of the above-mentioned attributes, be consistent throughout the presentation, that is, use the same attribute for the same type of information throughout.

When placing text on visuals, include only the essential elements of concepts. State ideas as though they were headlines. A visual is not meant to give the entire idea but rather to serve as a focus to assist the audience in following your presentation. Visuals can also be helpful to the presenter as a guide to the oral presentation.

Sans-serif font: Arial	Generally easier to read online
Serif font: Times New Roman	Easier to read in a print format

Figure 8-2 • Comparison of sans-serif and serif fonts.

Audiences should be able to get the point of the visual within the first five seconds after it appears. It is argued that a presenter should be quiet for those five seconds to allow the audience to grasp the point. To accomplish this, it is necessary to limit the text. One way to determine whether you have too much information on a visual image is to place the information on a 4 × 6 inches card and try to read it from a distance of about 5 – 6 feet. Never write the presentation on a series of slides that are intended to be read to the audience. Audiences can read faster than a speaker can talk and may become torn between reading ahead and listening. This practice leads the speaker to pay more attention to the slides than to the audience, and the audience to ignore the speaker.

IMAGES

A study at Wharton Research Centre demonstrated that visual messages have a large effect on retention: at three days, 10% of the text in bullet points was remembered, but 50% of illustrations were remembered (The Numbers on Why You Need Visuals, 2000). The message is to use pictures, graphs, or tables whenever it will illustrate better than words. Several sources of presentation quality images are available. Clip art, or small drawings that have already been created and are part of the presentation program, is one source of images; more clip art is usually available on the vendor's Web site. Additionally, images and sounds that can be used for noncommercial presentations or in a class can be found on the Web. Right clicking on most images on the Web will allow you to copy the image to the clipboard from where it can be placed in a presentation. You may even drag them into a Microsoft® program if using Internet Explorer® version 7. If the presentation will be used commercially, check the copyright information[1] for any images, sound, or video. Many types of clip art and other Web images have limitations on how they can be used. While buying a package

of clip art, one should be sure to read the fine print before purchasing the software to be certain they are royalty free.

Images are placed on a slide the same way that they are inserted into a word processor; use the Insert tab and proceed from there. Dragging an image will easily move it to where you want it on the slide. To resize the image, you need to select the image, place the mouse pointer on either the square or the circle on its square border, and drag. Dragging when the mouse pointer is on a corner will keep the proportions of the image; dragging while it is on a side will skew it.

Besides inserting images, slide creation packages provide drawing tools that allow one to create drawings, which can be used on slides or copied to another program. The drawing can also be saved, although in some presentation programs it will be saved as a slide. On a slide, images can be **cropped**; that is, the sides of the picture can be moved inwards to show only a smaller part of the image, a process that does not delete any of the image, but just makes the covered part invisible. If you want to use only a small portion of an image and you are using Vista®, you can use the Sniping tool found under Accessories. This tool will allow you to select any portion of an image, copy it to the clipboard, and place it anywhere. With this tool, the resulting image consists of only the selected part of the original.

Occasionally, an image may not project well. To prevent this from marring a presentation, check the appearance of the slide in the Play or Show view before committing to using the visual in the presentation. Generally, if an image looks good in playback mode, it will project well, but if possible, check the image with the projection equipment and the version of the presentation software that will be used in the presentation.

Although using a scanned image, a clip art, or images from the Internet makes it possible to include very detailed pictures, these images can sometimes confuse the learner. For example, in presenting information about blood circulation through the heart, a detailed picture would probably not aid the understanding as

---

[1] Copyright and fair use are discussed in Chapter 26.

much as a schematic drawing that only depicts the four chambers and the veins and arteries leading into and out of the heart.

When adding images, remember that the point of visuals is to communicate a message to the audience. Clip art can be appropriate if it emphasizes that message; when it is only used to enliven a slide, it seldom adds much to the presentation. A little variety, especially when it pertains to the message, can be helpful, but be careful not to distract the audience.

CHARTS AND TABLES

A table or chart is often clearer in communicating meaning than text. When using a table, one is limited in the size that can be created. Presentation software provides the ability to import a graph or data directly from a spreadsheet as well as the ability to copy and paste the graph. Be certain, when using either of these, that you use them to accurately convey information.[2] A detailed table or chart does not project well enough to be read by an audience. Instead print the chart or table and use it as a handout.

SPECIAL EFFECTS

Although one can add special effects independent of the visuals, those that are made possible by presentation software are often not available if the slides are put on the Web, especially if they have been converted to a pdf file. When doing a computer slide show, especially when using special effects such as sound and video clips, the complete presentation should be tested on the equipment that will actually be used during the presentation itself. Moderation should be used with any special effects. Like images, special effects can be helpful to some messages, but they become distracting when used inappropriately. You want the audience paying attention to your message, not wondering what special effect they will be assaulted with next.

Color

Although color can be used to draw attention to a feature, it should never be used as the only distinguishing characteristic. As with fonts, it is important to be consistent in using color. When an audience grasps the implications of a given color, the visuals are more easily comprehended. Although the eye can perceive millions of colors, screen colors should be limited to about six, which is all that the eye can track in one glance (Faioloa & DeBloois, 1988).

Color, like text fonts, also has an emotional appeal. Red can be seen as exciting or as the color of fire and blood, whereas green is usually seen as calming. The meaning of colors varies with cultures. Purple may indicate spirituality, mystery, aristocracy, and passion in some cultures; in others it may symbolize mourning, death, nausea, conceit, and pomposity (Morton, 1998).

Color combinations should be selected such that they are compatible but offer a contrast. When placed on top of one another, some colors, such as red on black, give a three-dimensional appearance that may make an object appear closer than the background. Additionally, objects sometimes appear larger in one color than in another. Reading accuracy is best when the colors used for background and text are on the opposite sides of the color wheel. Keep in mind that 9% of the population has some kind of color perception problem, usually a deficiency in discriminating red from green. When using a **gradient background** (Figure 8-3), it is imperative to use a very readable text and to test the slide for readability. Many of the backgrounds that are

Figure 8-3 • A gradient background.

---

[2] The use of charts is discussed in Chapter 9.

provided with presentation programs are gradient backgrounds.

Sound

Sound can be added by recording it using a microphone attached to the computer and special software, or through a sound file. Some sound files can be found on the Internet, whereas others can be purchased as software. After the file is selected, follow the directions prescribed by the presentation package you are using to attach the sound to a slide. The steps for adding sound to a presentation can be found by searching for "add sound" in the Help feature.

Video

Video clips are equally easy to insert. The video, however, must be in digital format instead of the analog mode used for ordinary videotape. Conversions from analog tape can be made, or cameras that record directly to the computer can be used. If one is planning to add video, limit its length to 45–60 seconds; any length beyond that may distract the audience. As with sound, before using video in a presentation, check the equipment. Make a copy of the presentation without video available in case the video portion of the presentation equipment fails on the day of the presentation.

Transitions

A transition is the way a slide makes its entrance. Presentation programs have available many different types of transitions. Some cause a slide to fade in; some cause the slide to appear first at the center, and then expand the view; and yet others cause the slide to sweep across the screen. Transitions can be dramatic, enhance your message, or distract the audience. The best rule is to use them sparingly. Avoid at all costs trying to dazzle the audience with multiple transitions.

Animation

The term animation, often referred to as Custom Animation, is used optimistically in the more well-known presentation software. Generally, animation takes the form of **progressive disclosure**, although some movement of objects is possible. Progressive disclosure is a technique in which one item at a time is revealed until all the items are displayed. When revealing bulleted points, those that have been discussed can be dimmed or converted to a different color while the current point takes center stage. The appearance of images can also be controlled with progressive disclosure. Additionally, using Custom Animation, you can make objects appear or disappear during a presentation.

Many options are available for how bulleted items will be progressively disclosed. Some of these options allow the item to slide in from any direction, bounce in, fade in, or even curve in. Like all options, this feature should be used judiciously. Animated gifs (a type of image files from the Web that show movement) can be used with many presentation programs. If the animated gif will be on the screen for a long time, it is a good idea to cover it up after a given time period – something that can be set to happen automatically. Movement on a screen can become very distracting. If using animation, be sure to check the animation on the computer that will be used for the presentation before the actual presentation. Unless you are using your own computer, do not plan a presentation around the movement in the image.

SPEAKER NOTES

As mentioned earlier, speaker notes are entered as text in either the Normal or the Notes view. They can be very helpful to you as a speaker to remember what you had in mind when you created a given slide. Although the notes are not seen when the slide is presented, they are connected to the slide in a way that allows them to be printed for use either as notes during the presentation or when rehearsing. Using a duplicate display, the notes can be shown on the presenter's computer while the audience sees only the slides. (Search the operating system for multiple monitors to find how to do this.)

CREATING A SHOW THAT ALLOWS FOR NONLINEAR PRESENTATIONS

When giving a presentation, you should be somewhat flexible. Some audiences may ask questions, others will not. A presenter can also misjudge the time needed for the presentation. By using the computer for the presentation, these eventualities can be handled easily. Depending on the program, the presenter can prepare a hidden slide to show if a specific question is asked or if time permits. One popular presentation program will advance (or retreat) to a specific slide when the number of the slide is typed followed by the Enter key. With this program, keeping a list of slide numbers while presenting will allow a presenter to easily show any slide in the presentation. Use the words "action settings" to search the Help contents to implement this feature.

Compatibility of Microsoft PowerPoint® Versions

Unfortunately, Microsoft PowerPoint® 2007 has difficulty with backward compatibility. Although you can open files created with earlier versions in the new version, you may lose some of the effects. If you create a slide show in Microsoft PowerPoint® 2007, but need to show it in an earlier version, you will need to save it as an earlier version. Be certain, however, to look at it with the earlier version before show time. To avoid these problems, download one of the free viewers at http://www.microsoft.com/downloads/details.aspx?familyid=048dc840-14e1-467d-8dca-19d2a8fd7485&displaylang=en and place it along with the slides on the flash disk that you will use to transport the file.

The Presentation

Although creating good visuals is part of a good presentation, it does not alone ensure a good presentation. To achieve that, one needs to be sure that the visuals and the presentation reinforce one another. To reach that goal, it is necessary to plan the visuals and the presentation together. A good presentation follows the rule of "tell'em"; that is, give the audience an overview of what you will tell them, tell them or present the information, then tell them what you told them by presenting a summary of the important points. Keep in mind that people will remember no more than five points at the most (Tips from all aspects of pulling off the successful presentation!, 2007). One suggestion in preparation is to write out your conclusion slide first, emphasizing your most important points, and build the presentation around that.

STORYBOARDING

The concept of **storyboarding**[3] originated with film, but is valuable in any presentation that involves visuals. A storyboard is just a plan for the visuals. It forces you to organize your thoughts and allows you to assemble your ideas into a coherent presentation. As with all projects, planning saves time! With a presentation package, you can outline your thoughts using a title and text on a slide. After you complete the first draft, use the Slide Sorter view to look at the presentation as a whole. This will help you to see where a rearrangement of slides would be helpful and make it easy to rearrange the order by dragging the slides to a new position. When you think things are in the correct order, go back to each slide and develop it into a meaningful communication tool. Expect to switch between the Slide Sorter view and the Design view many times while working on the actual visuals!

CREATING HANDOUTS

As stated earlier, rarely is a printed copy of slides alone, even with space for the audience to take notes, a worthwhile reason to destroy trees. Preparing a word-processed document using your notes and inserting appropriate illustrations is a much better use of paper. Complex information cannot be reduced to bullet points! To keep the audience's attention focused on your message, rather than reading the handout, provide the handouts after the presentation.

---

[3] Storyboarding has another meaning for standardized terminologies. In that context it means describing a case and pulling out the important points.

TRANSFERRING TO THE WEB

Although it is actually possible to transfer a computer slide show to the Web as an html or a pdf file, it is not a good idea. Remember that every medium is different, and the difference between a live slide presentation and a stand-alone Web presentation is huge. On the Web not only do the slides have to answer all questions, but they also need to be complete with all the information that readers need to have. Few slide shows meet this requirement. Bullet points do not! If the information needs to be posted to the Web, think about how it will be best presented. You may need to add audio to the slides, or a narrative text with embedded illustration(s) for those who learn best by reading, or both. You may want to review educational principles in Chapter 23 when considering posting something to the Web.

THE ACTUAL PRESENTATION

The moment has arrived; you have rehearsed the presentation until you know it cold. Despite this, hundreds of butterflies are tap dancing in your stomach, and you are wondering, "Will I remember what to say?" The title slide opens; you give the audience five seconds to read it – an eternity when you are the speaker. (Count, e.g., from 1001 to 1005.). Then you read the title, and give the audience an icebreaker, maybe an antidote about yourself or how you prepared for the talk, something light. Knowing that you want the audience to pay attention to the presentation, and not read ahead, you tell them that you will distribute handouts after the presentation. Your handouts are well thought out, are a narrative with occasional images, and will provide the reader with information months or years after your presentation is complete. With the introduction out of the way, you open the next slide and start to communicate your message.

By the third or fourth slide the butterflies are ending their dance, and the points on the slide remind you of the information you need to communicate. You make eye contact with various people in the audience, and the presentation is going smoothly – you are beginning to enjoy it.

A question is asked that requires you to diverge from the planned presentation. If this is a point that you thought might come up, you switch to your nonlinear presentation. You can even take the time to jot down the present slide number to return to it before you do this – audiences do not mind. If the question is something not planned for, but to which you need to respond, tap the letter "w" to make the screen white, or "b" to make it black, answer the question, tap enter to bring back the screen, and go on with the presentation. Then it is over! You made it – you are receiving thanks from the audience for sharing your knowledge.

Summary

The overuse of computer slides has led some to believe that we are dumbing down the message. Some believe that using bullet points forces presenters to "mutilate data beyond comprehension." (New York Times, 2003) and allows the speakers to not tie their information together. Nonetheless they are a ubiquitous feature of most presentations. Avoiding these pitfalls means giving attention to the real message and using visuals to aid the message, not substitute for it. Even a small presentation given to a group of colleagues will be better received if well thought-out visuals are used. As a nurse progresses up the career ladder, knowing how to make presentations that convey a solid message is an aid to advancement.

Although there are several vendors of presentation packages, including one free with *Open Office*, they all have similarities. Basically, they facilitate the job of creating good visuals by providing a constant background for the visual and tailored layouts. Any of these things, however, can be modified at any time. Although there are many options available, such as adding images or special effects such as sound, video clips, animation, and progressive disclosure, they should only be used to enhance the message. In the same vein, select colors, fonts, backgrounds, and layouts to extend a message.

All presentations need planning and organizing. Handouts should reflect what the audience needs to take away from the presentation, and not just the slides. Several issues are involved in creating a presentation: identifying key points, planning the visuals to be a partner, using good visual techniques, and preparing useful handouts. And finally, rehearsing!

APPLICATIONS AND COMPETENCIES

1. Compare the slides of the Gettysburg Address with the actual address at http://www.norvig.com/Gettysburg/index.htm. Do the slides convey the actual message?
2. Watch a presentation using computer slides and analyze the slides for:
   a. Whether the text is readable.
      i. Whether the background color shows text to best advantage.
      ii. Whether the font used is easily readable.
   b. Whether the content is enhanced or lost with the slides.
   c. Whether the presenter uses the visuals as a partner:
      i. Slides do not upstage the presenter.
      ii. Slides do not present a message different than what is being said.
      iii. Slides make the presentation easy or difficult to follow.
      iv. Images add to the message.
   d. Whether the slides could be used as handouts that would aid your understanding a month from today.
3. Open a presentation program, change the layout to blank, and insert one of the shapes or an illustration. Practice resizing it by selecting the object, and then placing the mouse pointer on first a circle at a corner and then a circle (square in PowerPoint® 2007 on a side. What happens to the image in each instance?
4. Experiment with different backgrounds and decide why or why not they would be effective in a specific type of presentation such as a research report, a class project, or a welcome speech. If they are not appropriate, how could they be modified to be more useful for your purpose?
5. How could you use a cartoon in a visual? What are some of the things that you would have to consider if you choose to do so?

6. You need to teach a class about a physiological process. On the Web find some illustrations that could be used in a noncommercial setting and insert it into a slide. (Search for "images of 'the process.'")
7. Create a three- or four-slide presentation on a topic of your choice.
   a. Add a background and use more than the title and bullet layouts.
   b. Use progressive disclosure (Search for animation to learn how).
   c. Add an image.
   d. Use the principles of good design mentioned in Table 8-1.
   e. Create a handout that would be appropriate for an audience reference six months after the presentation.

REFERENCES

Communicating Effectively with an Audience: Presenting with PowerPoint. Retrieved November 19, 2008, from http://www.lse.ac.uk/collections/TLCPhD/files/PresentationSkillsHandouts.pdf

Faioloa, T., & DeBloois, M. L. (1988). Designing a visual factors-based screen display interface: The new role of the graphic technologist. *Educational Technology, 28*(8), 12–21.

Kruchten, P. (2004, January 30). *Book review—the cognitive style of PowerPoint.* Retrieved November 19, 2008, from http://www.ibm.com/developerworks/rational/library/2051.html.

Morton, J. (1998). *Color, the chameleon of the web.* Retrieved November 19, 2008, from http://www.colormatters.com/chameleon.html.

New York Times. (2003, December 17). *PowerPoint makes you dumb.* Retrieved November 19, 2008, from http://www.unc.edu/~mumukshu/gandhi/gandhi/powerpoint.htm.

The Numbers on Why You Need Visuals. (2008). Retrieved November 19, 2008, from http://www.presentersonline.com/basics/visuals/needvisuals.shtml

Perry, W. (2008). Notes from the net nomad. *Computers, Informatics, Nursing: CIN, 26*(5), 247.

Prost, J. *8 Mistakes Made when Presenting with PowerPoint® and How to Correct Them.* Retrieved November 19, 2008, from http://www.frippandassociates.com/artprost2_faa.html

Springfield, E. (2007). PowerPoint pedagogy: Two usages, two pedagogical styles. *Computers, Informatics, Nursing: CIN, 25*(1), 15–20.

Tips from all aspects of pulling off the successful presentation! (2007). Retrieved November 19, 2008, from http://www.projectorreviews.com/effectivepresentations.php.

Tufte, E. (2003). *PowerPoint is evil: power corrupts. PowerPoint corrupts absolutely.* Retrieved November 19, 2008 from http://www.wired.com/wired/archive/11.09/ppt2.html.

CHAPTER 9

Spreadsheets: Making Numbers Talk

Learning Objectives

After studying this chapter you will be able to:

1. Identify differences between spreadsheet and word processing software.

2. Use computer conventions to create mathematical formulas to analyze data.

3. Develop basic competencies for use of spreadsheets to calculate numbers.

4. Explore functions specific to spreadsheets.

5. Design an appropriate chart to communicate a specific point.

Key Terms

Active Cell	Cumulative Chart
Area Chart	External Reference
Bar Chart	Freeze
Cell	Line Chart
Cell Address	Pie Chart
Cell Range	Spreadsheet
Chart	Stacked Chart
Column	Workbook
Combo Box	Worksheet

Numbers are often part of the information nurses need to manage. Computers, together with specialized software, provide freedom from the drudgery of manual calculations and make managing numerical information much easier. The first spreadsheet program, developed in 1979, greatly accelerated the acceptance of computers in the business world (Mattessich, n.d.). What is most remarkable about the first spreadsheet is that the design is so functional that few changes have been made to it over the years. Instead, many more features have been added, such as charts and components, which make it easier to enter formulas. The program design is intuitive and has remarkable similarities in spreadsheet vendor products.

Spreadsheets are not the only type of application program that simplifies managing numerical data. Other programs that assist in the management of numbers include financial management programs, tax preparation programs, and statistical software. Financial management software allows checkbooks to be balanced and the management of a personal budget, including providing help in categorizing items to facilitate tax preparation. Tax preparation software uses data from a financial manager or spreadsheet to create and print tax returns. Statistical software is designed with preset statistical functions to analyze data. While there are a variety of number-crunching software packages available, this chapter focuses specifically on spreadsheet competencies and applications.

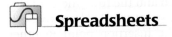

Spreadsheets

A **spreadsheet** is an electronic version of a table consisting of a grid of rectangles (cells) arranged in columns and rows. Each cell can be uniquely formatted to display numbers, text data, and formulas. Spreadsheet software is similar to word processing tables, but spreadsheets are specifically designed to crunch numbers and analyze data. Competency in the effective use of spreadsheets is an invaluable skill for nurses and other healthcare providers. Anytime numbers need to be crunched and analyzed, the electronic spreadsheet is the software of choice.

As when working with other computer applications, it is important that the user be able to identify the problem to be solved first. When beginning to use spreadsheet software, it's often most efficient to first draft out the design with a pencil and piece of paper. The paper and pencil design will assist the user to identify columns and field names and formulas. The computer should be used to calculate values from cell data.

Spreadsheet software, like word processing, is commonly bundled with other office software for purchase. Examples include Microsoft Excel, which is included with Microsoft Office, and Quattro Pro, which is included with Corel WordPerfect Office. Numerous free versions are also available such as OpenOffice.org Calc and Google Docs Spreadsheets™. What is the difference? Commercial software bundles are usually integrated, meaning that the various office products work together seamlessly. Vendor spreadsheet software includes features that may not be available in free versions. Examples include graphics samples; print formatting with custom headers and footers; formula wizards; dragging a cell data to copy data to other cells; and tools to expedite creating a series of numbers or words, such as the months of a year or a series of quarters of a year. If you don't have spreadsheet software on your computer, begin learning with a free version to visualize the features and functions. Figures 9-1 through 9-3 compare the menus of three popular spreadsheet applications.

The Spreadsheet Window

The spreadsheet window is similar in all application programs associated with a graphical user interface (GUI), which uses windows, icons, menus, and a mouse. At first glance, the main difference between a

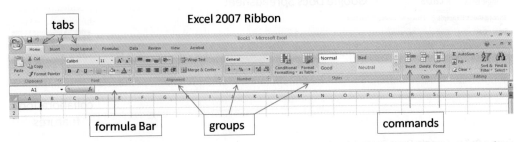

Figure 9-1 • Excel 2007 ribbon menu (Microsoft product screen shot reprinted with permission from Microsoft corporation).

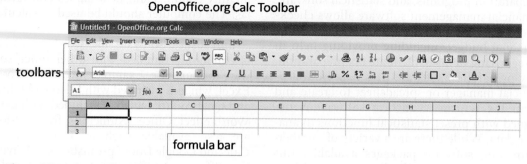

Figure 9-2 • Open office.org calc.

spreadsheet and a word processor seems to be that the document screen in a spreadsheet is only a table. Many of the features used in word processing are the same, such as file and edit. Some important differences, however, are for instance, formula and chart functions built into the menu options. By default, each spreadsheet file is actually a workbook containing one or more spreadsheets. The tabs at the bottom of each spreadsheet allow the user to provide meaningful names and differentiate between multiple spreadsheets in a workbook.

SPREADSHEET BASICS

The vocabulary of spreadsheets is simple. A **cell** refers to the rectangles in the table. A row is a horizontal group of cells, and a **column** is a vertical group of cells. **Cell address** is the name given to a cell, and it is derived from the

letter of the column and the row where it is located (similar to a street map). The **active cell** is analogous to the insertion point in other programs. It is the location where any information entered will be placed. Besides being visible in the table by bold lines, the contents of the active cell are mirrored in the formula bar. A **cell range** is a group of contiguous cells, for example, B11:D13. The range of A2 to B3 (Figure 9-4) would be expressed as A2:B3 or A2:B3; the formatting depends on the spreadsheet application publisher. Users can name ranges of cells and use this name in commands instead of the cell location to create formulas.

Two terms that may at first seem confusing are worksheet and workbook. A **worksheet** refers to one spreadsheet, whereas a **workbook** consists of one or more worksheets. Workbooks allow the user to have many worksheets open at the same time. Worksheets are identified by editing the tab name at the

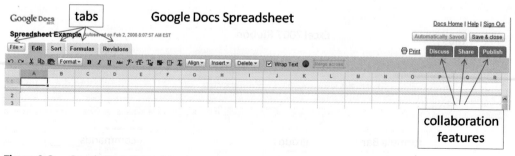

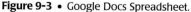

Figure 9-3 • Google Docs Spreadsheet.

Spreadsheet Basics

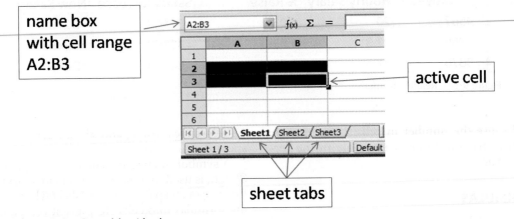

name box with cell range A2:B3

active cell

sheet tabs

Figure 9-4 • Spreadsheet basics.

bottom of the sheet. The user can change the order of the sheets, add, or delete sheets from a workbook. The number of columns and rows allowed in a worksheet varies according to the spreadsheet software publisher and version. For example, the size of a Microsoft 2007 Excel worksheet can be 16,384 columns by 1,048,576 rows. In contrast, Google Docs Spreadsheets will allow for 256 columns by 10,000 rows or up to 100,000 cells or up to 40 sheets (Google, 2007). The size of a spreadsheet should be designed for optimum use. When working on a project, keep the spreadsheet size as small as possible. A worksheet with data in 256 columns may be more manageable if it is broken down into several worksheets. The content of a spreadsheet is not confined to a table. Commercial products and some free products provide ways to include pictures (graphics). Commercial and free products provide a means to create charts (graphs) from data for analysis purposes. You have heard that a "picture is worth a thousand words"; charts can paint an impressive picture to assist in the analysis of complex data.

Commercial software spreadsheets that are designed for reuse can be saved as a template file. A template provides a pattern of content for software applications. Commercial software is often packaged with predesigned templates and/or provides a means to download template files from their Web site. For more information on the use of spreadsheet templates, check the software Help menu.

SPREADSHEET USES IN NURSING

Although spreadsheets are used extensively in healthcare for budgets and the management of financial records, they are useful whenever calculations are needed. For example, spreadsheets are commonly used for quality improvement of patient care. Nurses can monitor and analyze data for adverse events such as medication errors, patient falls, and hospital-acquired infections. Formulas, based on input data, can be used to calculate information such as length of stay, age, and gestation. Spreadsheets are also used for time and attendance information.

The real power of a spreadsheet is derived not only from the ability to organize and edit data but also from its ability to recalculate when a number in a referenced cell is changed. A referenced cell is the cell that is referred to in a formula. For example, in Figure 9-5, the cell F15 contains a formula. It references the cells C15, D15, and E15. Any changes made to the contents of either of these cells

	A	B	C	D	E
1	Employee #	Hourly Salary	% Raise	Salary Increase	New Salary
2	4567	20	0.03	=B2*C2	=D2+B2
3	7865	22.3	0.03	=B3*C3	=D3+B3
4	9876	21.5	0.03	=B4*C4	=D4+B4

Figure 9-5 • Relative formula.

will cause the number in cell F15 to change. Notice that the formula is visible in the formula bar.

FORMULAS

A spreadsheet formula is a mathematical equation that provides instructions to the computer for processing the data. Formulas can be either relative or absolute. When a relative formula is copied to another cell or range of cells, it adjusts to the move by changing the referenced cells (see Figure 9-5). An absolute formula uses the dollar sign ($) to signify that it will retain the specific column and/or row cell when moved. For example, in Figure 9-6 $F references column F;

$2 references row 2; and F2 references the specific cell address F2.

A symbol, such as the equals (=) sign or the @ sign, is used to indicate cell data in a formula. Errors can creep into a spreadsheet when entering formulas into cells. To prevent cell address entry errors, use the point and click method for entering cell addresses. After entering the symbol to indicate formula entry, put the mouse pointer on the first cell addressed by the formula and click with the left mouse button. The cell address will appear in the formula. Enter the necessary mathematical symbol, then point and click the next cell needed. When the formula is complete, tap the enter key. The formulas view in Figures 9-5 and 9-6 demonstrate the symbols used to enter the formulas.

Absolute Formulas

Values View

	A	B	C	D	E	F
1	Employee	Hourly Sal	Salary Inci	New Salary		% Raise
2	4567	20.00	0.60	20.60		3%
3	7865	22.30	0.67	22.97		
4	9876	21.50	0.65	22.15		

Formulas View

Press CTRL + ` (grave accent)

	A	B	C	D	E	F
1	Employee #	Hourly Salary	Salary Increase	New Salary		% Raise
2	4567	20	=B2*F2	=C2+B2		0.03
3	7865	22.3	=B3*F2	=C3+B3		
4	9876	21.5	=B4*F2	=C4+B4		

In this example, the % salary increase is 3% and noted in cell F2. The formula in C2 was copied to C3 and C4. The formulas in Column C reference the value in F2 using the $ sign (F2).

C2 is an example of an absolute formula. When the position of the cell that contains the formula changed, the absolute reference to cell F2 remained the same.

Figure 9-6 • Absolute formula.

An expression refers to the algebraic formula that contains symbols and characters to complete the formula operation. Functions refer to common predesigned formulas used in spreadsheet applications. Both commercial and free spreadsheet softwares include functions to expedite the accuracy of formula entry. Arguments are the specific values required by the formula. In computer terms, argument means the data that the user furnishes to calculate the formula value.

CREATING FORMULAS

The principles and symbols of formula calculation are identical in all computer programs. The characters used to communicate that the computer should perform a specific calculation, such as multiplying or dividing, are not necessarily the same as used on paper. An asterisk (*) is used to denote multiplication; if the familiar x is used, the computer would be unable to distinguish the character "x" from a multiplication symbol. A computer formula for the multiplication of 5 times 50 is 5*50.

The forward slash (/) located under the question mark key is used to denote division. To use the computer to divide 10 by 5, the formula is 10/5 (see Table 9-1). The results of division are not always a whole number (integer). Microsoft Excel 2007 formats numbers as "general" in decimal format by default. To format a number as an integer (whole number),

format the number with 0 decimal places. The integer is a rounded number, whereas a decimal provides accuracy to the specified decimal point.

The caret ($\wedge$) symbol located over the number 6 on the keyboard is used to represent an exponent (raises a number to another power). Calculation of body mass index (BMI) is an example for use of exponents in nursing. The formula for BMI when using pounds and inches is to divide the weight in pounds by height in inches squared and multiplied by a conversion factor of 703 (Centers for Disease Control and Prevention, 2007). For instance, if a person weighed 150 pounds and was 65 inches tall, the formula = [(150/65^2)*703] would result in a BMI of 24.96.

Order of Mathematical Operations

In performing arithmetical computations, computers follow the order of operations for mathematics. Three factors determine the order in which mathematical procedures will be performed:

▼ The kind of computation required.
▼ Nesting, or the placement of an expression within parentheses.
▼ Left-to-right placement of the expressions in the command.

The computer arbitrarily performs operations in the following order:

▼ Anything in parentheses is performed first.
▼ Exponentiation is done next.

TABLE 9-1 ● *Different Types of Arithmetic Division in Spreadsheets*				
			Answer	
Divide the Number	**By**	**As an Integer**	**Round to 2 Decimal Place**	**Round to 0 Decimal Place**
29	5	5	5.80	6
32	6	5	5.33	5
Formula		INT(29/5)	ROUND (29/5,2)	ROUND (29/5,0)
Spreadsheet		INT(B3/B5)	ROUND	ROUND
Example			[(B3/B5),2)]	[(B3/B5),0]

TABLE 9-2 ● *Acronym to Remember the Order in Which Computers Performs Calculations*					
Please	**Excuse**	**My**	**Dear**	**Aunt**	**Sally**
		Equal (Left to Right)		Equal (Left to Right)	
Parentheses	Exponentiation	Multiplication	Division	Addition	Subtraction

▼ Multiplication and division follow in left-to-right manner.

▼ Addition and subtraction are performed last.

These rules, which follow algebraic protocols, are used in all application packages that allow calculations including spreadsheets, statistical packages, and databases (see Table 9-2). When using the acronym (or mnemonic) in Table 9-2, remember that when two mathematical operations are equal, such as multiplication and division, the calculations are completed from left to right. There are a number of excellent review sites about the order of mathematical operations. An example is the Regents Exam Prep Center Web site at http://regentsprep.org/Regents/math/math-topic.cfm?TopicCode=orderop.

Other Spreadsheet Features

Besides the normal functions that can be applied across the board in most application programs, such as changing the font style and size or changing the color of the background or text, spreadsheets possess some unique characteristics that require specialized functions.

FORMATTING CELLS WITH TYPE OF CONTENTS

Contents in a spreadsheet cell are of two different types: numbers and text. Numbers, depending on what they reference, can be formatted in different ways and cell in a spreadsheet can be uniquely formatted. The default in all programs is no specific formatting, however, the cell will default to the type

of data that is entered. Commercial products and most free products allow for the following formatting: rounded or decimal; financial, currency, percent, date, and time. Commercial software includes formatting for exponents (scientific) and custom formatting for zip codes, telephone numbers, social security numbers, date, and time.

FREEZING ROWS AND COLUMNS

When there are more rows or columns in a spreadsheet than can be viewed on a computer screen, it is difficult to know what information is represented. Spreadsheets provide a way to **freeze** either the rows or columns or both. The term "freeze" means that you can keep one part of the spreadsheet visible while scrolling to another area on the spreadsheet. Free spreadsheet software usually allows the user to freeze rows, whereas commercial software allows for both. This feature is important for accurate data entry when the data refer to a heading in a column or row. To learn how to accomplish this task, use the Help menu. The name of the feature varies slightly according to the publisher but usually refers to "freezing" rows, windows, or panes.

USING AUTOMATIC DATA ENTRY

Sometimes spreadsheet design requires sequential data such as numbering 1–10, days of the week, months of the year, or quarters in the year. Commercial spreadsheet software includes a feature that allows the user to make a few entries and then have the computer complete the series. This feature works with a series of skipped numbers such as 2, 4, 6. The term for this feature varies according to the software publisher but usually refers to "fill."

USING DATABASE FUNCTIONS

Both commercial and free spreadsheets are capable of some database functions such as sorting data. The newest commercial products include features to assure that valid or correct data is entered into the cells. For example, one way to ensure that valid data is entered is to use a drop-down list (**combo box**). For example, you can limit data entry for a column heading of gender to two choices, male and female. Commercial software provides many other spreadsheet features such as a Forms view of data. Database features in spreadsheet software are not as robust as a true database, but they are functional for many simple operations. A spreadsheet, or any range of cells, can be easily imported to most database software for more extensive data manipulation. Any data that are structured in a table format, whether a spreadsheet, a table in a word processor, a statistical package, or database, can be easily passed (imported/exported) from program to program.

LINKING CELLS AND WORKSHEETS FROM OTHER SOURCES

There are times when a user will want to reference (link) to a cell or a cell range in a spreadsheet located in another workbook. Use of an **external reference** to the workbook is less prone to error than trying to check the other sheet, copying the value(s), and entering it into a formula. When cells are linked, if the value is changed in the linked cell, the change will be visible in the worksheet containing the referenced cell. Entire spreadsheet tables can often be linked in companion office software such as the word processor or database software. This feature is easy to use and is a very powerful tool to ensure data consistency. Use the spreadsheet Help menu for more information on this feature.

DATA PROTECTION AND SECURITY

In healthcare we often use spreadsheets to provide data protection and/or security. Data protection refers to locking cells to prevent the user from changing the cell value. This feature is very helpful to prevent accidental changes to cell text, numbers, or formulas. Security means that the user has to provide a password(s) to view and/or to edit the spreadsheet. Free online spreadsheets such as Google spreadsheets should not be used to store confidential data since the spreadsheets are stored online in a public domain. Use spreadsheets to enter confidential data only if there is a way to provide security. Only password-protected spreadsheets should be stored on public domains such as the shared healthcare agency or educational agency shared server. Check with your Health Insurance Portability and Accountability Act (HIPAA) security official if you have any questions about the security of your file(s).

 Tips for Better Spreadsheets

Designing a spreadsheet that effectively communicates does not happen by adopting a casual approach. Spreadsheets should be carefully designed and organized to make them useful. Design a spreadsheet on a piece of paper before using spreadsheet software. If the data needs to be sorted for analysis, make sure that only one value is entered into the cell. For example, if you need to sort by last name, create separate headers for first name and last name. Increase the row height rather than leaving blank rows between data. This tip is particularly important when formulas are with a range of cells.

It is best to use a separate worksheet for each table in a workbook. If you design a worksheet to include more than one table, make sure that if you need to insert a new row or column, it does not change or corrupt other parts of the spreadsheet data. Name each spreadsheet to clearly identify the purpose or topic.

While designing a complex spreadsheet or workbook, include a table of contents with hyperlinks to the appropriate sections. Include explanations of any logic or assumptions on the first worksheet. Provide clear labels and instructions that all users will be able to understand. Other users rarely have the same viewpoint as the creator. When using a complex formula, especially one that references the results of other formulas, carefully test the formula with simple numbers. This is particularly important if the spreadsheet will be used with many different values.

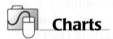

Charts

A **chart** is a graphical presentation of a set of numbers. "Chart" is the terminology used in spreadsheet software. Charts are used to communicate meaning that can be difficult to understand from a raw set of numbers. That said, research has shown that the ability to interpret charts is strongly affected by the viewer's expertise and understanding of the purposes of the different chart formats (Ancker, Senathirajah, Kukafka, & Starren, 2006). Charts should be created keeping in mind the user's ability to interpret the data.

Creating charts using a computer is relatively easy. A computer can create any type of chart, whether or not it communicates anything meaningful. Using charts appropriately involves knowing the message that needs to be communicated and selecting the type of chart that best accomplishes the goal accurately and efficiently (Few, 2004a). Although spreadsheets, word processors, databases, and presentation packages all facilitate the creation of charts, spreadsheets have the most powerful chart creation tools. Perhaps the biggest plus for creating charts in a spreadsheet is that if the numbers in the cells used to create the chart change, the chart automatically reflects the change.

CHART BASICS

To construct a meaningful chart, it is necessary to understand the chart basics vocabulary. Table 9-3 and Figure 9-6 can assist with the task. It is important to use the types of charts appropriately. The chart should assist the viewer to understand data, but not ever distort the meaning of data.

Types of Charts

Spreadsheets take the drudgery out of creating charts as well as present the option for creating not only many different types of charts, but of making them three dimensional, changing the orientation for the horizontal (x) axis to that of a vertical position, and combinations of all these factors. Each of these features can

TABLE 9-3 ● *Chart Basics*	
Term	**Meaning**
x axis	The horizontal axis (line) of a bar, line, or scatter graph, generally represents time values, categories, or division.
y axis	The vertical axis (line) of a bar, line, or scatter graph, most often used to represent amounts.
Data	Numbers without meaning; those that are unprocessed.
Data series or set	A set of numbers that will be represented in the chart, usually on y axis, or a group of items that will be represented on x axis.
Axis title	The title for the information displayed on an axis.
Graph title	A description of the graph used to title the graph.
Legend	The visual representation of each item in the data series. Maybe a color, shape, or both.
Data point	The point where a number is plotted. It is the intersection of its value on the x and y axes.
Data labels	Labels that show the actual value of specific data, or the data points.
Two-dimensional chart	A chart that represents data on the x and y axes.
Three-dimensional chart	A chart that adds a third axis, referred to as the z axis. Can be very misleading, use only when there is need to communicate an added dimension.

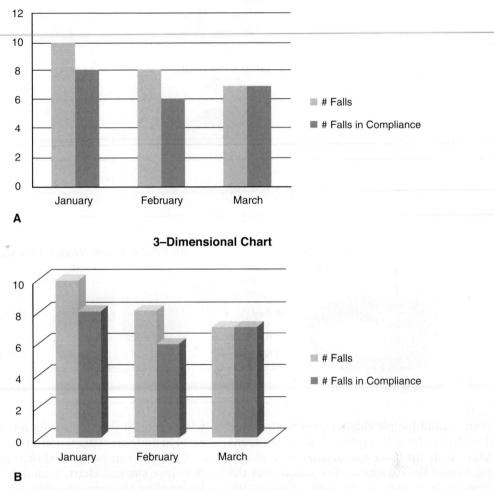

Figure 9-7 • Two- and three-dimensional charts.

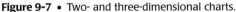

emphasize objects in the chart that may misconstrue the true meaning of the base numbers. Compare the two- and three-dimensional charts in Figure 9-7. In which does the figure for April stand out? Most of these variations can be used in all charts. When using these variations, be certain that they reflect the point that needs to be communicated. As a user of charts, be aware that these distortions exist. Although spreadsheet software provides many different chart types including pie, column, bar, line, stock, surface, doughnut, bubble, and radar; this section will focus on the four

main types of charts: pie, column, bar, and line charts.

Pie Charts. **Pie charts** are used to communicate the proportion of various items in relation to the whole. They are designed to show percentages, not amounts. A pie chart may also be used to show a proportional relationship between a slice and a whole. To clearly communicate percentages, use six or less sectors. Color and shading of the pie sectors should emphasize the chart message (Duffy & Jacobsen, 2005). Figure 9-8 illustrates different types of pie

Shift:	# Falls:
Day	15
Eve	13
Night	25

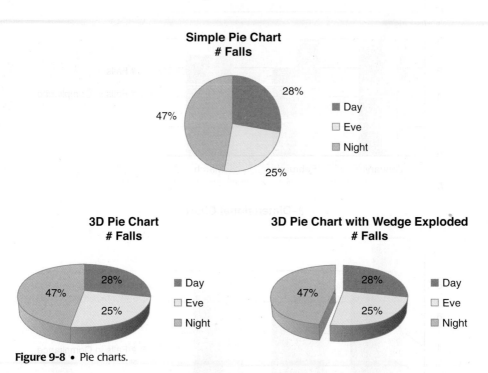

Simple Pie Chart
 # Falls

28%
47%
25%
■ Day
☐ Eve
▨ Night

3D Pie Chart
 # Falls

28%
47%
25%
■ Day
☐ Eve
▨ Night

3D Pie Chart with Wedge Exploded
 # Falls

28%
47%
25%
■ Day
☐ Eve
▨ Night

Figure 9-8 • Pie charts.

charts. All of the pie charts represent the same data. Notice how the exploded view chart looks larger than the three-dimensional and simple pie views. The explosion view can distort the viewer's perception of the data. Without the percent values, it is difficult to determine which slice is largest in both the exploded wedge and the three-dimensional pie.

Column and Bar Charts. Column charts are used to depict changes over time or to show comparisons. Placing amounts on the y axis meets the common expectation that an upward movement is associated with an increase in amount, whereas a downward movement indicates a decrease. When the horizontal x axis is used for the passage of time, the most effective form of communications is achieved when the earliest time is placed on the left and time elapses to the right. To prevent a distortion of value, it is best if the longitudinal y axis starts with a zero. If the y axis does not start with a zero, include an explanation in the chart.

Columns can be stacked or made cumulative. In a **stacked chart**, each data set uses as its baseline the previous data set. A stacked chart can also be a 100% chart in which each data set is a percentage of the whole. In a **cumulative chart**, the data accumulate for each series. Figure 9-9 is a cumulative chart.

Bar charts are generally associated with comparisons of amounts. Figure 9-10 depicts several types of bar charts that compare the number of births for January to June. If the bar chart is seen in color, use bright and darker colors to emphasize key data. If all of the bars are bright and/or dark, the message will be confusing (Few, 2004b). The simple bar chart shows the total number of births each month, whereas the cluster, stacked, and 100% formats allow comparisons of the number of vaginal and cesarean births each month.

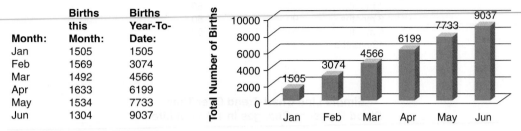

Month:	Births this Month:	Births Year-To-Date:
Jan	1505	1505
Feb	1569	3074
Mar	1492	4566
Apr	1633	6199
May	1534	7733
Jun	1304	9037

Figure 9-9 • Cumulative chart.

Month:	Vaginal:	Cesarean:	Total Births:
Jan	1505	1505	1505
Feb	1569	3074	3074
Mar	1492	4566	4566
Apr	1633	6199	6199
May	1534	7733	7733
Jun	1304	9037	9037

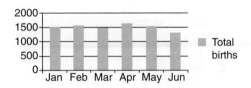

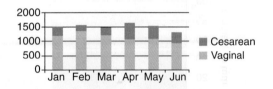

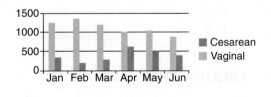

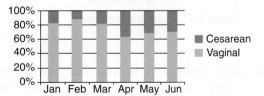

Figure 9-10 • Bar charts.

Line and Area Charts. Line charts also show amounts, but their emphasis is on communicating changes in data over an elapsed time period, as opposed to the comparisons repre-

sented by a bar chart. **Area charts** are similar to line charts, but the color and visual display makes the data differences clearer. Figure 9-11 shows line and area charts to depict the change

Age:	Systolic BP:	Diastolic BP:
Birth	69	55
14 days	77	54
1 month	85	52
3 months	90	50
6 months	91	53
12 months	91	55

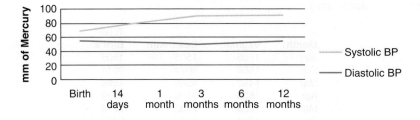

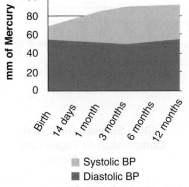

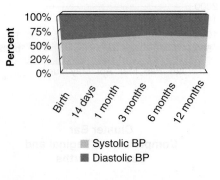

Figure 9-11 • Line and area charts.

in blood pressure during the first year of life. The simple line chart depicts the changes in the average systolic and diastolic blood pressures during the first year of life. In the area chart, both the systolic and diastolic start at zero. In the 100% area chart, the diastolic is seen as a percentage of the systolic. The area and 100% area charts show clearly the changes in pulse pressure.

CREATING THE CHART

Computer applications programs allow the creation of many types of charts. The first task in creating any chart is to select the cells that represent the data to be charted. After the appropriate cells have been selected, click on the chart tool and select the types of chart that will best represent those data. Commercial

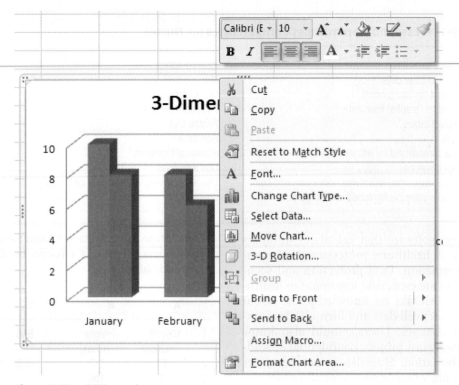

Figure 9-12 • Editing a chart.

spreadsheet software provides a preview of how the chart will look before the final selection is made. If you are using free software and do not like the chart, delete it and begin again. Both commercial and free spreadsheet software provide a way to create and edit the chart title and legends. Commercial software includes the ability to modify fonts and colors used in the chart. Once you have clicked on the icon to indicate that you have finished, the chart appears on the spreadsheet. A completed chart can always be resized, moved, or edited (see Figure 9-12). To edit the chart, right click the object that needs to be changed to obtain a drop-down menu of choices.

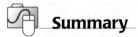 **Summary**

Spreadsheet programs have taken much of the drudgery out of calculations and deserve a place on every nurse's desktop. Nurses should all demonstrate essential spreadsheet competencies (see Box 9-1). Spreadsheets have much in common with other office application programs including word processing, presentation software, and database software. The basic structure in a spreadsheet is a table, with a column of numbers on the left side and a row of letters at the top. The letters and numbers provide a way for each cell to have a corresponding name. The principles and symbols for formula calculation are the same as all other computer programs.

Although spreadsheet software can make managing numbers easier, if spreadsheets are not carefully designed and used, they can create a great amount of misinformation. Users should use spreadsheets to perform calculations from data. Formulas should be scrutinized for accuracy to avoid misinterpretation of data. As with all computer use, nurses should use common sense when interpreting computer numerical and chart outputs; this includes understanding the assumptions that various models use. Given thoughtful use,

---

Box 9-1 • Essential Spreadsheet Competencies for Nurses

Conditional formatting

Copy data to other cells

Create formulas using words

Create charts (graphs) from data

Create pivot tables

Date/time

Design a spreadsheet for efficient use

Financial functions

Format cell data using font styles, font sizes, and color

Format cells using backgrounds and borders

Insert graphics

Manage text

Merge cells

Password protect

Resize a cell

Sort data

Statistical functions

Use templates

Use wizards to guide you through complex calculation operations

---

spreadsheet software that calculates numbers can assist all healthcare professionals in managing information. Data protection and security features are especially important in healthcare. Users should be knowledgeable about how to protect cell data and formulas from inadvertent changes. Users should also know how to password protect confidential spreadsheet information. Spreadsheet competencies and skills are valuable assets for all nurses.

APPLICATIONS AND COMPETENCIES

1. Identify at least three differences between a word processor and a spreadsheet.
2. Use spreadsheet software to calculate a baby's gestational age at the time of the mother's prenatal visit. Copy the column headers and dates below. Type the formula in C2 and then copy the formula to cells C3:C5.

	A	B	C
1	Prenatal Checkup Date	Baby's Due Date	Baby's Gestational Age (Weeks)
2	1/1/2009	9/1/2009	={[(B2-A2)-280]/7}*-1
3	9/2/2009	2/20/2010	
4	4/1/2010	9/1/2010	
5	1/20/2011	2/20/2011	

3. Calculate the BMI using the data in the table below. Copy the column headers and data below. Type the formula in C2 and then copy the formula to cells C3:C4. Format the BMI to one decimal point.

	A	B	C
1	Weight (pounds)	Height (inches)	BMI
2	67	110	=[(B2/A2^2)*703]
3	70	150	
4	75	200	

4. In a spreadsheet, create a formula to calculate the number of intravenous (IV) drops per minute when the IV tubing is calibrated to 20 drops per minute, the time for the infusion is eight hours, and the total volume to be infused in 1,000 mL.
5. Calculate the ages of patients on admission to your nursing unit. Copy the data from the table below onto a spreadsheet. Format the cells C2:C4 as YY. Type the formula in C2 and then copy the formula to cells C3:C4. Type the formula noted in cell C5 to determine the average age of the patients.

	A	B	C
1	Admission Date	Birth Date	Age
2	9/16/2010	11/10/1985	=B2–C2
3	4/5/2011	11/17/1971	
4	4/27/2011	4/27/1950	
5			=AVERAGE(D2:D4)

6. You recently implemented a new intervention to prevent patient falls. Copy the data noted below on a spreadsheet. Use the Fill feature to create columns with the months of the year. Design a chart to show the changes in the number of falls. Use the Help feature when necessary.

	Jan	Feb	Mar	Apr	May	Jun
Number of Falls	25	31	35	10	12	30

7. You want to show the percentage of all visits to your emergency department during each shift. For the month of May, you had 600 visits on the day shift, 1,000 visits on the evening shift, and 400 visits on the night shift. Design a chart depicting the data.

8. You want to show the changes in the number of pounds gained each month of pregnancy from month 3 to month 5. You have the average number of pounds gained in each month (2 pounds in month 3, 5 pounds in month 5) for 300 pregnant women. Design a chart to show the changes over time.

REFERENCES

Ancker, J. S., Senathirajah, Y., Kukafka, R., & Starren, J. B. (2006). Design features of graphs in health risk communication: A systematic review. *Journal of the American Medical Informatics Association, 13*(6), 608–618.

Centers for Disease Control and Prevention. (2007, May 22). *About BMI for adults*. Retrieved November 22, 2008, from http://www.cdc.gov/nccdphp/dnpa/bmi/adult_BMI/about_adult_BMI.htm

Duffy, M. E., & Jacobsen, B. S. (2005). Organizing and displaying data. In B. H. Munro (Ed.), *Statistical methods for health care research* (5th ed., pp. 16–27). Philadelphia: Lippincott Williams & Wilkins.

Few, S. (2004a). Common mistakes in data presentation. *Intelligent Enterprise, 7*(12), 34.

Few, S. (2004b). Elegance through simplicity. *Intelligent Enterprise, 7*(15), 35.

Google. (2008). *Getting to know Google docs: Size limits*. Retrieved November 22, 2008, from http://docs.google.com/support/bin/answer.py?answer=37603

Mattessich, R. (n.d.). *Spreadsheet: Its first computerization (1961–1964)*. Retrieved November 22, 2008, from http://www.j-walk.com/ss/history/spreadsh.htm

Databases: Creating Information From Data

Learning Objectives

After studying this chapter you will be able to:

1. *Describe a database.*

2. *Use Boolean tools in searching a database.*

3. *Explain the role of databases in improving patient care.*

4. *Describe methods of discovering knowledge in both relational and large databases.*

5. *Differentiate methods of viewing data in a database.*

6. *List some steps in creating a database.*

Key Terms

Aggregated Data
Atomic Level
Attribute
Boolean Logic
Child Table
Data
Database
Database Management
    System (DBMS)
Database Model
Data Mining
Data Warehouse
Entity
Field
Flat Database
Form

Hierarchical Database
Knowledge Discovery (KDD)
Lookup table
Network Model
Query
Record
Relational Database
Report
Secondary Data Use
Scope Creep
Sort
Structured Query
    Language (SQL)
Table
Virtual

Does hospitalization of patients whose diabetes is newly diagnosed prevent future hospitalizations for diabetic complications? Do certain approaches to pain management shorten hospital stays? Is the incidence of preventable illnesses lower in children whose mothers received postpartum visits from a nurse? The literature can provide some answers to these questions, but true evidence-based practice requires clinical **data**. The clinical data that could be used in conjunction with the literature to answer these questions are recorded, but are very infrequently used to answer these questions.

Nursing and Databases

As a nurse you are concerned with improving patient care. In the past we have looked to experience and experts to help us in this area. The electronic patient record, however, will allow us to add patient documentation data to this equation. Although a paper medical record provides a wonderful individualized record for one patient, because most of the data lacks structure, it is difficult to retrieve, which makes comparisons with similar patients exceedingly difficult. As a result, we are not yet aware of the richness that lies embedded in patient care data.

When we think about documentation and patient care, we think of one patient. We carefully record patient care information in the proper place in the patient's record and use it to care for this patient at this time Any thought of using data **aggregated**[1] from many medical records to answer clinical questions and gain a broader understanding of a condition is generally discarded because the location of most of the data in paper records makes this type of data retrieval difficult.

The electronic patient record, however, changes this equation. With electronic records, we can retrieve data that will provide answers to the questions at the beginning of this chapter and many others. Given the long history of the use of paper records, it is not surprising that even when data are in an electronic format and could be used to answer clinical questions, we are unaware of the possibilities for using these data. This picture will change only when we gain an understanding of how a **database** works and how one can manipulate data to provide information. This chapter will provide a beginning view of the principles behind storing, retrieving, and manipulating data that could be used to create knowledge from data in an electronic record. Experimenting with, and expanding on, these ideas in a real database will further your ability to employ evidence-based care.

Learning about databases will also guide you to see a use for databases in the many reports that modern healthcare demands. To illustrate some of the potential, we will present an example of a current use for a database in nursing. As you may be aware, as of October 1, 2008, the Center for Medicare and Medicaid Services (CMS) no longer paid for care for patients with nosocomial urinary tract infections (UTIs). To be a successful hospital, it will be necessary to develop and implement protocols to keep these infections to a bare minimum. To do this requires data. UTIs are sometimes caused by indwelling catheters and may or may not be caused by the agency that treats them.

For our example, let's pretend that your agency is a tertiary care hospital and admits patients from other hospitals, long-term care facilities, and directly from home. Your nurse manager wants to find out how many patients arrive with UTIs, and how many develop them after they arrive. She assigns you to do a monthly report with this data.

To do this, you will need to track the data. You could do this with a word processing **table**, a spreadsheet, or a **relational database**. The tool that you use to create this database, however, determines the answers that you can get from the data. A word processing table will allow you to count instances as will a spreadsheet. A spreadsheet will also permit some searching and reordering of the **records**. Both of these, because there may be the same data entered in more than one place, may lead to errors. A well-designed relational database, however, not only prevents data duplication, but also provides maximum searching with multiple variables. It allows processed, selected data to be exported into a spreadsheet, a statistical package, or word processing software and to be presented in many different ways – all without reentering a piece of data more than once. Past experience has also shown you that once the data is collected and reported, the nurse manager will want more answers. Therefore, you decide that the best choice is a relational database.

A database is a collection of data that are organized or structured in such a way that data

---

[1] Aggregated data are discussed in detail in Chapter 1.

that is in the key field of the master UTI table with the description, "Foreign Key." When this data is identical in both the tables, the information from the records in them can be tied together, or related.

Notice that the field type in the foreign field that matches the AutoNumber field is numeric. Fields that are related must be of the same type, and a numeric field that contains only long integers matches the AutoNumber type of field. Numeric fields serve other purposes too. Among many things, they can be used in calculations the same as in a spreadsheet and added for totals for a report page or the entire report. A text field can contain any type of data, but is limited to 255 characters, including spaces. If a field will contain more than 255 characters, use a Memo field. Date/Time fields allow "date calculations." In this database, the date fields will allow us to calculate the LOS when the time as well as the date is entered in this field. The "Yes/No" field type is a logical field, that is, only yes or no can be entered.

By looking at the table in Figure 10-1 again, we realize that the data that we want in the field "Where the patient is admitted from" is limited to four possibilities: long-term care facility, emergency department, home, or another acute

care facility. To make data entry easier we create a **lookup table** that has these entries and relate this table to that field in the design view. When this is done, a data enterer selects from a list instead of typing in an entry. Whenever possible, the designer should create a list of possible data entries to be used as a lookup table. This makes it easier for the data enterer and ensures that correct, identical, data will be entered in the field.

Full table relationships, as opposed to lookup table relationships, are created in the relationship window by dragging the key field in the Master Infections table to the matching field in the Antibiotics table, which is the table that may or may not contain a record that matches a record in the Master Infections table. This type of relationship that you see pictured in Figure 10-3 is a one-to-many relationship. That is, a record in the main, or Master Infections table, may have none, or an infinite number of matching records in the antibiotics table. This type of relationship is symbolized in the relationship window by the infinity sign (∞) next to the antibiotics, or subordinate table. Notice that each table name is preceded by the suffix "tbl." It is good practice in a database to precede each object with a prefix designating its type.

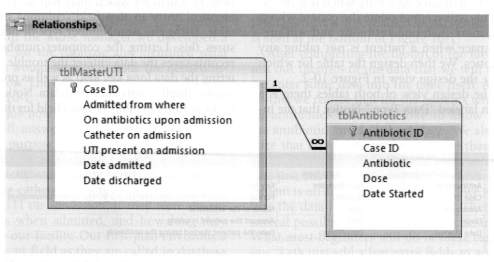

Figure 10-3 • Relationship between tables.

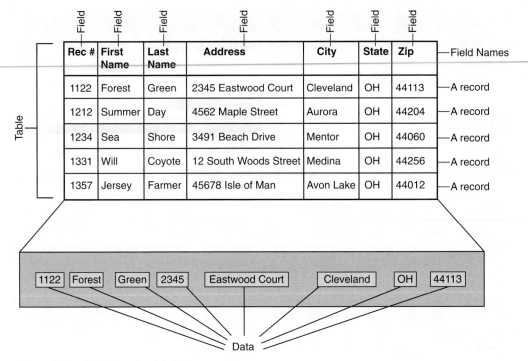

Figure 10-4 • Anatomy of a database.

 ## Overview of Databases

Let's digress for a minute and use a different example to look at the overall anatomy of a database table. Figure 10-4 shows the names of the objects in a database table and Table 10-1

TABLE 10-1 • *Database Phenomena*	
Database Term	**Definition**
Data	Facts without meaning, e.g., the number 37.
Field (**attribute**)	Smallest structure in a database.
Field name	The label applied to a field.
Record (**tuple**)	All the information about a single "member" of a table
Table (**entity** or file)	A collection of related information. A table consists of records, and each record is made up of a number of fields.

Words in parentheses are the names that database professionals use for these items.

provides the terminology that database professionals use for these objects. Data is always stored in a table; other views as well as data manipulations are **virtual** and use data from the tables. This makes it possible to use a piece of data many times, even though it has only been entered once. This concept also underlies healthcare information systems, although data storage is more complex.

FORMS

Although stored in a table, data entry is not confined to the table view. Data entry can be made easy by creating a **form** view that shows all the fields related to that record for which data must be entered, regardless of the base table in which this data will be stored. To ease data entry in our UTI Infections database, we create the data entry form seen in Figure 10-5. Notice the "drop-down" list for the field "Admitted from where?" When the data enterer clicked the black triangle at the end of the

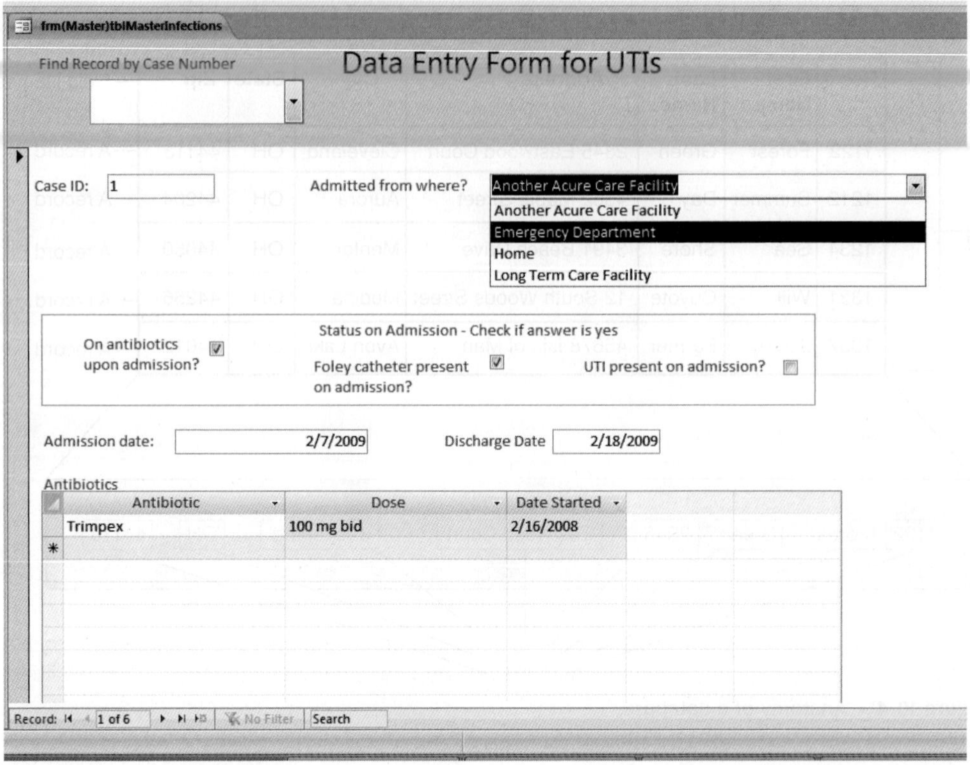

Figure 10-5 • Data entry form.

blank field, this list, which is from a lookup table, appeared. Now all the data enterer does is to point and click the correct choice. Notice that the logical fields all have checkboxes for data entry, again forcing answers to conform to given choices and making data entry easier. Because we knew that different people would be entering data, we included instructions on the form for the data enterer. Forms are not only useful for data entry, but can be used to view or print data for one record.

In the upper left corner of the entry form is a box that allows a data enterer to search for a case by number. It is strongly suggested that the person in charge of this database have some way of finding the data that belongs to a specific case. This could be a separate table with the name of the patient, or the medical record number, or this information could be included in the master table. This information, of course, needs to be kept locked up to comply with Health Insurance Portability and Accountabilty Act (HIPAA) regulations. Tables can be locked so that a password is required to open them.

REPORTS

Reports are another view of data and, like forms, can present information from more than one table as well as from queries. Figure 10-6 shows one report that is possible from the data that was gathered in the UTI database. By using "date arithmetic" the computer calculated the LOS for patients. We also organized the report by reporting the data for the type of facility from which they were admitted. Once this report is constructed and saved, when run, it reports the data that is currently in the table, not the data that was there when it was created. Thus time spent creating a well-designed report is paid back many times.

LOS for February 1 to February 18, 2009 for UTIs

Admitted from where	Date admitted	LOS
Another Acure Care Facility		
	2/7/2009	11
Emergency Department		
	2/8/2009	10
	2/12/2009	3
Home		
	2/8/2009	3
Long-Term Care Facility		
	2/13/2009	8
	2/18/2009	4

Figure 10-6 • UTI report by facility admitted.

Reports may include graphs[2] as well as permit calculations on data. Reports should be designed in such a way that the information will be easy for the person who needs the report to understand. If a person is used to a given format for paper reports, the data from a database can be presented in a report styled to match that format even when the data input screens do not match the old paper input.

SAVING DATA IN A DATABASE

Unlike other application programs, databases save a data entry as soon as the insertion point is moved from the record in which the data was entered. This has several implications. Once you make a change to a record and leave it, consider the change permanent. It is possible to undo one change, but only the last change made. Deleting a record, however, is permanent; there is no redo. When using a database, the only things that you need to save are objects such as a table or form after you create them. Entering data into a table or form does

---

[2] See Chapter 9 for information about graphs. Graphs can be used in spreadsheets and databases as well as pasted or linked into a word processing document.

not change the basic design; hence, they do not need to be saved after data is entered. The only time you need to save is after you create an object, or after you make a change to the object in the design mode. When you close this object, you will be prompted to save. Some databases, such as Access®, save all the objects such as tables, forms, reports etc. as one file. If you want to send a piece of a database that you have created, such as just a table, to someone, you will need to send the entire file, or copy the piece to another database and send that.

Basic Database Searching

We've looked at all the basic objects in a database except a **query**. Queries are one of the characteristics that give databases their power. The ability to create information from the data in a database is limited only by the ingenuity of the query creator. Because querying is such a powerful and important tool in all electronic databases, not just relational ones, we will leave our example, and look at searching, which is a type of querying.

With the progression from paper to electronic library catalogs, as well as Web search

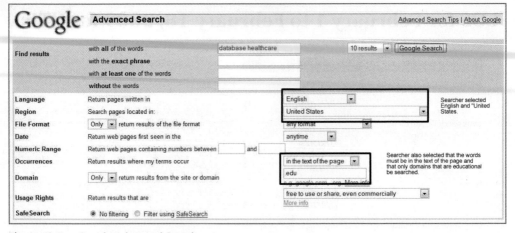

Figure 10-7 • Google Advanced Search.

tools, most of us have had experience with some type of database searching. You have probably searched the Web for something, or needed references on a specific subject and used an electronic bibliographic catalog to find them.[3] In asking for this information, you created a query, or a set of conditions that the located records should meet. When you clicked the Search button, the search tool looked for references that met the criteria you stated in the query.

BOOLEAN LOGIC QUERYING

Sometimes simple queries produce too many results. To further refine a search, it is necessary to use the advanced features of a search tool. For example, one searcher was told that there was a Web page[4] from an educational institution that described the use of databases in healthcare. Because using just those two words retrieved too many links, she narrowed her search using the Google™ Advanced Search tool. In the illustration in Figure 10-7, you can see that she set criteria to return pages with the words "database" AND "healthcare." When two words are entered in the Search

box, Google, and many other catalog search tools including many bibliographical ones, assume that the searcher means to find sources that have both words, even if separated. (This does not apply to searching in a relational database.) To locate links in which these two words appeared as a phrase, the user would have put quotation marks around them.

Searching in any database uses what is called **Boolean logic**, which is named after the 19th century mathematician George Boole. It is a form of algebra in which matches are either true or false. That is, the data in the field either is a match or is not. There are three concepts that make up Boolean logic: "And," "OR," and "Not." "And" searches require that all specified terms be returned. By specifying that both database AND healthcare needed to be present, our searcher was using the Boolean "And" to narrow the search. If the user had selected the choice "At least one of the words," this would have been an "OR" search and would have returned not only records with both terms, but also those in which only one term appeared. What criteria would you use and where would you enter it in Figure 10-7 if you wanted to see Web pages for healthcare, but NOT databases?[5] Searching a database

---

[3] An in-depth look at searching bibliographical databases is seen in Chapter 12.

[4] A Web page is not peer reviewed. Information there should be carefully evaluated using the information in Chapter 11.

[5] You would enter "database" in the field "without the words" on the upper-left side of Figure 10-7 and delete it from the "with all the words" field.

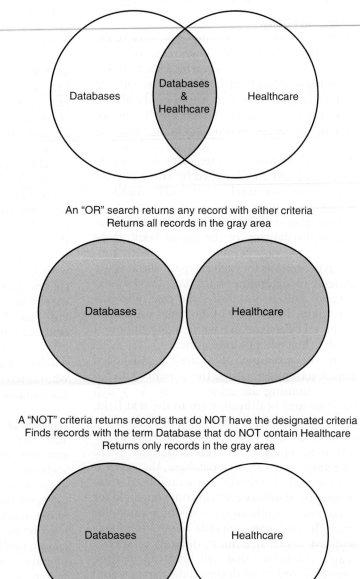

An "AND" search only returns records in which BOTH criteria are met
Returns only records in the gray area

Databases

Databases
&
Healthcare

Healthcare

An "OR" search returns any record with either criteria
Returns all records in the gray area

Databases

Healthcare

A "NOT" criteria returns records that do NOT have the designated criteria
Finds records with the term Database that do NOT contain Healthcare
Returns only records in the gray area

Databases

Healthcare

Figure 10-8 • Boolean Logic.

created with Microsoft Access or any other database from a office suite has the same feature of stating the criteria for the records you wish see; however, they add many other query abilities (Figure 10-8).

RECORD REQUIREMENTS

If data are to be searchable, there are several requirements that it must meet. The data must be structured, there must be a category for the data that is to be searched, and the terms used for a given meaning must be standardized.

Structured Format

To allow specialized searching, data must be organized in a way that allows criteria to be matched to the data in a given field such as title. If a bibliographical database were just full text with no organization, you would not be able to state that you wanted to search only in the author or title areas. When data is organized by categories, it is said to be structured data. In a structured format the categories into which data are placed are identified by labels like the field names we used in our UTI database. Additionally, there must be agreement about exactly what data matches the label. In bibliographical databases, or the phone book, these decisions are easy because there are fairly universal definitions for each category and it is not difficult to determine what data they should contain. This is not always the case, which is why in the design view of the tables we created in the UTI database, we wrote a description of the data that belongs in each field.[6]

In the example of Google™ Advanced Search tool given earlier, the searcher entered criteria limiting the search to sites in which database and healthcare were in the text field. When searching, the search engine ignored the other fields and searched only the data in the text field, ignoring the title and links fields. The more structure to a database, the easier it is to set search criteria. For example, if a demographic database contains only one field for name and it holds all the parts of a name, for example, first name, middle name (or initial) and last name, it is more difficult to specify search conditions that will bring up just the correct record. Well-designed databases would include at least two fields for name, first and last name and often one for the middle name and another for the salutation. If you have ever filled out a form on the Web that asks for demographic information, you will have noticed

that you are asked to enter the different parts in different boxes. Each piece of data that you enter is then stored in the field with that label. For example, first name is stored in the first name field.

Contains a Field for the Data.   You can only search for data in the fields that the database contains. For example, an electronic record for an obstetric labor and delivery unit would probably contain a field for data about the type of birth such as vaginal, Cesarean, forceps. It would also contain fields, or probably fields in related tables, to record any complications such as postpartum hemorrhage as well as date and time fields. From this database you could learn how many Cesarean births occurred in the month of October 2008. You could not, however, answer the question, "Do women with red hair have more postpartum hemorrhages than brunettes or blondes?" because there is no field to record the color of a parturient's hair. In the UTI database you could not find out which units the patients were on because this data is not in the current form of the database. (In real life it certainly would be, but we wanted to keep this simple to make understanding easier.)

Terminology Used to Enter Data Is Standardized. You may have experienced frustration in searching an electronic database or for help in a software program using a term that has meaning to you, but that returns no results. Computers, as you remember, are black-and-white instruments. When your term is not one used by the database that you are searching, it cannot find it. For this reason, in electronic bibliographic databases it is necessary to use terminology that has been agreed on by all to have the same meaning. For example, if the agreed upon term for aspirin is acetylsalicylic acid, if you enter the term "aspirin" or ASA, all synonyms for acetylsalicylic acid, as a search word, you will not be able to find any references.

To meet this criteria, when entering data, the terms used must be standardized. To provide this standardization, many electronic databases limit the terms that can be used to

---

[6] In some databases, when in the data entry mode and the insertion point is in a field, the information in the description column for that field can be seen in the lower-left corner of the screen.

First Name	Last Name	Unit	Surgery	LOS
Star	Bright	2 West	ORIF - Rt hip	6
Will	Coyote	2 East	Lt hip arthroplasty	7
Summer	Day	2 West	Rt hip arthroplasty	4
Jersey	Farmer	2 East	ORIF - Rt hip	3
Spring	Flower	2 West	ORIF - Lt hip	3
Forest	Green	2 East	ORIF - Rt hip	4
Tiffany	Light	2 West	Lt hip arthroplasty	3
Misty	Mountain	2 West	Rt hip arthroplasty	6
Tuesday	Night	2 West	ORIF - Lt hip	4
Sea	Shore	2 West	Lt hip arthroplasty	3
Glen	Springs	2 East	Lt hip arthroplasty	3
Mark	Time	2 East	Lt hip arthroplasty	4
Storm	Wave	2 West	Rt hip arthroplasty	4
Caspar	White	2 East	Rt hip arthroplasty	3
Pearl	White	2 West	Rt hip arthroplasty	4

Figure 10-9 • Patients, surgery, and LOS sorted on last name.

enter data just as we did in the UTI database. In the example of aspirin given above, if you try to enter aspirin when the agreed upon term is acetylsalicylic acid, the computer may tell you that this term is not acceptable and ask you to enter another term.[7] In the UTI database we decided that there would only be four entries allowed in the "admitted from where" field and limited those by using a lookup table. We also decided to limit entries in the "date admitted" and "date discharged" field to dates so we could do date arithmetic. This limitation was accomplished by the database program when we made the field type a Date/Time field.

Today many regulatory agencies from The Joint Commission to the government require that hospitals submit electronic data about their patients. These data, which must be standardized, are used for many things, including identifying healthcare needs. When an electronic patient record does not contain fields for the independent actions of nursing, nursing care cannot be analyzed, and there is no indication that nursing care is part of hospital

care. Reaching conclusions on incomplete data often results in poor decisions.

Manipulating Data

We have discussed different ways of viewing data in a table and some requirements for searching a database including Boolean Logic searching. Relational databases also provide the ability to reorder records, a process known as sorting as well as additional ways of searching, or querying.

SORTING

When data is entered in a database, a record is created. The records are often not entered in the order in which they need to be viewed. This can be overcome by sorting the records on a given field, either alphabetically, or numerically. Sorting is just rearranging the records in a table based on the data in a field or fields in a table. The simplest **sort** is a primary sort; that is, the records are re-sorted based on one field. An example would be reordering records in a database based on last name to produce a table like the records in Figure 10-9.

[7] Standardized terminology is discussed in Chapters 16 (national and international) and 17 (nursing).

First Name ▾	Last Name ▾	Unit ▾	Surgery ▾	LOS ▾
Glen	Springs	2 East	Lt hip arthroplasty	3
Mark	Time	2 East	Lt hip arthroplasty	4
Will	Coyote	2 East	Lt hip arthroplasty	7
Jersey	Farmer	2 East	ORIF - Rt hip	3
Forest	Green	2 East	ORIF - Rt hip	4
Caspar	White	2 East	Rt hip arthroplasty	3
Tiffany	Light	2 West	Lt hip arthroplasty	3
Sea	Shore	2 West	Lt hip arthroplasty	3
Spring	Flower	2 West	ORIF - Lt hip	3
Tuesday	Night	2 West	ORIF - Lt hip	4
Star	Bright	2 West	ORIF - Rt hip	6
Pearl	White	2 West	Rt hip arthroplasty	4
Storm	Wave	2 West	Rt hip arthroplasty	4
Summer	Day	2 West	Rt hip arthroplasty	4
Misty	Mountain	2 West	Rt hip arthroplasty	6

Primary Sort is Unit · Secondary Sort on Surgery · Tertiary Sort on LOS

Figure 10-10 • Primary, secondary, and tertiary sort.

Databases, however, are not limited to sorting on just one field. One can have primary, secondary, tertiary, and even further levels of sorts, each built on the groupings provided by the sort one level above it. In a tertiary sort, the records will first be sorted in a primary sort so that those that have similarities in the sort field are listed together; then another sorting is done on another field on records in each group created from the primary sort (the secondary sort); finally, a tertiary sort on another field of each group from the secondary sort. For example, a primary sort is performed on all patients in a hospital by the type of surgery; then the records are reordered within each type of surgery in a secondary sort so that those from the same unit within each type of surgery are together. The records, for a tertiary sort, are further reordered so that the records on a given unit for each type of surgery are reordered by the primary surgeon. In the example in Figure 10-10, the primary sort is the patient unit, the secondary sort is the type of surgery, and the tertiary sort is the LOS. This type of grouping is most useful in producing reports that need to look at a given characteristic within various groups. The report in Figure 10-6 was produced by a primary sort of the records into the type of facility from which the patient was admitted.

TABLE 10-2 • *Mathematical Operators for Querying*		
Operator	**Query Criteria in Age Field**	**Returns from a Table with Data in the Age Field**
> (greater than)	>50	Records in which the entry in the age field is greater than 50
<(less than)	<50	Records in which the entry in the age field is less than 50
<> (not equal to)	<>50	Records in which the entry in the age field is any number but 50
≥ (greater than or equal to)	≥50	Records in which the entry in the age field is greater than or equal to 50
≤ (less than or equal to)	≤50	Records in which the entry in the age field is less than or equal to 50
Between	Between 30 and 40	Records in which the entry in the age field is between 30 and 40 (inclusive)
Null, or blank (field is empty)	Null (or blank)	Records in which the entry in the age field is empty.
Count, sum, average, standard deviation, minimum, maximum, and others	Make a selection from a drop-down list.	Does a calculation based on the term selected. For text fields, only the count function, which counts the number of times a given term appears, is available. Numeric fields are open to all types of calculations.

QUERIES

A query is the most powerful tool in a database. You have seen the results of a Boolean query in bibliographic databases. There are many other ways that queries can be used to manipulate data. Queries can produce a subset of records on the basis of fields that meet given criteria, or they can report on the entire database. Additionally, queries can be performed on the results of another query. The only limiting factors are the data available, the user's imagination, and the ability to use the criteria selectors of Boolean algebra and the symbols referred to as mathematical operators. (This is not as complicated as it sounds, keep reading! ☺).

The mathematical operators in Table 10-2 may be used in combination with each other or with Boolean Logic. The patient table that is part of Figures 10-9 and 10-10 has another related table that contains the nursing diagnoses for each patient. This allowed the nurses on that unit to see how many times each nursing diagnosis occurred in this given set of patients.

To accomplish this, they used the "count" function and created the table in Figure 10-11. They also wanted to see the average LOS and standard deviation for each of these patients. Using those functions on the LOS field, they created the table in Figure 10-12. On finding the average LOS to be a little over four days they became curious about what the nursing diagnoses were for those patients whose LOS was greater than four days. Using the greater than operator, with the number 4 (>4), they created a query that produced the table you see in Figure 10-13. They used this information to study their care plans and see if they could improve care for these nursing diagnoses.

It is possible to have data downloaded from a large information system in a way that it can be manipulated to answer questions such as those above. Although some of the examples used in this chapter included identifying information about fictitious patients to help clarify the examples, data downloaded from a healthcare agency database should not contain any

Nursing Diagnosis	CountOfNur
Altered role performance - work	1
Altered tissue perfusion	1
Colonic constipation	4
Fear	1
Impaired home maintenance management	3
Impaired physical mobility - Level 1	4
Impaired physical mobility - Level 3	9
Impaired physical mobility - Level 4	2
Ineffective breathing pattern	5
Ineffective management of theraupeutic regin	1
Pain	4
Potential for impaired tissue integrity	1
Potential impaired tissue integrity	2
Powerlessness - Low	2
Risk for altered parenting	1

Figure 10-11 • Number of patients with each nursing diagnosis.

Unit	AvgOfLOS	StDevOfLOS
2 East	4.00	1.55
2 West	4.11	1.17

Figure 10-12 • Average and standard deviation.

LOS	Nursing Diagnosis
7	Colonic constipation
7	Impaired physical mobility - Level 4
7	Pain
6	Impaired home maintenance management
6	Impaired physical mobility - Level 1
6	Pain
6	Risk for altered parenting
6	Impaired physical mobility - Level 3
6	Pain

Figure 10-13 • Nursing diagnosis patients LOS greater than four.

data that would allow individual patients to be identified.

Effective querying involves not necessarily the technical skill to construct a query, but instead the cognitive component that allows us to see the possibilities. When we can communicate exactly what information we want from data, a technical person can construct the query. One way to get this cognitive component is to create and use small databases. Using data that you have entered, or a database that you have designed, creates a situation in which you can see more of the possibilities for getting answers.

One caveat, when you design a query, always test it with a subset of data for which you know the answers to test if it actually works as desired. Include in this subset, outliers that might or might not conform to your query. The best way to learn how to query is to play with the data by querying. You may have to try several different times to get the desired answer. This is not unusual; this author has seen database professionals work hard to enter just the right criteria to produce the answers they needed. Because ultimately the database designer is responsible for answers that are produced, testing a query with a small subset of data holds true especially when someone else, unfamiliar with the data, constructs the query.

Database Models

In our UTI example, we used a relational **database model**. The term "database model" refers to the way in which the data/tables in a database are organized. Several models exist: hierarchical, network, flat, relational, and object oriented. Each has advantages and disadvantages. The choice of which model to use is based on the tasks that the database must perform. Today, many operational databases, instead of belonging to one class, have characteristics from more than one model.

FLAT DATABASE

A **flat database** is a database in which the data are all in one table. It is exemplified by a spreadsheet worksheet and is the simplest database model. The address book in a word processor is another example of a flat database. Flat databases are very simple to construct and use, but they have limitations when it comes to tracking items that belong in a record when there are more than one of the same item. For example, if one wanted to track the infections that occurred in a unit using a flat database, one would need to enter two records for each patient that had more than one pathogen causing the infection. This duplicates data and wastes memory, but more importantly, creates errors in data manipulation when the person doing data input does not enter identical information for the same field in the new record.

HIERARCHICAL DATABASE

The **hierarchical database** was an early database model. This type of database (see Figure 10-14) is a database with tables that are organized in the shape of an inverted tree like a taxonomy or the file structure of a disk as described in Chapter 4. In this organizational plan, often called a tree structure, records are linked to a base, or root, but through successive layers. In Figure 10-14, the Record Number table would be the root table. The Demographics table would be a child of the root, as would the LOS table. Nursing Diagnosis and Surgery would be the children of the parent LOS table and the grandchild of the Record Number. Each child in a hierarchical database can have only one parent, whereas a parent may have none, one, or many children. The difficulty with the hierarchical structure is that it is hard to link data from one branch of the tree with another (e.g., Nursing Diagnoses with Demographics). Because of its structure, this model results in redundant data and cannot support complex relationships (Hernandez, 2003).

Network Model

The **network model** of database organization was developed in part to address some problems with the hierarchical model (Hernandez,

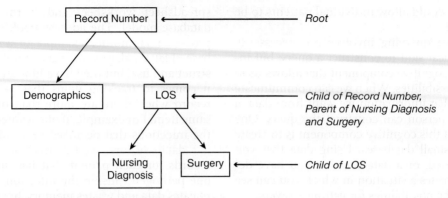

Figure 10-14 • Hierarchical database model.

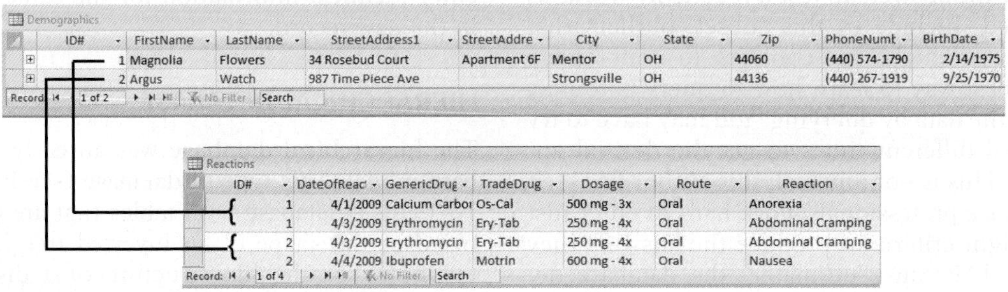

Figure 10-15 • Relational database model.

2003). The basic structure is similar to that of the hierarchical model, but the trees can share branches. If Figure 10-14 were a network database, you would see a line indicating a relationship between demographics and all the tables at lower levels. Additionally, the Demographics table would be able to connect with both the Nursing Diagnosis and Surgery table.

Relational Database Model

To review, in a relational database model there can be two or more tables that are connected by identical information in fields in each table that are called key fields. This allows the data in a record from one table to be matched to any piece or pieces of data in records in another table. How the tables are related can be clearly seen in Figure 10-15. The number 1 in the key field of "ID#" from the master, or Demographics, table is matched to the

number 1 in the records in the drug reactions table; likewise the number 2. Thus, data from the record with 1 in the key field in the demographics table is connected with the data that has the number 1 in the ID# field of the reactions table.

In Figure 10-15, the key field for the reactions table is not shown because it is automatically populated when a new record is entered. Fields that populate themselves do not need to be visible in a form view of a record. However, including one in the table design for **child tables** is an excellent idea because it preserves the ability to further develop the database. Databases have a habit of "**scope creep.**" That is, when those who want information see what they can learn from the data, they ask for more information. A good database designer will anticipate this reaction and provide for expansion in the original design (see Table 10-3).

TABLE 10-3* • *Relational Database Terms

Some Other Relational Database Terms

View	A look at the data; these vary according to the requirements of the user. Tables, forms, queries, and reports are all different views of data.
Database Management System (DBMS)	A software application that provides tools for creating a database, entering data, retrieving, manipulating, and reporting information contained within the data.
Form	A view of data that often shows only fields from one record. Very useful for data entry. Can be printed.
Query	Search function for a relational database.
Parameter query	A query that when run asks the user to specify data for a given field so that only records that match that "parameter" are returned.
Report	Often used for printing information from data in a table(s) or query, it provides data organized to fulfill user need.
Primary key	The key field in the master (parent) table.
Foreign key	A field that contains data identical to that in the master table, but is in the detail (child) table.
Validation table (lookup table)	A table that provides a list of allowable entries for a field that is linked to that field. The data in the drop-down boxes in the Google™ Advanced Search are an example.

The table in Figure 10-16 is an example of a query that matched the UTI infections table and the antibiotics table from the UTI database using the key fields. Notice that there are two entries for case number 6. This is because, although there is only one entry in the master infections table for this case, there are two entries in the antibiotic table. This query created a flat table from the two tables to provide an answer of what antibiotics the patients were taking.

In the relational model, queries can be used as a basis for a report. Queries, like reports, always produce their information on the basis of the current data in the tables, not the data that was there when they were created. It is often desired to routinely, such as monthly, have a query answer a question using specific criteria in a given field; for example, what were the medical diagnoses for a specified nursing diagnosis in January 2009. To meet this need, a query can be designed so that when run, it asks the user to specify criteria for a field, such as the month and year for the date field. These are called parameter queries. To print out monthly reports in our UTI database, we will create a parameter query that when run, asks us for the dates for which we wish information. Then we will design a report to be based on the results from only the query data – a report that will ask for desired parameters when run. In this way the same report can be used every month, but instead of showing all the data in the table, it will only show the information

qryAntibiotics

Case ID	Admitted from where	Antibiotic
1	Another Acute Care Facility	Trimpex
6	Long-Term Care Facility	Bactrim DS
6	Long-Term Care Facility	Amoxicillin

Figure 10-16 • Query from two tables.

diverse data from sources that one would not think of relating that is specifically structured for query and analysis. Developing a data warehouse involves processes that extract the data, then clean and date it. It is not a process that is done in a vacuum. It is imperative that this be done with someone who is familiar with the data. Barriers that impede the large-scale use of data mining in healthcare are the lack of integrated medical data repositories such as those that can be made possible by regional health information organizations (RHIO)[9], guidelines for the secondary use of medical data (Harrison, 2008), and differing work processes among healthcare facilities that make it difficult to maintain clean and useful data (Gillespie, 2000).

ONLINE ANALYTICAL PROCESSING

Online Analytical Processing (OLAP), or Fast Analysis of Shared Multidimensional Information (FASM), performs real-time analysis of data stored in databases. Despite the name, one does not have to be online to use it. Not nearly as powerful as data mining, it is a faster way of analyzing information. OLAP provides a multidimensional analysis of various types of data as well as the ability to do complex calculations and sophisticated data modeling ("What is OLAP?" 2008). The final result can be as simple as frequency tables, cross tabulations, or descriptive statistics, or more complex such as the removal of outliers, or other forms of data cleansing (StarSoft Inc., 2006).

STRUCTURED QUERY LANGUAGE

Structured Query Language (SQL) is the name of the coding that is used for querying in many databases. It is an ANSI (American National Standards Institute) standard computer language for retrieving and updating data in a database. It is used by Microsoft Access™ as well as with the more powerful

Oracle™ relational DBMS. Many different versions of SQL are available, but to comply with the ANSI standard they must support such major query keywords as Select, Update, Delete, Insert, Where, and others (W3 Schools, 2008).[10]

Summary

Databases are the underpinning of all healthcare information systems. Data at the atomic level are the basis for the tables that are the structure on which a database is built. There are several different database models: hierarchical, network, object oriented, flat, and relational. The databases that come in the professional version of Office software suites are a hybrid combination of the object-oriented and relational models, but they primarily use the relational model. In a relational database, the records in tables are related by a key field that is present in both tables. Getting data into a database, including a healthcare information system, is one of the most difficult tasks involved with databases. This is why a database designer should try to make it as simple as possible through the use of forms and entry selections.

Information is produced from a database by querying. Boolean and mathematical operators can be used with criteria either singly or in combination. Before trusting query outcomes, results should always be tested with a subset of data for which the answers can be visually determined. When conclusions are drawn from data, it is advisable to consider whether all the data needed for that conclusion are present in the database.

Effective databases are planned on paper before being created on the computer. The first step is to identify what outcomes the database should provide. By using that information, the data necessary to meet these needs are determined, along with the methods for manipulating and reporting those data. These

---

[9] RHIOs are discussed in Chapter 16.

[10] In Microsoft Access™ if you click View when Queries are the active object, one of your choices is SQL View. Clicking that will show you the code that is executed when you run that query.

tblMasterUTI		
Field Name	**Data Type**	**Description**
Case ID	AutoNumber	Key field used for relating tables
Admitted from where	Text	Where the patient was admitted from
On antibiotics upon admission	Yes/No	Is patient currently on antibiotics, if so, what drug and when started
Catheter on admission	Yes/No	Does the patient have an indwelling catheter on admission?
UTI present on admission	Yes/No	Results of urinalysis on admission
Date admitted	Date/Time	Date patient admitted
Date discharged	Text	Date patient discharged

Figure 10-17 •

steps are iterative; it is often necessary to make corrections or additions to a prior step as planning progresses.

A well-designed database, whether a small one such as the UTI example or a large electronic patient record system, can perform many tasks. When electronic patient records become more prevalent, we will move beyond just using patient care data in a primary way, that is, only for the care of one patient, and use it in a secondary way, or for purposes other than the primary one for which it was collected. To effectively use this data we will need the skills for effective querying. One difficulty with today's electronic patient records is the lack of identifiable, retrievable in an aggregated form, nursing data in which we can link problems, interventions, and outcomes. This puts nursing at a disadvantage in improving our practice as well as preventing nursing data from being considered in planning healthcare. As was pointed out in this chapter, if data is not in the database, it cannot be used to answer questions. Missing data leads to erroneous conclusions.

APPLICATIONS AND COMPETENCIES

1. Look at Figure 10-17. Keeping data types in mind what is wrong with this design? What problems do you think this might create?
2. Search Google using the Advanced Search tool and specify
   a. files only in English,
   b. files from the country where you live,
   c. where the terms are in the text of the page that the pages returned only be from Web sites in the ".edu" domain.
3. You are searching a Web database with Boolean Logic searching. The returns are very few and you wish to expand the search. Which Boolean term will you use? Why?
4. With what database functions will terms with the same meaning, but that are synonyms instead of identical, interfere?
5. List some clinical conditions that it would be possible to investigate by importing data from a healthcare information system. What data would you need?
6. In the database below, identify a field, field name, and record.

Patient	Unit	Pathogen
Sylvia Forest	2A	Streptococcus

7. What is a function of a key field?
8. What fields would be needed in a database that has data at the atomic level to record the five (include pain) vital signs?
9. You have a table with the fields in the table below. Reduce the fields in this table to atomic level and create a new design that would accommodate BPs taken at hours other than those in the present design.

Name	Date	8a BP	12p BP	4p BP	8p BP

10. What questions could you ask of a database with the following data? Which of the Boolean or mathematical operators would you use for the query?

First Name	Last Name	Primary Medical Diagnosis	Nursing Diagnosis

11. Plan a database to provide information for a topic of your choosing. Keep it simple!
12. Discuss the limitations of a database.
13. Evaluate the data that is collected by an information system for identifiable nursing-sensitive data.

REFERENCES

Gillespie, G. (2000). There's gold in them thar' databases. *Health Data Management, 8*(11), 40–42, 44, 46, 48–50, 52.

Harrison, J. H., Jr. (2008). Introduction to the mining of clinical data. *Clinics in Laboratory Medicine 28*(1), 1–7.

Hernandez, M. J. (2003). *Database design for mere mortals.* 2nd ed. Boston: Addison Wesley.

Lashenko, A. (n.d.). *Database models.* Retrieved November 21, 2008, from http://www.unixspace.com/context/databases.html

Safran, C., Bloomrosen, M., Hammond, W. E., Labkoff, S., Markel-Fox, S., Tang, P. C., et al. (2007). Toward a national framework for the secondary use of health data: An American medical informatics association white paper. *Journal of the American Medical Association, 14*(1), 1–9.

StarSoft Inc. (2006). *Data mining techniques.* Retrieved November 21, 2008, from http://www.statsoft.com/textbook/stdatmin.html

Two Crows Corporation. (1999). Introduction to data mining and knowledge discovery. Retrieved November 21, 2008, from http://www.twocrows.com/booklet.htm

W3 Schools. (2008). *Introduction to SQL.* Retrieved November 21, 2008, from http://www.w3schools.com/sql/sql_intro.asp

What is OLAP? Retrieved November 21, 2008, from http://www.olapreport.com/fasmi.htm

UNIT III

Information Competency

CHAPTER 11 The Internet: One Road to Health and Evidence-Based
            Practice Information
CHAPTER 12 Finding Knowledge in the Digital Library Haystack
CHAPTER 13 Mobile Computing: Finding Knowledge in the Palm
            of Your Hand

John Paul Getty once said, "In time of rapid change experience is our worst enemy." Healthcare continues to stay in the midst of rapid change. As a result, nurses have an obligation to proficiently use information and health literacy skills, as well as computer technology skills. These skills are not only important for nurses' personal growth but also for their professional growth. In clinical practice, nurses will not only need to stay current in their knowledge, but also guide patients and families in accessing quality healthcare information from the plethora of Web health sites. Information literacy is a lifelong journey that requires repeated practice to obtain proficiency. Some of the skills needed to achieve this type of literacy are critical thinking and the ability to find new, reliable information pertinent to the clinical practice; computer skills are just one small component.

Chapter 11 opens this unit with an exploration of evidence-based practice (EBP) using the untold millions of resources found on the Internet while focusing on the essential skills for discovering valid and reliable health information in the literature and on the Internet. Chapter 12 guides the user to develop the essential information search competencies necessary to discover knowledge embedded in online library resources and digital databases. Chapter 13 focuses on the use of handheld mobile devices, such as PDAs and smart phones in educational and healthcare settings.

CHAPTER 11

The Internet: One Road to Health and Evidence-Based Practice Information

Learning Objectives

After studying this chapter you will be able to:

1. *Interpret the relationships between information literacy, health literacy, and information technology skills.*

2. *Discuss the impact of healthcare consumer information literacy on patient care and education.*

3. *Identify the essential elements for validating nursing knowledge on the Internet.*

4. *Differentiate a scholarly nursing article, from an article in a magazine, newspaper, newsletter, or Web site.*

5. *Compare and contrast the quality and quantity of evidence-based nursing resources found on the Internet with those in library databases.*

6. *Discuss how to identify evidence-based practice nursing resources on the Internet.*

7. *Identify three stumbling blocks that interfere with the adoption of evidence-based resources in nursing practice.*

Key Terms

Evidence-Based Nursing
Evidence-Based Practice (EBP)
Ezine
Flesch-Kincaid Grade Level
Flesch Reading Ease
Health Literacy
Information Literacy

Information Technology Skills
Nursing Knowledge
Peer-Reviewed Article
Readability
Scholarly Nursing Journal

There was a time when scholarly health information was found only in printed journals, textbooks, and brick and mortar libraries. The nonprofessional healthcare consumers were dependent on healthcare providers for all their information needs. The advent of the Internet in the 1990s leveled the playing field so that the consumer had access to much of the same information as the healthcare professional. The caveat is that the Internet has empowered consumers to take ownership of their health but without the benefit of advanced education and training to interpret the meaning of most of the information. The brick and mortar libraries continue to be essential resources for healthcare knowledge and EBP, but now include access to the Internet as well as digital library catalogs. This chapter will focus on the essential skills for discovering valid and reliable health information on the Internet for nursing and other healthcare professionals.

According to a 2007 report from the Pew Foundation, 73% of Internet users with a disability or chronic condition have searched the Internet for information on a disease or medical problem. That percentage was up from 63% in 2006 (Fox, 2006). Of the eighty-five million Americans who searched for health information, only 15% stated that they always check for the source and date of the information (Fox, 2007). In essence, the general public is turning to the Internet for health information but most need assistance to evaluate and effectively use the information. If the general public is learning to be information literate, it behooves those of us in the healthcare profession to stay one step ahead. We must be able to guide the healthcare consumers to make decisions about the care that they receive. Healthcare providers must develop information literacy, health literacy, and information technology skills to identify valid and reliable health information on the Internet and interpret the findings to improve patient care outcomes.

Information and Health Literacy

Information literacy refers to the awareness that there is a "need to know" information, the ability to find it, analyze it for validity and relevance, and interpret it for use. **Health literacy** is a subset of information literacy. Health literacy is "the degree to which individuals have the capacity to obtain, process, and understand basic health information and services needed to make appropriate health decisions (National Forum on Information Literacy, 1989). Both information and health literacy are learned competencies that require repeated practice over time to develop expertise. According to the American Library information, literate individuals should be able to demonstrate the six competencies listed in Box 11-1 (American Library Association, 2000).

HEALTHCARE PROFESSIONAL INFORMATION AND HEALTH LITERACY

As a result of the rapid changes in healthcare developments and information technology,

---

Box 11-1 • Information Literate Competencies

The information literate individual is able to:
- Determine the extent of information needed
- Access the needed information effectively and efficiently
- Evaluate information and its sources critically
- Incorporate selected information into one's knowledge base
- Use information effectively to accomplish a specific purpose
- Understand the economic, legal, and social issues surrounding the use of information, and access and use information ethically and legally.

Source: Reproduced with permission from American Library Association, 2008.

---

information and health literacy skills are necessary for nurses and other healthcare professionals to continue lifelong learning (American Library Association, 2000; Cheek & Doskatsch, 1998). The American Association of Colleges of Nursing (AACN) recommends that nursing curricula include information seeking, sorting, and selecting; critical thinking; and information and healthcare technologies (American Association of Colleges of Nursing, 2005). As a result of these recommendations, nursing programs are beginning to focus on teaching these essential skills.

Faculty have chosen to teach literacy skills using specific learning modules in a variety of ways. Courey, Benson-Soros, Deemer, and Zeller reported findings of research done with 57 first-semester associate-degree nursing students. They reported a comparison of evaluation of students' skills at the beginning of a semester, before a one-day interactive collaborative module, and at the end of the semester. At the end of the semester, the associate-degree students expressed increased knowledge about the access of professional nursing literature; however, they also expressed a less positive attitude toward the need to stay current (Courey, Benson-Soros, Deemer, & Zeller, 2006).

Ku, Sheu, and Kuo reported a similar study conducted with 77 RN–BSN students studying women's health in Taiwan. The program was conducted over a four-month period and integrated into the course content. Their study focused on changes in the following skills: searching and screening, integrating, analyzing, applying, and presenting. With the exception of presenting skills, the researchers found a significant difference between the group that had information literacy education and the one that did not (Ku, Sheu, & Kuo, 2007).

Grant and Brettle reported a study conducted with 13 masters and PhD students studying nursing, occupational therapy, and physiotherapy in England. They used interactive Web-based tutorial delivered over a 12-week period to teach information skills as part of an EBP module. Although the study was very small, there was a significant difference between pre-training and post-training scores (Grant & Brettle, 2006).

Perhaps the associated degree first-semester students did not have enough domain knowledge about nursing to fully appreciate the need to stay current with nursing literature. The RN–BSN and graduate students would have had both domain knowledge and nursing experience to appreciate the importance of nursing information literature. Moreover, the learning content for the RN–BSN and graduate students was delivered over time, providing opportunities for skill building, feedback, and practice. The results of the studies indicate that information and health literacy skills cannot be learned by reading a book or listening to a lecture. Nursing and other healthcare professionals must have domain knowledge, clinical experience, functional understanding of search skills, and be able to analyze, integrate, and apply knowledge to practice. The skills are best learned with repeated practice using a variety of search settings over time.

Pluses for Healthcare Professional Information and Health Literacy

Synthesizing the results of a literature search is an important tool for improving the quality of patient care, as well as the first step in any research study. Research has shown that the information provided by literature searches changes clinical decisions. Literature findings provide information to justify, question, and improve patient care. Synthesis of literature leads to new knowledge, design of solutions, implementation, and evaluation methods. Knowledge from literature findings allows the nurses to empower the healthcare consumers so that they can be partners in their own care. The positive patient care outcomes from nursing and medical research support the Joint Commission requirements for access to knowledge-based information resources. Information literacy is essential for evidence-based nursing practice.

CRITICAL THINKING

Critical thinking supports information literacy. It is a difficult concept to define. It is a little like good nursing care, we know it when we see it, but defining it in objective terms is complex. Consequently, it has been defined from several different perspectives. Some say it is thinking about thinking. Others believe critical thinking is purposeful, goal directed, and that it requires the use of cognitive strategies to increase the probability of a desired outcome. Breivik (1991, p. 226) related information literacy as an initial component to the continuum of critical-thinking skills stating, "In this information age, it does not matter how well people can analyze or synthesize; if they do not start with an adequate, accurate, and up-to-date body of information, they will not come up with a good answer." Critical thinking is a tool that does not exist until it is used. It has two components: skill sets to process and generate information, and the intellectual commitment to use those skills to guide behavior. Critical thinkers approach a problem from multiple angles and in a logical manner. A vital part of critical thinking includes asking questions, knowing when one needs more information, developing and applying a plan for acquiring this information, and using the plan to generate knowledge. This plan can encompass searching for information in established databases, creating a database for the purpose of creating information and knowledge, or both. Either way, the result is directed toward improved outcomes based on information and knowledge.

KNOWLEDGE GENERATION

Integrating evidence-based literature with clinical information results in new knowledge. Knowledge generation has two parts. In terms of clinical informatics, it refers to the knowledge that is developed from converting nursing data into information and reinterpreting it. Some clinical information systems are designed with decision support systems that automate knowledge generation from clinical data. From the research perspective, knowledge generation starts with the application of the steps of information literacy – identifying, retrieving, appraising, and synthesizing nursing literature to solve nursing problems in new and better ways. Recognition of the nurse's role as a knowledge worker evolves from understanding both parts and their relationships to nursing practice. Information literacy and informatics are keys to knowledge work and generation.

KNOWLEDGE DISSEMINATION ACTIVITIES

When data is changed from information into knowledge by nurses, it maintains value only if it is also shared among the others in the profession so that it makes an impact across practice settings. Knowledge sharing allows nurses to influence not only nursing, but to drive health policy and influence interdisciplinary health practices. The computer is a tool that facilitates knowledge dissemination in multiple ways. In a broad sense, raw data can be transferred between settings to facilitate use in different ways by different nurse groups.

Once data is changed into information and interpreted, the findings can be published for dissemination across the profession. This can be accomplished by desktop software:

- Word processing to create a manuscript
- Presentation and graphics programs to develop drawings or create a presentation or poster presentation
- Spreadsheets to aggregate data and create graphs
- Databases to query, aggregate data, and create reports
- Web development software to create Web documents
- Statistical software to analyze quantitative data
- Email to collaborate and share nursing knowledge
- Wikis and blogs to interact using Web-based professional collaboration on nursing knowledge.

The maturation of professional nursing practice is dependent on the development and dissemination **of nursing knowledge.** Whether information is shared between two nurses or more widely shared across the members of the profession, information technology can speed the dissemination process.

HEALTHCARE CONSUMER INFORMATION AND HEALTH LITERACY

The information literacy level of the healthcare consumer is a significant factor for the nurse providing patient education and discharge planning for acute and chronically ill patients. Noncompliance with treatment and care regimes is often a sign of literacy problems. Noncompliance is associated with higher costs of healthcare that is particularly associated with treatment and medication errors. Patients with literacy problems are often embarrassed and hide their problems (Schloman, 2004). In addition to gaining personal information and health literacy, the nurse must be able to assess those same skills with the patient to plan and implement effective care and teaching.

In a 2003 study of health literacy of 19,000 adults, the U.S. Department of Education found that 36% of the adults had only basic or below basic literacy skills. Adults who were 65 or older had lower average literacy skills than any of the other age groups; 29% had below basic skills and 30% had basic skills. (Kutner, Greenberg, Jin, & Paulsen, 2006). To address the literacy issue and improve patient outcomes, the National Work Group on Literacy and Health recommends that patient education materials be written at no higher than a fifth-grade reading level. In addition, healthcare providers should incorporate nonwritten materials into patient education (National Work Group on Literacy and Health, 1998).

Initial patient assessments often include questions about learning styles and educational levels. One research study found that a straightforward approach for clinicians to identify those with limited or marginal health literacy skills was to simply ask how confident the patients were completing medical forms on their own (Wallace, Rogers, Roskos,

Holiday, & Weiss, 2006). Limited skills were defined as reading at sixth grade or lower and marginal skills were defined as reading at the seventh- to eighth-grade levels.

The Pfizer Clear Health Communication Initiative (Pfizer, 2006) provides a Web site at http://www.pfizerhealthliteracy.org/ with comprehensive information about the health literacy problem. The Web site includes a white paper "Eradicating Low Health Literacy: The First Public Health Movement of the 21st Century," references, a health literacy quiz, and a checklist for providers. Although Pfizer is a commercial pharmaceutical company, the Web site was developed with the purpose of improving patient outcomes. The site references the National Assessment of Adult Literacy Study, published by the National Center for Education Statistics, and the National Patient Safety Foundation, a nonprofit organization.

Box 11-2 • Tests Document Readability and Improve it

This free online software tool calculates various readability measurements like Coleman Liau index, Flesch-Kincaid Grade Level, ARI (Automated Readability Index), SMOG. Document readability is the indication of number of years of education that a person needs, to be able to understand the text easily on the first reading. Comprehensions test and skills training.

Tool is made primarily for English texts but might work also for some other languages.

It displays also complicated sentences (with many words and syllables) as suggestion what you might do to improve its readability.

Number of characters (without spaces):	589.00
Number of words:	127.00
Number of sentences:	9.00
Average number of characters per word:	4.64
Average number of words per sentence:	14.11

Indication of the number of years of formal education that a person requires to easily understand the text on the first reading.

Gunning Fox Index:	7.53

Approximate representation of the U.S. grade level needed to comprehend the text:

Coleman Liau index:	9.39
Flesch-Kincaid Grade level:	7.94
ARI:	7.47
SMOG:	7.47
Flesch Reading Ease:	63.28

List of sentences which we suggest you should consider to rewrite to improve readability of the text:

- That makes them very sensitive, and they may react strongly to things that you are allergic to or find irritating.
- In a severe asthma attack, the airways can close so much that your vital organs do not get enough oxygen.

TABLE 11-1 • *Health Information Web Site Check List*

• Source	Who is the Web site sponsor? Who is the Web site owner?
	Who is the author? Are the author's credentials noted? Is the author an expert in the subject area? Is the author qualified to write the information?
	What is the author's affiliation?
	Is there a link that will allow the user to contact the author?
• Funding	Is the site a not-for-profit site?
	Is there any commercial funding?
	Are there any potential conflicts of interest?
	Are there any advertisements on the site, if so, are they clearly labeled?
• Validity and quality	Is the date that the site was last updated clearly specified?
	Is the purpose of the Web site clearly stated?
	Is the information accurate and referenced to current scholarly nursing and medical resources?
	Is the information up-to-date?
	Is the information peer reviewed or verified by a qualified editor?
	Is the site free from content and typing errors?
	Is the information free from bias and opinion?
	Are all the links to quality reputable resources?
	Are all the links functioning?
• Privacy	Does the site include a privacy statement that is easily understood?
	Does the site meet a recognized privacy standard such as "Health on the Net" (http://www.hon.ch/)?

education programs; government sponsored and not-for-profit health and disease specialty organizations; nursing professional organizations and continuing education resources; and evidence-based nursing resources. This list is not meant to be all inclusive, but serves to provide the wide scope of resources designed to enhance nursing practice.

LAWS, RULES, AND REGULATIONS

Several sites relate to laws, rules, and regulations. The National Council of State Boards of Nursing (NCSBN) (https://www.ncsbn.org/index.htm) includes links to all U.S. state boards of nursing and also includes information about the National Council Licensure Examination (NCLEX). Each state board of nursing site includes clearly stated laws, policies, and rules and regulations. The state board of nursing Web sites also provide services for license verification and license renewal online. Other regulatory Web sites include the Joint Commission (http://www.jointcommission.org/), the Centers for Medicare and Medicaid (CMS) (http://www.cms

.hhs.gov/), and individual state departments of health and human services.

GOVERNMENT AND NOT-FOR-PROFIT HEALTH AND DISEASE SPECIALTY ORGANIZATIONS

Government sponsored and not-for-profit health and disease specialty organizations include quality information that enhances nursing knowledge. The National Institutes of Health (NIH) (http://www.nih.gov/) has links to the associated 27 specialty institutes and centers providing information to the latest research, clinical trials, and grants to promote health. The Centers for Disease Control and Prevention (CDC) (http://www.cdc.gov/) provides statistical data, information about diseases and disease control, and online disease control and prevention journals. CDC Wonder (http://wonder.cdc.gov/) provides searchable online databases with public health data, morbidity tables, and Healthy People 2010. The Agency for Healthcare Research and Quality (http://www.ahrq

.gov/) provides information on EBP, grants, research, and quality and patient safety issues.

SCHOLARLY JOURNALS AND JOURNAL ARTICLES

Although libraries provide the most comprehensive nursing and medical knowledge, some nursing and medical journals and full-text scholarly journal articles are also available on the Internet. True online journals publish all of their articles online with no print version. They feature peer-reviewed articles and maintain an archive of the articles. Some online journals are indexed in nursing bibliographic databases such as Cumulative Index to Nursing and Allied Health Literature (CINAHL) and Medline. Most feature articles in HTML format, but some use portable document format (PDF), which requires Adobe Acrobat Reader to use.

Online Journals

There are a small but growing number of free online nursing journals. The *Online Journal for Issues in Nursing* (OJIN) at http://www.nursing world.org/MainMenuCategories/ANAMarket place/ANAPeriodicals/OJIN.aspx, first published in June 1996 by Kent State University College of Nursing Faculty in conjuction with the American Nurses Association (ANA), is now sponsored by the ANA. The focus of OJIN is to provide different views on current topics relating to nursing practice, research, and education. OJIN is peer reviewed and indexed in both CINAHL and Medline. The *Online Journal of Nursing Informatics* (OJNI) at http://eaa-knowledge.com/ojni/index.htm focuses on topics relating to nursing informatics. OJNI is peer reviewed and indexed in CINAHL. *BMC Nursing,* at http://www.biomedcentral.com/bmcnurs/ is a peer-reviewed open-access journal that publishes research on topics relating to nursing research, training, practice, and education.

Open access journals have limited copyright/licensing restrictions and allow anyone with an Internet connection to download, copy, and distribute the articles. Access to full-text articles from other medical journals is available from Free Medical Journals at http://www.freemedicaljournals.com/ and BioMed Central at http://www.biomedcentral.com/browse/journals/. The MERLOT Journal of Online Learning and Teaching (JOLT) at http://jolt.merlot.org/ is a peer-reviewed journal, with articles about the scholarly use of multimedia resources in education. All BioMed Central journals and JOLT are classified as open access.

Factors Affecting Online Journals

Several factors are associated with online journals. One difficulty with online journals is the perception that the quality of their content is lower than that of print journals. Some bibliographic indexes still categorically refuse to index such journals. Part of this perception may result from the great variability in online journals; part is a belief among some academics that only print journals have peer-reviewed articles. This perception is changing as the realization that online journals can be and are peer-reviewed permeates faculty.

Writing for publication in an online journal can present a dilemma, given that most writers are members of academic faculties who need publication in recognized journals to gain promotion and tenure. Promotions are made both on the number of articles published and the reputation of the publishing journal. This makes publishing in an online journal risky for faculty who are seeking tenure. These perceptions can affect the quality of writers, and therefore the quality of the articles these writers produce.

Another difficulty with online journals is nurses' lack of awareness that the journals exist. Although nurses in all specialties need to be information literate, many are not. A person who has not learned how to use the Web is limited to print journals. In addition, search engine results don't necessarily make a distinction between a scholarly print journal with a Web presence, a true online journal, ezine, or newspaper. **Ezine** is a term for an electronic magazine; however, ezines may also

other healthcare information found on the Internet, the variation in quality is tremendous. The first step toward approaching a search for evidence-based care is to determine what you want to learn. Some of the most comprehensive Web sites are found in libraries and educational EBP centers. Clinical practice guidelines are available from government and educational Web sites in the United States, Canada, England, and Australia. Table 11-2 was designed to provide a starting point for nurses and healthcare professionals beginning to learn about EBP.

TABLE 11-2 ● Evidence-Based Practice Information on the Internet	
Evidence-Based Practice Topic	**Web Sites and URLs**

EBP/Medicine
• Definition
• History
• Recommendations
• Terminology
	Crossing the quality chasm: A new health system for the 21st century
	   http://www.iom.edu/?id=12736
	Health professions education: A bridge to quality
	   http://www.nap.edu/catalog.php?record_id=10681
	EBP (Interactive Tutorial) http://www.biomed.lib.umn.edu/learn/ebp/
	Netting the evidence http://www.shef.ac.uk/scharr/ir/netting/
	Center for Evidence-Based Medicine http://www.cebm.utoronto.ca/
	NOAH http://www.noah-health.org/en/ebm/

Evidence-Based Nursing • Definition • History • Challenges • Other Resources	Sigma Theta Tau International http://www.nursingsociety.org/default.aspx Introduction to evidence-based nursing http://medical.lib.uci.edu/ebp.html Academic Center for Evidence-Based Nursing http://www.acestar.uthscsa.edu/default.html Evidence Based Nursing http://www.hsl.unc.edu/services/tutorials/ebn/splash.htm Joanna Briggs Institute: Evidence-based nursing http://www.joannabriggs.edu.au/about/eb_nursing.php NurseScribe http://www.enursescribe.com/evidencebased.htm
Evidence-Based Care Competencies	*Health professions education: A bridge to quality* http://www.nap.edu/catalog.php?record_id=10681 Academic Center for Evidence-Based Practice http://www.acestar.uthscsa.edu/default.html

Clinical Practice Guidelines	AHRQ Clinical Practice Guidelines Online http://www.ahrq.gov/clinic/cpgonline.htm
	AHRQ National Guideline Clearinghouse http://www.guideline.gov/
	CDC: The Community Guide http://www.thecommunityguide.org/
	Nursing Best Practice Guidelines (Registered Nurses of Ontario)
	   http://www.rnao.org/Page.asp?PageID=861&SiteNodeID=133
	Canadian Medical Association: INFOBASE http://mdm.ca/cpgsnew/cpgs/index.asp
	Joanna Briggs Institute: Best Practice Information Sheets
	   http://www.joannabriggs.edu.au/pubs/best_practice.php

Research • Types of research How to read How to find How to evaluate How to use	Evidence-based nursing http://www.hsl.unc.edu/services/tutorials/ebn/splash.htm Netting the evidence http://www.shef.ac.uk/scharr/ir/netting/ What is critical appraisal? http://www.jr2.ox.ac.uk/Bandolier/painres/download/whatis/What_is_critical_appraisal.pdf Nursing research: Show me the evidence (blog) http://evidencebasednursing.blogspot.com/
Online Databases	The Cochrane Collaboration (abstracts) http://www.cochrane.org/index.htm University of Minnesota: Bio-Medical Library http://www.biomed.lib.umn.edu/help/guides/EBM Netting the Evidence http://www.shef.ac.uk/scharr/ir/netting/
Handheld Computer Evidence-Based Care Resources	National Institute of Nursing Research: Video/Audio/Podcasts http://www.ninr.nih.gov/NewsAndInformation/PodCastMultimedia/ Center for Evidence-Based Medicine http://www.cebm.utoronto.ca/ University of Minnesota: Bio-Medical Library http://www.biomed.lib.umn.edu/help/guides/EBM

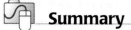
Summary

Nurses and healthcare providers have an obligation to become proficient in the use of information and health literacy skills, as well as information technology skills for several reasons. Nurses should be able to guide the patients and their families to obtain health information using the Internet. Health information on the Internet should be held to a much higher standard than any other information because inaccuracies have the potential to impact patient injury, illness, and death. Nurses must be able to assess patient and family information literacy skills, including their ability to read and understand information. To match written health teaching learning materials with the patient's health literacy skills, nurses need to be able to test written resources using readability statistics.

Information literacy is a skill that must be introduced in the undergraduate nursing program. As with all skills, it must be practiced in a variety of settings over time. Expertise in health literacy depends on the development of nursing domain knowledge, experience, information technology skills, critical thinking, and knowledge dissemination skills. Information literacy is an integral component of evidence-based nursing practice.

EBP is recommended by the Institute of Medicine and by professional nursing organizations to improve patient care outcomes. In theory, EBP is widely accepted, but practice of EBP is not universal in all education and clinical practice settings. Knowledge deficits about how to access, search, and synthesize literature findings has slowed implementation. Moreover, nurses in some clinical settings prefer to consult colleagues seen as having clinical expertise rather than analyze clinical and literature findings.

The good news is that abundant health information and EBP resources are available on the Internet. The Internet opens endless learning opportunities to nursing and healthcare providers who use analytical skills to scrutinize online resources for value.

APPLICATIONS AND COMPETENCIES

1. Discuss the differences between the relationships between information literacy, health literacy, and information technology skills. Give examples of each and describe the significance to nursing.
2. Identify the impact of healthcare consumer information literacy on patient care and education in one of your local healthcare agencies.
3. Analyze a patient education brochure using readability statistics. After completing the analysis, would you recommend continued use of the brochure for patients? Why or why not?
4. Identify a Web site with nursing knowledge and identify the essential elements for validating the knowledge.
5. Find healthcare examples for each of the following and discuss the differences:
   * online scholarly nursing article
   * article in a nursing magazine
   * newspaper
   * newsletter
   * Web site
6. Identify one EBP nursing resource you found by searching the Internet. Explain how you were able to determine the quality of the Web site.
7. Identify any stumbling blocks that interfere with the adoption of evidence-based resources in nursing practice in your clinical or healthcare agency work setting. Discuss how those stumbling blocks could be successfully addressed.

REFERENCES

American Association of Colleges of Nursing. (2005). *Position paper: Nursing education's agenda for the 21st century.* Retrieved January 4, 2008, from http://www.aacn.nche.edu/Publications/positions/nrsgedag.htm

American Library Association. (2000). *Information literacy competency standards for higher education.* Retrieved January 4, 2008, from http://www.ala.org/ala/acrl/acrlstandards/standards.pdf

Breivik, P. S. (1991). Information literacy [Electronic version]. *Bulletin of the Medical Library Association, 79,* 226–229. Retrieved January 11, 2008 from http://www.pubmedcentral.nih.gov/picrender.fcgi?artid=225527&blobtype=pdf

Cheek, J., & Doskatsch, I. (1998). Information literacy: A resource for nurses as lifelong learners. *Nurse Education Today, 18*(3), 243–250.

Committee on Information Technology Literacy, & National Research Council. (1999). *Being Fluent with Information*

Technology. Retrieved January 5, 2008, from http://www.nap.edu/html/beingfluent/

Courey, T., Benson-Soros, J., Deemer, K., & Zeller, R. A. (2006). The missing link: Information literacy and evidence-based practice as a new challenge for nurse educators. *Nurse Education Today, 27*(6), 320–323.

Fox, S. (2006). *Online Health Search 2006.* Retrieved July 21, 2007, from http://www.pewinternet.org/pdfs/ PIP_Online_Health_2006.pdf

Fox, S. (2007, October 8). *E-patients with a disability or chronic disease.* Retrieved January 4, 2008, from http://www.pewinternet.org/pdfs/EPatients_Chronic_ Conditions_2007.pdf

Grant, M. J., & Brettle, A. J. (2006). Developing and evaluating an interactive information skills tutorial. *Health Information and Libraries Journal, 23*(2), 79–86.

Greiner, A. C., & Knebel, E. (Eds.). (2003). *Health professions education: A bridge to quality.* Washington, DC National Academy Press.

Ku, Y. L., Sheu, S., & Kuo, S. M. (2007). Efficacy of integrating information literacy education into a women's health course on information literacy for RN-BSN students. *The Canadian Journal of Nursing Research, 15*(1), 67–77.

Kutner, M., Greenberg, E., Jin, Y., & Paulsen, C. (2006). *The health literacy of America's adults: Results from the 2003 National Assessment of Adult Literacy* (No. NCES 2006-483). Washington, DC: U.S. Department of Education. National Center for Education Statistics.

National Forum on Information Literacy. (1989). *Definitions, standards, and competencies related to information literacy.* Retrieved January 4, 2008, from http://www.infolit.org/definitions.html

National Work Group on Literacy and Health. (1998). Communicating with patients who have limited literacy skills: Report of the National Work Group on Literacy and Health [Electronic version]. *Journal of Family Practice, 46.* Retrieved January 5, 2008, from http://findarticles.com/p/articles/mi_m0689/is_n2_v46/ ai_20331148/pg_1

Pfizer. (2006). *What is clear health communication?* Retrieved January 5, 2008, from http://www .pfizerhealthliteracy.org/

Schloman, B. F. (2004). Health literacy: A key ingredient for managing personal health. *Online Journal of Issues In Nursing, 9*(2), 6.

Sigma Theta Tau International. (2002, December 12). *Evidence based nursing position statement.* Retrieved January 3, 2008, from http://www.nursingknowledge .org/Portal/CMSLite/GetFile.aspx?ContentID=78260

Sigma Theta Tau International. (2004). *Virginia Henderson international nursing library.* Retrieved January 6, 2008, from http://www.nursinglibrary.org/portal/Main .aspx?PageID=4002

Stevens, K. R. (2005). *ACE: Learn about EBP.* Retrieved November 19, 2008, from http://www.acestar.uthscsa .edu/Learn_model.htm

Wallace, L. S., Rogers, E. S., Roskos, S. E., Holiday, D. B., & Weiss, B. D. (2006). Brief report: Screening items to identify patients with limited health literacy skills. *Journal of General Internal Medicine, 21*(8), 874–877.

CHAPTER 12

Finding Knowledge in the Digital Library Haystack

Learning Objectives

After studying this chapter you will be able to:

1. *Compare nursing knowledge found in online library databases with that found using the Internet.*

2. *Discuss library bibliographic databases useful to nurses.*

3. *Demonstrate effective literature search strategies to support evidence-based practice.*

4. *Describe the use of personal reference management software.*

Key Terms

Advanced Search
Evidence-Based Care
Factual Database
Index
Keywords
Knowledge-Based Database
Medical Subject Headings (MeSH)

Meta-Analysis
Personal Reference Manager
Randomized Controlled Trials
Research Practice Gap
Seminal Work
Subject Heading
Systematic Review

Given the vast amount of published information, it is impossible to know everything applicable to nursing practice. According to Barnard, Nash, and O'Brien (2005, p. 505), "the amount and complexity of information nurses are expected to manage continues to increase exponentially." Library online resources provide a pivotal gateway to knowledge discovery. All nurses and healthcare providers must proactively develop and practice information search competencies to improve patient care and promote the scholarship of nursing. Without effective information search competencies, knowledge remains embedded in the digital haystack.

To assist with information searches, librarians created digital **index** guides to the literature. The index guides are produced as bibliographic databases, which can be searched electronically. Bibliographic databases have replaced print card catalogs and annual print indexes of the periodical literature. Electronic databases, not limited by paper, are generally more flexible and provide more information than print indexes. A user can retrieve information from electronic databases in the form of citations, abstracts, and in some cases, even full-text journal articles or full-text books. Many types of information and media resources are indexed in online databases.

 ## Digital Library Basics

There are two types of digital databases: knowledge based and factual. **Knowledge-based databases** index published literature. **Factual databases** replace reference books with searchable and updatable online information, for example, drug and laboratory manuals. Knowledge-based databases focus on areas such as health sciences, business, history, government, law, and ethics. Furthermore, each database is specialized by the number and type of resources (e.g., journal or book names) indexed, the span of years indexed, and the words that the database uses to describe the resources for searching purposes.

Libraries purchase electronic databases from library vendors. Library vendors market and package their databases into bundles containing two or more separate databases. Libraries, therefore, may offer different electronic resources depending on the vendor and the database bundle that the library purchased. Each bundle of databases comes with a search interface window that identifies the vendor name. A few examples of library venders that package health science databases are EBSCO, Ovid, and ProQuest. Access to databases is essential for clinical nurses and nursing students to stay current in the profession and to provide **evidence-based care.** Nurses should discuss their needs with their librarian to ensure access to the specific health science databases that allow them to improve clinical practice. Searching online bibliographic databases is a skill demanded of all healthcare professionals. An index system used to file or catalog references provides the mechanism for library searches. Electronic databases are indexed, or searchable, by many different attributes such as title, author name, and year. Given that, unlike print catalogs, only one entry

for a source is needed; there are many other ways to search an online bibliographic database. **Keywords** are used, and searchers may designate if this word or words should be searched for in a title, abstract, often even the text, or all of these. Searchers can also limit searches to finding sources by language, by age of subjects of a research article, by type of article, and by years of publication, and in some databases to finding only those sources that provide full text. There may be times when it is helpful to search more than one database at a time; this is called a federated search.

Most library vendor search windows allow users to select a citation format and to save the search results. If there is an option for saving with a specific citation format, there will be a drop-down menu with the common formats such as American Psychological Association (APA), Modern Languages Association (MLA), and American Medical Association (AMA). Search findings can be printed, emailed, and saved as a file onto the personal computer (PC).

 ## Personal Reference Managers

Library database search findings can often be exported into a personal reference manager. A **personal reference manager** refers to database software that allows the user to create a personal collection of citations. Most library database interfaces include an export feature that allows the user to download citation information into a commercial personal reference manager. There are a number of commercial products available, for example, EndNote®, ProCite®, Reference Manager®, and RefWorks. The citation information saved in commercial software can include hyperlinks to the associated resources on the PC, such as digital versions of articles, Web sites, or graphics.

Personal reference managers that include the import/export feature provide an efficient means of managing citation information. However, reference managers integrated into word processing software may not have the import/export feature. For example, Microsoft® Word 2007 and OpenOffice.org Writer 2.3X both include reference manager features; however, each citation must be keyed in separately.

Personal reference managers are also available free online. Zotero at http://www.zotero .org/ is a very powerful open source personal reference manager. Once downloaded it is an extension in the Firefox 2.0 Web browser (Zotero, 2008). Zotero allows the user to save citation information from most library bibliographic databases and certain Web sites, such as Amazon.com and the New York Times. Other features include note taking, the ability to hyperlink to files and images, and automatically capture screenshots of Web pages. Zotero personal libraries can be imported into EndNote and RefWorks. Zotero works with Microsoft Word 2007 as a plug-in so that users can cite and create reference lists in a Word document. Once the plug-in is installed, Zotero will be visible from the Add-In tab in the Ribbon menu. Zotero is also compatible with OpenOffice after downloading and installing the OpenOffice extensions. Zotero also works with Google docs. Figure 12-1 shows a screen shot of Zotero.

CiteULike at http://www.CiteULike.org/ is a free online personal reference manager service that allows users to store, organize, and share citation information (CiteULike, n.d.). Users must register for an account with a login and password. Building an online library of personal citations is fairly easy. All you have to do is to enter the hyperlink of the reference. You can import and export references from CiteULike to proprietary software.

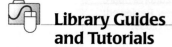 **Library Guides and Tutorials**

Even the most experienced library patrons can benefit from library guides and tutorials because the technology development for library resources continues to change rapidly. Lifelong learning for professional nursing must begin with demonstrated competencies in use of digital library searches to discover new nursing knowledge. Nursing knowledge,

including evidence-based practice (EBP) findings, should be quickly integrated into clinical practice to improve patient outcomes. Fortunately, there are numerous library guides and tutorials available on the Internet. The most efficient way to develop/improve library competencies is with the assistance of a librarian. Qualified librarians have a master's or doctoral degree and have specialized in an area of library science. The focus of their expertise and continuing education is to assist users in accessing and utilizing library resources.

Just-in-time learning using online library guides and tutorials is also an efficient way to develop/improve library information competencies. The guides and tutorials address how to use the specific library facility, how to search using **medical subject headings (MeSH)**, how to use a vendor search interface, and how to use a specific database. To learn how to use a library facility, use the Internet to find the library's homepage. Information on a library Web page generally includes the hours of operation, links to services and departments, information on how to find books and journals, and links to help resources such as guides and tutorials.

SUBJECT HEADINGS

Subject headings refer to standardized terms used to index or catalog reference materials. Each library chooses a standard subject authority of thesaurus for all of its cataloging. Libraries using the National Library of Medicine classification use the MeSH.

SEARCHING USING MESH TERMS

Each library database also uses a "controlled vocabulary" of terms (subject headings) to index the materials so that the database can be searched. MeSH refers to the controlled vocabulary of terms used to index materials in PubMed and MEDLINE databases. Cumulative Index to Nursing and Allied Health Literature (CINAHL) subject headings follow the MeSH structure (CINAHL, 2006). Since CINAHL and MEDLINE are two primary databases with nursing literature it is important to understand the

---

Box 12-2 • Examples of Stop Words

After	Be	Like	Said	Through
Also	Do	Make	Should	To
An	Each	Many	So	Use
And	For	More	Some	Was

Some vendor search engines, such as EBSCOhost, Ovid, or ProQuest, allow the user to restrict online searches to peer-reviewed articles in scholarly journals, articles with references, articles with abstracts, research articles, or full-text articles. Peer-reviewed articles are excellent resources to support nursing knowledge. A journal is a scholarly publication that provides peer-reviewed articles.[2] In contrast, articles in magazines, newsletters, and newspapers should serve as points of information and entertainment, but never be used to support nursing knowledge.

Bibliographic Databases Pertinent to Nursing

There are numerous databases with information that is pertinent to nursing. Essential ones with a focus on nursing and health-related topics are CINAHL, MEDLINE/PubMed, Cochrane Library, and PsycINFO. Although there may be some overlap in the journals and resources these databases index, there are important differences that may affect the search outcome. Furthermore, there are variations for each of the databases for each library system; some include only citations and abstracts and others contain varying numbers of full-text documents. Unless you are an experienced researcher, consult with a reference librarian to assist with refining your search question and selecting the best databases to search. See Table 12-2 for a list of databases according to nursing topic. The databases discussed in this

table are commonly available through most medical and academic libraries.

USING A SPECIFIC LIBRARY DATABASE

Most vendor search interfaces and online libraries provide links to guides and tutorials for specific databases within the collection. Unfortunately, at the present time there is no universal standard for indexing health science search terms; each library database is unique. Unless you have expertise in using a particular library database, it is critical that you review a guide and tutorials first. The nuances in the search terminology and methods can be very tricky, especially for novice student nurses who are in the process of learning terminology. Table 12-3 provides the location of the tutorials for many of the bibliographic indexes that nurses need.

CINAHL

When researching a nursing topic, the CINAHL database is an excellent place to start. This database includes citations and abstracts for more than 500 nursing journals and 400 allied health journals dating back to 1982 (CINAHL, 2006). CINAHL Plus with Full-Text database includes full-text articles in addition to citations and abstracts. The subject headings use the National Library of Medicine MeSH structure. To identify search terms, click *CINAHL Headings* in the Menu bar and enter the word or phrase you are searching to get a list of the associated subject headings. CINAHL may also include selected full-text documents such as nursing journal articles, evidence-based care sheets, book chapters, newsletters, standards of practice, and nurse practice acts.

---

[2] See Chapter 11 for more information on the peer-reviewed process.

TABLE 12-2 ● *Discovering Nursing Knowledge in Library Databases*

Topic of Search Question	Examples of Databases to Search	Topic of Search Question	Examples of Databases to Search

Nursing	CINAHL
	Cochrane Library
	ProQuest Nursing and
	  Allied Health Source
	PubMed/MEDLINE
		Patient teaching	MedlinePlus
			HealthSource:
			  Consumer Edition
			Consumer Health Complete
			Micromedex CareNotes™

Biomedical research	PubMed/MEDLINE EMBASE CINAHL		CINAHL
		Psychosocial	PsycINFO PsycARTICLES
Education	ERIC CINAHL		Sociological Abstracts Sociological Collection
Legal/ethical	LexisNexis Academic CINAHL PubMed/MEDLINE		Cambridge Scientific Abstracts CINAHL
Management	ABI/Inform CINAHL		
Oncology	PubMed/MEDLINE National Cancer Institute & PDQ CINAHL		

MEDLINE

When researching a biomedical research topic that crosses healthcare disciplines, use MEDLINE in addition to CINAHL. MEDLINE, a service made available through the National Library of Medicine (NLM), is unique from proprietary library databases because it is also a free service that is accessible on the Internet through PubMed. The NLM is the largest medical library in the world. MEDLINE provides access to over 5,000 journals worldwide and includes a comprehensive collection of citations from biomedical articles dating back to the 1950s. You can access MEDLINE through PubMed on the Internet at http://www.ncbi.nlm.nih.gov/PubMed/ PubMed includes citations to literature not yet included in MEDLINE in addition to other services. PubMed Central allows access to free full-text articles (National Institutes of Health, 2007).

PubMed provides a variety of free services. NLM Mobile at http://www.nlm.nih.gov/mobile/ provides software applications for

TABLE 12-3 ● *Online Help for Specific Library Databases*

Online Help for Specific Library Databases	URL
CINAHL	http://support.ebsco.com/training/flash_videos/CINAHLBasicSearching.html
Cochrane Library	http://www3.interscience.wiley.com/aboutus/demo/
PsycInfo	http://scientific.thomson.com/tutorials/psycinfo2/
PubMed/MEDLINE	http://www.nlm.nih.gov/bsd/disted/pubmedtutorial/ http://www.nlm.nih.gov/bsd/viewlet/search/subject/subject.html (MeSH) http://www.ncbi.nlm.nih.gov/sites/entrez?db=mesh

Palm™ and Pocket PC handheld computers.[3] PubMed for Handhelds at http://pubmedhh .nlm.nih.gov/nlm/ is a Web site designed specifically for use with handheld computers. My NCBI at http://www.ncbi.nlm.nih.gov/ entrez/cubby.fcgi? provides the ability to save user information and preferences and store searches, and automatically emails search information (National Library of Medicine, 2007) on designated topics to users after they register and receive a login and password.

COCHRANE LIBRARY

The Institute of Medicine (IOM) (2001, p. 145) challenged us in 2001 to implement "systematic approaches to analyzing and synthesizing medical evidence for both clinicians and patients." The Cochrane Collaboration, founded in 1993 by Dr. Archie Cochrane, was recognized by the IOM as a model for synthesizing evidence to inform healthcare decision making. The Cochrane Library, available through Wiley InterScience, is considered a gold standard for meta-analysis of medical research. Access to the library may be through the library digital database listing or by using a login and password provided by your local library. The Cochrane Library is online at http://www3.interscience.wiley.com/cgi-bin/ mrwhome/106568753/HOME? The Cochrane library is available free in many countries. For example, it is available free for residents of the state of Wyoming in the United States.

Cochrane reports are useful to nursing students, practicing nurses, and nurse researchers. Nursing students and practicing nurses may not have the confidence and experience to analyze research without assistance of faculty or nurse researchers. The Cochrane Library provides access to systematic reviews of the best research evidence. A systematic review is designed to reduce three types of bias inherent in individual research studies: selection, indexing, and publication (South African Cochrane Centre, 2007). Selection bias is based on a per-

son's point of view. Indexing bias is caused by limited searches to limited databases or search terms. Publishing bias results when searches are limited to certain publications or languages. The process of systematic reviews is known as meta-analysis, which means that the results of multiple, similar research studies are carefully reviewed and analyzed.

PYSCINFO

Because nursing is a holistic profession, some questions are best answered with information from searches of psychosocial databases, such as PsycINFO and PsycArticles. PsycINFO, a service of the APA, provides citations and abstracts for psychology and psychosocial aspects of other disciplines dating back to the 19th century (American Psychological Association, n.d.). PsycArticles provides access to full-text articles.

 ## Embarking on the Quest for Knowledge

The quest for knowledge is a five-step process. The process is cyclical and iterative rather than linear. In other words, the researcher may go back and forth through the steps. The process really never stops because new knowledge is continually being generated.

QUESTIONING PRACTICE: RECOGNIZING AN INFORMATION NEED

The first step in the quest for knowledge is recognizing an information need. Questioning practice may be difficult, but Medicare nonpayment for higher costs of care resulting from preventable hospital-acquired injuries such as patient falls and infections from medical errors has been a wake-up call for healthcare (Centers for Medicare & Medicaid Services, 2007). Healthcare practices must change to make patients safe, and nurses must be involved in searches for solutions to improve care practices.

As an example of a quest for knowledge, consider conducting a literature search for

---

[3] See Chapter 13 for more information on handheld computers.

information on *prevention of patient falls.* The search question is "How can patient falls be prevented in nursing?" Notice that the broad topic, *patient falls,* is narrowed using the terms *prevention* and *nursing.* A common search mistake is that the search topic is too broad. Take a few moments to write out the search question to focus on the topic. Although it is best to carefully define the information need before beginning the search, it is possible to allow the search engine to assist by allowing you to choose terms from a list of search terms.

SEARCHING FOR APPROPRIATE EVIDENCE

The literature search process is an essential skill that nursing professionals must learn and practice. It is a vital step in discovering nursing knowledge and developing EBP. The quest for new nursing knowledge involves discovering, understanding, analyzing, and applying findings from literature. The process for conducting a literature search must be systematic and comprehensive (Conn et al., 2003). Subject headings are used to develop search strategies that will lead you to the most useful information on your search question. Although ideas for changes in clinical practice may come from regular reading of the literature, it is still necessary to search for more information to determine whether the information in the original article is supported by other articles and warrants a change in clinical practices.

While searching, first determine the library databases that are most appropriate for the evidence for which you are searching and then identify the search terms that match that database. Selecting the most appropriate database(s) is just as important as the search strategy. If you are looking for peer-reviewed scholarly literature, use the online databases for libraries serving populations engaged in healthcare and education, and search databases and indexes such as CINAHL, MEDLINE, Cochrane Library, and ERIC. If you are looking for patient teaching resources, use the online library databases and the Internet, especially MedlinePlus (http://www.nlm.nih.gov/medlineplus/), an NLM resource, which is designed for consumers. It is important to remember that a comprehensive search must never be limited to the Internet or online library full-text resources. Although a wide range of information resources may be found online, libraries, librarians, and bookstores are vital to help borrow or purchase the knowledge-based resources needed for nursing education and practice. If a search finds resources that your library does not have, it is often possible to obtain these from interlibrary loan.

For the *patient fall* example, we used the CINAHL Plus with Full-Text database and EBSCO search interface window. After opening the database, the Advanced Search tab was selected (see Figure 12-2).[4] The phrase **advanced search** is misleading because the search tools really allow users to clearly define

---

[4] See your librarian if you need help gaining access to the database.

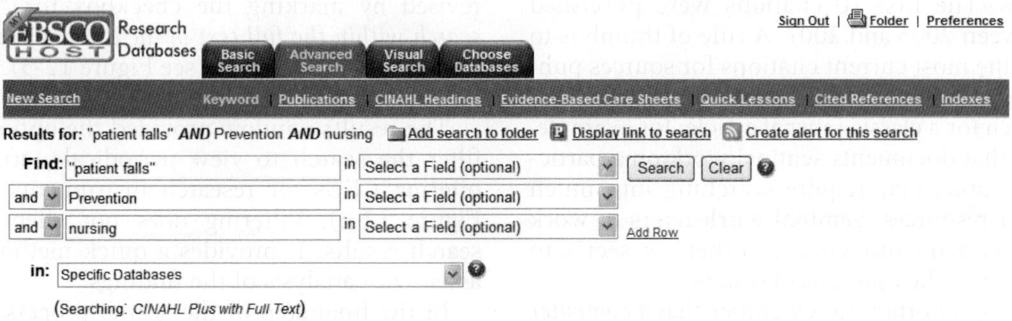

Figure 12-2 • Advanced search – selecting search terms.

Narrow Results by Subject

Accidental Falls

Inpatients

Aged

Patient Safety

Risk Assessment

Middle Age

Female

Male

Risk Factors

Nursing Assessment

Figure 12-3 • Narrowing the search.

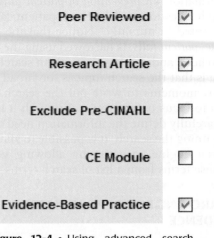

Figure 12-4 • Using advanced search checkboxes.

the search. The Subject Terms checkbox (if it is available) or CINAHL Headings can be used for assistance with search terms. In this example, patient falls was entered with double quotes to find only "patient falls" as a phrase. A goal for an effective search is a return of about 50 results.

The search was run in early 2008. There were 52 results; the most recent article was published in 2007. Using the option of further narrowing the search by clicking *Risk Assessment* in the "Narrow Results by Subject" (see Figure 12-3) window produced 18 citations. The first 10 citations were published between 2003 and 2007. A rule of thumb is to use the most current citations for sources published within the past three to five years. A search for a classic journal article, for example, one that documents seminal work on a particular topic, may require searching into much older resources. **Seminal work** refers to work that is frequently cited by others or seems to influence the opinions of others.

It is important to remember that a *computer* determined the results of the search on the basis of search terms. Although critical thinking is required for each step in the search process, it is especially important to analyze the information from the search results to make sure that it provides the appropriate evidence to answer the information need. Is the purpose of the search to advance nursing knowledge, advance EBP, or both? In order to set further limits on the search, the checkboxes for peer-reviewed, research article, and evidence-based practice in the Advanced Search menu were marked (see Figure 12-4).

In the fall prevention example, the initial search used keywords. After the citations and other information from the initial search were reviewed, it was determined that the search should be expanded using the same search terms in the full text of the articles. The search was revised by marking the checkbox for *"Also search within the full text of the articles"* in the Advanced Search menu (see Figure 12-5). The new search resulted in 34 citations.

The results window provided the option to filter the search to view periodicals, articles offering CEUs, or research instruments (see Figure 12-6). Filtering does not affect the search results. It provides a quick method to assist with analysis of the findings.

In the final step of the search process, the citation information is saved or downloaded

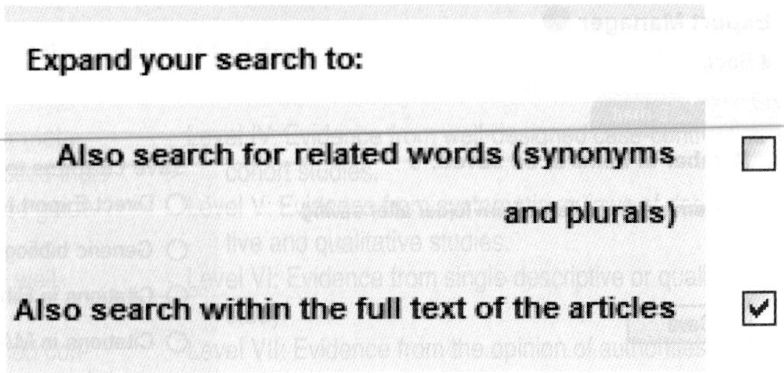

Expand your search to:

Also search for related words (synonyms and plurals) ☐

Also search within the full text of the articles ☑

Figure 12-5 • Further modifying the search.

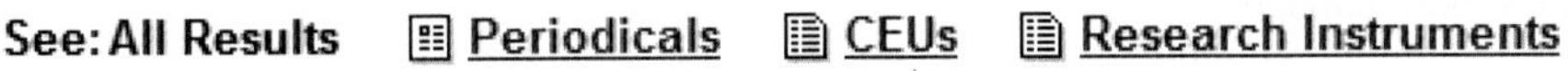

See: All Results   📄 Periodicals   📄 CEUs   📄 Research Instruments

Figure 12-6 • Filtering the search.

for use in the analysis and summary of the literature search. The EBSCO search window allows the user to save results of searches to a search folder. Once the search is completed, the search folder should be clicked for options (see Figure 12-7). When the search folder is opened, the user can print, email, save, and/or export the selected citations from the results of the search (see Figure 12-8).

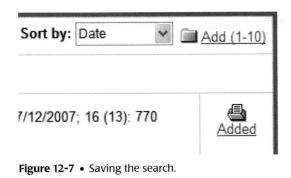

📂 Folder has items.

Sort by: Date ▾   📁 Add (1-10)

7/12/2007; 16 (13): 770   📄 Added

Figure 12-7 • Saving the search.

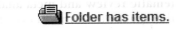

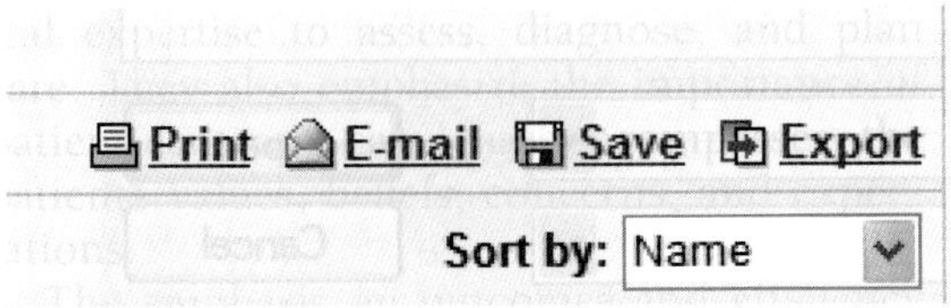

📄 Print 📧 E-mail 💾 Save 📤 Export

Sort by: Name ▾

Figure 12-8 • Saving options.

Personal Reference Manager Software

The Export Manager in EBSCO can be used to format the search findings for export into a commercial product personal reference manager (e.g., EndNote, ProCite, or Reference Manager) by clicking the Save tab.[5] For the patient fall example discussed in the preceding text, clicking the Save tab prompted the file format export option. The radio button next to "Direct Export to EndNote, ProCite, or Reference Manager" was checked so that the file could be exported into EndNote (see Figure 12-9). After the EndNote "HIS-Converted library" was selected from the browse menu on the PC, all the citation information was downloaded instantaneously from the library database (see Figure 12-10).

CRITICAL ANALYSIS OF THE LITERATURE FINDINGS

Critical analysis of the literature findings is the point in the process where new knowledge is discovered. The first step is to select citations for articles that are possibly relevant to the information need and then obtain a full-text version of the articles. Review of the article abstract,

[5] If using the Zotero extension in the FireFox Web browser, clicking the folder icon to the right of the URL will prompt the user to select citations for download in the Zotero personal reference manager.

skills. Findings from nursing research suggest that challenges to wide adoption of EBP in nursing persist. The problem is complex, ranging from access to knowledge resources, attitudes toward research, and information literacy knowledge and skills (Pravikoff, Tanner, & Pierce, 2005). Other barriers to evidence-based nursing include lack of time, lack of sufficient staff, and difficulties in interpreting statistics and research writings (Hannes et al., 2007; Thompson, McCaughan, Cullum, Sheldon, & Raynor, 2005).

Access to resources is a challenge. Joint Commission requires facilities to have knowledge resources available in the healthcare facility; however, access to digital libraries resources is not universally available 24 hours a day, 7 days a week. Recommendations from the IOM and professional nursing organizations are unified in the definition of EBP as being the best evidence currently available, yet there is no universal recommendation about what constitutes resources (e.g., library databases) of best practice. As a result, the available library resources for nursing programs and healthcare providers vary. Access to information and knowledge resources is improving, but is not yet universal for all nursing programs and clinical settings (Penz & Bassendowski, 2006). The Cochrane Library is recognized as the gold standard for systematic reviews and meta-analysis research findings, but Wyoming is the only state in the United States that has free access to it.

The culture of clinical practice settings may not support or value information-seeking practices and current research (Mohide & King, 2003). Culture of clinical practice refers to situations in which management, physicians, and other nurses do not value or support information seeking and research. Another challenge to the adoption of EBP is that nurses prefer to obtain their information from another colleague, especially if they see that person as a nursing expert (Penz & Bassendowski, 2006). Often in the fast pace of providing healthcare, nurses prefer to ask another nurse whose opinion they value rather than search for answers themselves.

Nursing research on the challenges for adoption of evidence-based care reveals the complexity of the problem. A 2006 quantitative survey of 568 nurses (Sigma Theta Tau International, 2006) revealed unsettling results. Twenty-four percent of the nurses reported a low familiarity with EBP. The majority (66%) stated that the primary challenge for finding and using EBP is time to search and analyze findings. Almost half (45%) of the nurses indicated that finding and using EBP was difficult because they have difficulty interpreting and analyzing the findings because of the way they are written.

A recent study by Pravikoff et al. (2005) revealed 10 personal barriers to the adoption of EBP; the most significant was the lack of value in clinical settings for research. The other nine barriers related to access of research resources, lack of research skills, lack of information literacy skills, and lack of information technology competencies. The study revealed six different institutional barriers; the primary one was the presence of goals with a higher priority. Other organizational barriers related to staffing issues, budget, organizational perceptions about nurses preparation for EBP, and organizational perceptions about the unrealistic use of research.

A qualitative research study done in Belgium indicates that the barriers to evidence-based nursing may be universal (Hannes et al., 2007). The study revealed characteristics related to five themes: doctors, patients, families, management, and supervisors. There were two subthemes for nurses' discomfort: 1) Nurses did not feel comfortable questioning doctor's opinions and 2) they were uncomfortable making suggestions that conflicted with the wishes and preferences of patients and families. Nurses who were concerned with quality of care found themselves at odds with management/supervisors that were perceived to be more concerned with reducing costs. The finding, lack of knowledge and skills, was very similar to that of the research reported by SSTI and Pravikoff.

Summary

The two types of library databases – knowledge based and factual – provide an essential gateway to knowledge discovery. Information search competencies and the use of a personal bibliographic reference manager are essential skills for all nurses who use online library databases to extract nursing knowledge. Effective use of online library databases provides unlimited opportunities to discover knowledge that will improve patient care.

The CINAHL, PubMed/MEDLINE, Cochrane Library, and PsycINFO databases are just a few knowledge-based databases vital to nursing knowledge discovery. The process of searching for knowledge is a skill that is learned only with repeated practice. The process is cyclical and iterative, but not linear. There are five steps in this process: 1) defining a search topic based on an information need, 2) searching for evidence embedded in the literature, 3) critically analyzing and summarizing the literature, 4) implementing the findings into practice, and 5) evaluating the results of implementation by asking additional questions or discovering new questions.

Improving patient care and reducing healthcare errors require that nursing and hospital administrators, clinicians, educators, and nursing students adopt a culture of care that uses evidence-informed nursing practice. To this end, nurses must be proactive in breaking down the challenges and barriers to adopting EBP. It also requires that nurses self-assess their knowledge needs in locating and evaluating research and identify strategies for gaining the skills needed for competency in this area. Additionally, administrators must see that clinicians have the necessary time, training, support, and access to knowledge resources needed for EBP.

APPLICATIONS AND COMPETENCIES

1. Indexing an article:
   a. Find a peer-reviewed nursing journal article, either online or in your library or personal collection.
   b. Create an electronic document using word processing software or spreadsheet software. (Use a piece of paper if a computer is not available.) At the top of the document note the author name, date, article title, journal title, and source. Create a four-column table using the following column headings: My Subject Terms, CINAHL Subject Terms, MEDLINE Subject Terms, and Cochrane Library Subject Terms.
   c. Read the article and write the subject terms you think it includes in the first column.
   d. Do an author/title search in each of the three databases and note the subject terms in the corresponding columns.
   e. Discuss your analysis of similarities and differences of subject terms for the three databases.
2. Finding databases:
   a. Look for five databases that are pertinent to nursing knowledge in your library and health system Web sites.
   b. Create an electronic document using either word processing or spreadsheet software.
   c. Develop a five-column table using the following column headings: Library Databases, Bibliographic Database, Bibliographic with Full-Text Database, Factual Database, and How Information can Support EBP.
   d. Complete the matrix noting the database name, type(s), and EBP implications.
   e. Discuss your findings.
3. Searching a Database:
   a. Choose a search topic related to a current patient care question.
   b. Plan a search strategy for CINAHL, MEDLINE, and one of the other databases described in this chapter. Note the subject headings on a worksheet similar to the one used in the first exercise.
   c. Execute the search in each of these databases.
   d. Compare and contrast your results.
4. Searching for EBP:
   a. Identify a nursing outcome that needs improvement in your health system.
   b. Plan search strategies to identify relevant translation literature, evidence summaries, and original research.
   c. Execute these searches and evaluate results.
   d. Discuss how the cited publications might help you prepare a clinical guideline to facilitate needed changes in practice.

5. Searching for bibliographic management software:

a. Conduct an online search for bibliographic management software.

b. Read recent articles and reviews discussing bibliographic management software, both online and in journal articles that you retrieve through searching.

c. Investigate the availability of online tutorials and support for specific products.

d. Based on your research, designate a bibliographic management software package that best meets your needs and discuss the rationale for the choice.

REFERENCES

American Psychological Association. (n.d.). *PsycINFO.* Retrieved October 1, 2007, from http://www.apa.org/psycinfo/

Barnard, A., Nash, R., & O'Brien, M. (2005). Information literacy: Developing lifelong skills through nursing education. *Journal of Nursing Education, 44*(11), 505–510.

Centers for Medicare & Medicaid Services. (2008, November 21). *Hospital-acquired conditions.* Retrieved November 22, 2008, from http://www.cms.hhs.gov/hospitalacqcond/

CINAHL. (2006, January 19). *CINAHL databases.* Retrieved November 22, 2008, from http://www.ebscohost.com/cinahl/

CiteULike. (n.d.). *A free online service to organise your academic papers.* Retrieved January 31, 2008, from http://www.citeulike.org/

Conn, V. S., Isaramalai, S., Rath, S., Jantarakupt, P., Wadhawan, R., & Dash, Y. (2003). Beyond MEDLINE for literature searches. *Journal of Nursing Scholarship, 35*(2), 177–182.

Dobbins, M. (2007). Journey to evidence-informed nursing practice: Understanding the process as an iterative loop [Electronic version]. *Reflections on Nursing Leadership, 33*(2). Retrieved January 9, 2008 from http://www2.nursingsociety.org/RNL/2Q_2007/columns/dobbins.html

Hannes, K., Vandersmissen, J., De Blaeser, L., Peeters, G., Goedhuys, J., & Aertgeerts, B. (2007). Barriers to evidence-based nursing: A focus group study. *The Australian Journal of Advanced Nursing, 60*(2), 162–171.

Institute of Medicine, & National Academy of Sciences. (2001). *Crossing the quality chasm: A new health system for the 21st century.* Washington, DC: National Academies Press.

Melnyk, B. M., & Fineout-Overholt, E. (2005). *Evidence-based practice in nursing & healthcare: A guide to best practice.* Philadelphia, PA: Lippincott Williams & Wilkins.

Mohide, E. A., & King, B. (2003). Building a foundation for evidence-based practice: Experiences in a tertiary hospital. *Evidence-Based Nursing, 6*(4), 100–103.

National Institutes of Health. (2007, April 16). *PubMed Central (PMC).* Retrieved October 2, 2007, from http://www.pubmedcentral.nih.gov/

National Library of Medicine. (2007, September 19). *PubMed overview.* Retrieved October 2, 2007, from http://www.ncbi.nlm.nih.gov/entrez/query/static/overview.html

Penz, K. L., & Bassendowski, S. L. (2006). Evidence-based nursing in clinical practice: Implications for nurse educators. *Journal of Continuing Education in Nursing, 37*(6), 251–254; quiz 255–256, 269.

Pravikoff, D. S., Tanner, A. B., & Pierce, S. T. (2005). Readiness of U.S. nurses for evidence-based practice. *American Journal of Nursing, 105*(9), 40–51; quiz 52.

Sackett, D. L., Rosenberg, W. M. C., Gray, J. A. M., Haynes, R. B., & Richardson, W. S. (1996). Evidence-based medicine: What it is and what it isn't [Electronic version]. *British Medical Journal, 312,* 71–72. Retrieved January 13, 1996, from http://pkuebm.bjmu.cn/files/EBM%20what%20it%20is%20and%20what%20it%20is%20not.pdf

Sigma Theta Tau International. (2006). *2006 EBP study: Summary of findings.* Retrieved January 3, 2008, from http://www.nursingknowledge.org/Portal/CMSLite/GetFile.aspx?ContentID=78260

South African Cochrane Centre. (2007, January 29). *What is a systematic review?* Retrieved January 20, 2008, from http://www.mrc.ac.za/cochrane/systematic.htm

Thompson, C., McCaughan, D., Cullum, N., Sheldon, T., & Raynor, P. (2005). Barriers to evidence-based practice in primary care nursing – Viewing decision-making as context is helpful. *Journal of Advanced Nursing, 52*(4), 432–444.

Valente, S. M. (2003). Research dissemination and utilization improving care at the bedside. *Journal of Nursing Care Quality, 18*(2), 114–121.

Zotero. (2008, January 25). *Quick start guide [Zotero Documentation].* Retrieved January 31, 2008, from http://www.zotero.org/documentation/quick_start_guide

CHAPTER

13

Mobile Computing: Finding Knowledge in the Palm of Your Hand

Learning Objectives

After studying this chapter you will be able to:

1. *Discuss the uses of handheld computers in healthcare.*

2. *Describe the strengths and weaknesses of personal digital assistants (PDAs) and smartphones.*

3. *Discuss data security issues associated with the use of handheld computers.*

4. *Identify handheld software appropriate for nurses to use in the clinical setting.*

5. *Identify handheld software appropriate for students to use in the learning setting.*

Key Terms

Beaming	Piconet
Bluetooth	PIM
Cell Phone	QWERTY Keyboard
e-Book	RAM
Flash Memory	ROM
Handheld Computer	Smartphone
Hotspot	Synchronization
PDA	WiFi

The development of wireless technology has radically changed the way we do business worldwide. Communication devices are no longer tethered to a cord in the wall. Batteries supplement electricity requirements. As a result, nurses and other healthcare providers can use mobile devices such as the personal digital assistant (**PDA**) and smartphone at the point of need. Most PDAs come with an assortment of personal information management (**PIM**) software, such as contact information, a calendar, and a clock. The large storage capacities of mobile devices allow for storage of electronic books (**e-books**) reference material, graphics, videos, and other data files. Connectivity using synchronization software, beaming, Bluetooth, **WiFi** (wireless fidelity), and cellular phone lines allows for transfer of information from mobile devices to personal computers (PCs) or health information clinical systems. The possibilities for effective use of handheld mobile computing in education and healthcare are endless.

PDA and Smartphone Basics

The **PDA** is a small handheld computer. All PDAs use an operating system (OS), and most allow the use of third-party software applications. The **cell phone** is a shortwave wireless communication device that has a connection to a transmitter. The word "cell" refers to the area of transmission. Cell phones, like landline phones, require a paid subscription to the transmission service provider. **Smartphones** are a combination of a PDA and a cell phone. This chapter will focus on handheld mobile devices, such as PDAs and smartphones. The common term "**handheld computer**" is used in this chapter to refer to all handheld mobile devices. The information will include differences in features for each device, as well as examples of the use of these devices in educational and healthcare settings.

History of PDAs and Smartphones

The PDA concept was developed in the early 1980s with the Psion (Medindia, 2007). The first PDAs were designed primarily as personal information managers (PIMs) that included electronic telephone books and appointment calendars. The Newton MessagePad, developed by Apple in 1983, was the first popular PDA that featured a touch screen and handwriting capabilities. However, the Palm Pilot, introduced by U.S. Robotics in 1996, was light, fit in the palm of the user's hand, and featured Graffiti handwriting recognition software. It also had much better handwriting recognition than the Newton. As a result, it quickly dominated the market by 1999. Apple discontinued production of the Newton in 1998. The Pocket PC, introduced by Microsoft in 2000 (HPC: Factor, 2007), offered a compact version of the Windows OS. It gave users the privilege of having more than one application open at the same time. They could also view or edit Microsoft Office documents. The Pocket PC is

growing in popularity with users, capturing the market with 54.2% of the OS shipments in the second quarter of 2006 (Cellular-News, 2006).

The first smartphone, known as "Simon," was introduced by IBM in 1993. The smartphones combined features of the cellular telephone and PIM software. In 1999 (3Com Public Relations, 1999), Palm released the QUALCOMM pdQ, which featured a cell phone and the Palm organizer. The smartphone of today is a miniature computer that includes multiple software programs, documents, music, video, Internet access capability, and a telephone. Smartphones fall into two categories: they are primarily either a cell phone with computer application features or a PDA that can also be used as a phone. The phones of today provide Internet access using cellular phone connections, or WiFi, or both. All smartphones require a subscription to a cellular phone provider. They are popular with users who do not want to carry a PDA and phone as separate devices. They are growing in popularity because cellular providers offer them at substantially discounted rates over stand-alone PDAs with the same features. A variety of PDAs and smartphones are available through manufacturers including Palm®, Hewlett-Packard Company, Research in Motion Limited, and Apple® (see Figure 13-1).

The iPod®, a PDA introduced by Apple in 2001, dominated the music player market with more than 100 million devices sold in less than six years (Thompson, 2007). The iPod® uses Apple iTunes software to transfer music, video, or other applications quickly to the device. In a short time since the iPod's® inception, a number of generations have been released. The iPod® Touch and the iPhone™ were both released in 2007. The iPod® Touch provides a screen size close to the width and length of the device including touch screen icons, and WiFi access to the Internet. The iPhone™ looks almost identical to the iPod® Touch, but it is also a cellular phone. The size of the storage drives and the simplicity for transferring audio, video, and data have made the iPod® a favorite media device for users of all ages.

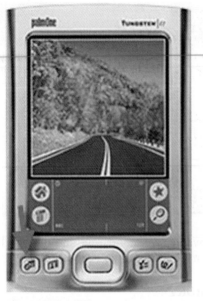

Figure 13-1 • PDA.

Understanding Handheld Computer Concepts

There are similarities and differences between PCs and **handheld computers**. Handheld computers do not necessarily have the same OS as the PC. Even if the OSs differ, mobile computing software is designed for interoperability (the devices work together). There are hardware differences between handheld computers and PCs, and it is important to understand these differences. Hardware variations include display, battery, memory, synchronization and connectivity, and data entry devices. Synchronization and connectivity using beaming, Bluetooth, WiFi, and cellular phone line connections are data transfer functions common to handheld computers.

HANDHELD COMPUTER OPERATING SYSTEMS

The OSs of PDAs and smartphones determine the functions and software capabilities. The OSs include Garnet OS (formerly Palm OS),

Windows Compact Edition (CE), Symbian, Linux, Apple, and Research in Motion (RIM), the Blackberry proprietary OS. The iPod® and iPhone™ use the Mac OS X proprietary OS. Android is the OS for the Google smartphones.

The Palm Garnet OS is popular in the healthcare arena because it is simple to use. Many electronic nursing and medical reference resources, free, and shareware (available for a small fee) medical software applications are developed for the Garnet OS. The Windows CE has a growing popularity among healthcare providers because it resembles the Window desktop OS. Numerous nursing and medical reference software applications are available for Windows CE, though less freeware and shareware. A growing number of medical software applications are available for the RIM Blackberry OS, although commercial, free, and shareware applications trail behind the Palm and Windows CE OSs (Budd, 2007).

There is limited nursing and medical software for the newest OS, the Mac OS X, and Google Android. The Mac OS X, originally designed to allow sharing of music, provides access to numerous free audio and video podcasts through the iTunes store or any iPod® server for the iPod®. It is inevitable that nursing and medical resources will be developed now that the Apple OS allows for wireless connection to the Internet. The Google Android OS, released in 2008, is a Linux – open software platform designed to rival the Mac iPhone™.

DISPLAY

Handheld computers have a liquid crystal display (LCD) like the laptop PCs. Many handheld computers also provide a touch screen for data input. The screen display size and resolution differ from PCs. The screen display size on handheld computers ranges from 1.74 to 3.5 inches (see Table 13-1). Resolution is an important consideration – the higher the numbers, the sharper is the image. A sharp screen image is a factor to consider if the user needs to view video, for example, of physical assessment or nursing procedures.

TABLE 13-1 ● *Examples of Screen Resolution and Display Size Differences for PDAs and Smartphones*

Classification	Mobile Device	Screen Resolution	Display Size (in inches)
Apple Smartphone	Apple iPhone™	320 × 480	3.5
Palm PDA	Palm T|X	320 × 480	2.5
Palm Smartphone	Palm Treo	320 × 320	1.74
Windows Mobile PDA	HP iPac	240 × 320	3.5
Windows Mobile Smartphone	Samsung Blackjack	320 × 240	2.3

BATTERY

All handheld computers operate using battery power.[1] Earlier Palm devices used replaceable alkaline (AAA) batteries that lasted several weeks. Most mobile devices now use rechargeable (nickel-metal hydride, nickel-cadmium, lithium ion) batteries. Factors that shorten battery life are multitasking features (Pocket PC), increased memory, a color display (standard for today's PDAs), audio, backlight display, and Bluetooth/WiFi connections (Cornelius & Gordon, 2007). If the battery is

removable, a second one should be charged and made available as a replacement.

MEMORY

PDAs and smartphones use three types of built-in memory – read-only memory (**ROM**), random-access memory (**RAM**), and built-in flash memory. Flash memory is also available as expansion cards, as shown in Figure 13-2. The ROM stores the OSs and standard applications such as contacts, calendar, and notes. The RAM stores all of the add-on applications and data files and requires a small amount of continuous battery power. RAM memory is volatile; hence, if the battery power is depleted, all of the data stored in RAM is lost. Some

[1] See Chapter 2 for more information about batteries.

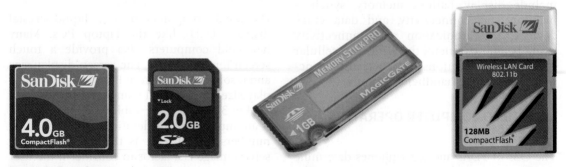

Figure 13-2 ● Flash memory cards.

devices use flash memory instead of RAM because flash memory is nonvolatile, meaning that the applications and data will not disappear if the battery power is depleted.[2]

Unlike the PC, non-Apple PDAs and smartphones do not have a hard drive. Many mobile digital devices have expansion slots for removable **flash memory** cards for software and data storage. Removable memory, commonly used by mobile devices, includes Secure Digital (SD) cards, Compact Flash (CF) cards, and Memory Sticks (MSs). A few PDAs also accept a universal serial bus (USB) flash drive. Flash memory cards are useful for storing e-books, photographs, video, and music. The price of flash memory has plummeted. Today a 2 gigabyte (GB) SD card can be purchased for less than $20.

In contrast to Palm and Windows Mobile devices, the Apple iPod® Classic comes equipped with a very large hard drive. In fact, the iPod® Classic is available with a 160 GB hard drive. The iPod® Nano, iPod® Touch, and iPhone™ use flash memory instead of a hard drive (Apple, 2007). The Apple devices were designed primarily to deliver music and video, so it makes sense that they are designed with large storage capacities.

DATA ENTRY

Many devices allow for data entry using a stylus or the touch of a finger (iPod® Touch and iPhone™) on a touch screen. **QWERTY keyboard** data entry is available in all smartphones and many PDAs (see Figure 13-3). QWERTY refers to a keyboard layout common to the PC and typewriter and comprises the first six letters on the top row of letters. Depending on the mobile device, data entry is enhanced using a navigation button and thumbwheel for scrolling. Mobile devices may also include a microphone and an audio recorder. Smartphones usually include a camera with a zoom lens that can be used to capture pictures and video clips.

[2] See Chapter 2 for more information about Flash memory.

Unless there is a separate keyboard especially designed for the mobile device, it is easier to enter large amounts of data using a PC, rather than the mobile device, and then synchronize the file with the mobile device. It is simple, however, to enter data such as a new appointment or contact on a mobile device. Office software such as Documents to Go (http://www.dataviz.com/) or Windows Office Mobile (bundled with some versions of Windows Mobile 6) allows users to create or edit Microsoft Word or Excel files on the mobile device. Google Docs allows for word processing and spreadsheet solutions (http://docs.google.com/m) on mobile devices.

SYNCHRONIZATION

Mobile devices are designed to **synchronize** with the PC using proprietary software so that all of the files on the two computers coincide. The Palm devices use HotSync and Windows Mobile devices use Windows Mobile for data transfer between the mobile device and the PC. The Apple devices use iTunes, a free download, to transfer data. PIM contact information (names, phone numbers, and addresses) is transferred to mobile devices using software such as Microsoft Outlook or Palm Desktop.

CONNECTIVITY

Depending on the mobile device, there are several ways these devices can connect with other devices or the Internet. Connectivity features include beaming, Bluetooth, WiFi, and cellular phone line. Bluetooth and WiFi expansion cards are available for those devices that have an expansion card slot but do not have this built-in feature of connectivity.

Beaming

Beaming allows for wireless, very short-ranged (3 feet), infrared (IR) transmission of information to other beam-enabled devices with the same OS. The beaming feature is used to share files, such as contact information and calendar, or documents such as Word or Excel,

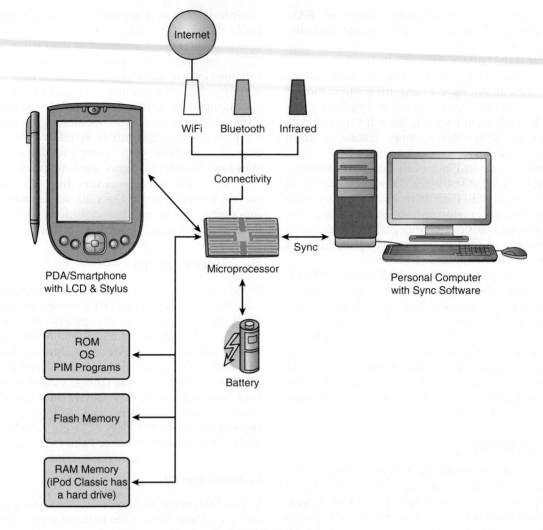

Parts of a PDA/Smartphone

Figure 13-3 • Parts of a PDA/smartphone.

with another mobile device. To use beaming, both mobile devices must have an IR port and the beaming feature enabled.[3] You select the file that you want to share and then select *beam* from the menu (see Figure 13-4). Check your user's manual for the exact procedure to use with your device.

---

[3] See Chapter 2 for more information about infrared (IR) ports.

Bluetooth

Bluetooth allows for wireless, short-ranged (32 feet), low-powered radio frequency connection to other Bluetooth-enabled devices. When Bluetooth is enabled on the mobile device and paired with another Bluetooth device, a personal area connection (PAN) or **piconet** is created (Layton & Franklin, 2007). There are several uses of Bluetooth. Bluetooth can be used to synchronize a mobile device with a PC or print to a Bluetooth-enabled

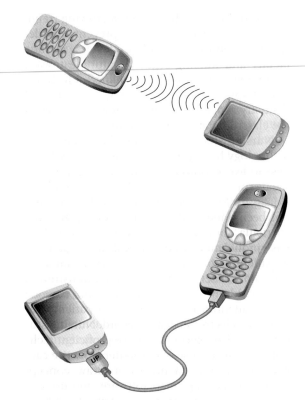

Figure 13-4 • Beaming data using infrared.

multiple users to access wireless printers and the Internet. WiFi networks are fairly simple to set up using a software wizard that comes with the purchase of a wireless router.

"Hotspot" is a term used to identify a WiFi-enabled area so that you can use your WiFi-enabled mobile device to connect to the Internet. You can find Hotspots at public libraries, most colleges and universities, coffee shops, airport terminals, and hotels. Not all Hotspots are public; many are encrypted for security reasons and require the user to enter an access code or pay a fee for access. WiFi security, like Bluetooth, is an important issue. For example, hospitals that use WiFi have very secure encrypted systems. Setup information for routers used in home wireless networks includes methods to address security issues.

Smartphones can connect to the Internet using regular cell phone networks. Smartphone users who use this connection should be aware of their "connection package" agreement to avoid paying high fees for large data downloads. Users who need to access the Internet using the cellular phone network, as opposed to WiFi, should have unlimited minutes as part of their cellular service agreement.

Uses of PDA in Nursing

There are benefits and shortcomings of the use of handheld computers in nursing, although many argue that the benefits far outweigh the shortfalls. Time saving and time management are often mentioned in the literature as positive outcomes after infusing PDAs in nursing education and clinical settings. Instead of looking up information in several printed textbooks, the nursing students can query the handheld mobile device, which can hold numerous textbooks. Patient safety and error reduction are also benefits. The ease of looking up reference information (see Table 13-1) improves confidence and prevents errors in the clinical setting. Unlike the printed counterpart, reference **e-books** can be updated and subscriptions renewed. Finally, the PDAs are easy for nursing students and other healthcare

printer. Bluetooth headphones allow the user to listen to music, podcasts, and other audio media. Bluetooth headsets provide hands-free use of smartphones for phone calls. Security is always a potential issue for wireless use, so it is a good idea to have the feature turned off when it isn't necessary to have the mobile device discoverable.

WiFi

WiFi networking is another means of mobile device connectivity. WiFi is an acronym for wireless fidelity, and it is an industry standard (Mitchell, 2007). It uses a router that supports WiFi standard 802.11 a, b, g, or n to form a local area network (LAN). The 802.11 b g standard is very common and inexpensive. The newer 802.11 n is an emerging standard that improves the range and speed of the wireless connection (Brain & Wilson, 2007). WiFi networking is popular with family homes because it allows

TABLE 13-2 ● Library Web Sites Designed for Handheld Computers

Library Sites Designed for Handheld Computers	Web Site Address
American University Library	http://www.library.american.edu/mobile/
Ball State University Libraries	http://www.bsu.edu/libraries/mobile/
Bobst Library, New York University	http://library.nyu.edu/mobile
Boston University Medical Center Mobile Library	http://med-libwww.bu.edu/mobile/index.cfm
Harvard College Library	http://hcl.harvard.edu/mobile/
National Library of Medicine (NLM)	http://pubmedhh.nlm.nih.gov/nlm/
University of Richmond Library	http://oncampus.richmond.edu/academics/library/mobile/
Western Kentucky University Libraries	http://www.wku.edu/library/tip/pda/

http://web.simmons.edu/~fox/pda/ (Fox, 2007). The site includes presentations and reports, links to Web sites designed for mobile devices, and much more. The Web site would be beneficial to both novice and expert handheld computer users.

Use of Handheld Computers in Clinical Practice

GENERAL NURSING CLINICAL PRACTICE

When nurses discover better ways to deliver patient care, they quickly adopt the new ways. The nursing literature has an abundance of information on how to purchase and use handheld computers. Nurses find handheld computers affordable and indispensable in various nursing practice clinical settings including the medical-surgical nursing unit, the operating room, and the emergency department. A growing number of clinical information systems incorporate the use of handheld computers for point-of-need documentation. Wireless synchronization allows for real-time documentation in the electronic medical record.

Personal Handheld Computers for Clinical Use

Many nurses in clinical practice purchase their own handheld computers to use electronic references to provide point-of-need information for decision making in practice. References commonly used by a clinical nurse include a nursing drug book, a medical dictionary, a nursing procedures manual, a handbook of diagnostics tests, and a health assessment handbook (see Table 13-3). The cost of the electronic references is comparable to the print version. The advantage of the electronic format is that when updates are available, they can be downloaded and saved to the mobile device so that the information is available at the point of care.

The American Association of Critical Care Nurses (AACN) offers a variety of critical care software, including the AACN Medicopeia and Critical Care Nurse Edition for the PDA. Nurses can choose to purchase a PDA with software already installed or to purchase and download software packages to install separately (American Association of Critical Care Nurses, 2007). The AACN PDA Web site empowers new PDA users with multimedia tutorials on PDA basics, clinical software, Adobe Acrobat, and PowerPoint. After completing the tutorials tests, AACN members can obtain free continuing education credit (Box 13-1).

Handheld Computers for Clinical Information Systems

The use of PDAs for bar code administration of medications is becoming more prevalent. Visualize a scenario. The nurses arrive for report from the 7 a.m. to 7 p.m. shift on the cardiac nursing unit. After the walking rounds report, each nurse picks up a wireless PDA, logs into the device, and uses a stylus to select assigned patients from the list of patients on the nursing unit. While planning medication

TABLE 13-3 • Examples of Handheld Computer Reference Resources

Examples of Handheld Reference Resources	Web Site Address
Skyscape Drug books, medical dictionaries, laboratory and diagnostic test books, NCLEX review manuals, and nursing procedure manuals	http://www.skyscape.com
Handango Many healthcare and office applications	http://www.handango.com/
CDC Podcasts and STD treatment guidelines	http://www2a.cdc.gov/podcasts/ http://www.cdcnpin.org/scripts/std/pda.asp
Epocrates Rx Drug database (free)	http://www.epocrates.com/
Pepid Reference resources for clinical nursing, oncology, and critical care	http://www.pepid.com/
Critical care AACN's PDA Center	http://aacn.pdaorder.com/welcome.xml
The Group on Immunizations of the Society of Teachers of Family Medicine Shots (free)	http://www.immunizationed.org/
Statcoder Coding and billing tools (free)	http://www.statcoder.com

administration for the shift, the nurse uses the real-time electronic medication administration record (MAR) to review the scheduled medications for each patient in preparation for organizing care. When administering the medication, the nurses follow the six rights of

medication administration (right drug, right patient, right dose, right time, right route, and right documentation) using bar coding technology by first scanning the bar code on the drug. In addition to asking the patients their names, the nurse also scans the identification band to verify that the correct patient is administered the medication. Afterwards, the nurse charts the drug administration by clicking a checkbox on the PDA MAR.

PDAs with a secure wireless connection to the clinical information system are being used in many healthcare facilities for medication administration. Because the PDA is wireless, the patient data are always up to date. As soon as a patient is admitted to a room, the patient's name shows up on the list of patients for that unit. When a medication is ordered and verified by the pharmacy, it shows up on the list of

---

Box 13-1 • PDAs and Nursing:
Words From a User

"When you use a PDA while providing clinical care, you have a remarkable resource in your hand." Edward Stern, RN. [From Hodson Carlton, K., Dillard, N., Campbell, B. R., & Baker, N. (2007). Personal digital assistants in the classroom and clinical areas. *Computers, Informatics, Nursing: CIN, 25*(5), 253–258.]

APPLICATIONS AND COMPETENCIES

1. Use a search engine, such as Google, to search for health science library PDA Web sites.
2. Check with your local library to see if they lend out mobile computing devices such as PDAs and iPods®.
3. If you have access to a PDA or smartphone, discuss the connection resources. Does the device have Bluetooth, beaming, or Internet capabilities? Explain the advantages and disadvantages of each type of connection.
4. Enter your name and contact information on a handheld mobile device and then beam the data to the device of a classmate.
5. Download a trial version of nursing reference software from the Internet. Use a search engine, such as Google, and enter the search terms: "nursing mobile software trial downloads."
6. Use the Internet to preview software that you might use on a mobile device. Discuss the similarities and differences between the printed book view and the electronic view.

REFERENCES

3Com Public Relations. (1999). *Press release: 3Com corporation acquires Smartcode Technologie*. Retrieved January 11, 2008, from http://www.palm.com/us/company/pr/1999/smartcode.html

American Association of Critical Care Nurses. (2007, August 24). *AACN's PDA center*. Retrieved November 2, 2008, from http://aacn.pdaorder.com/welcome.xml

Apple. (2007). *Apple*. Retrieved November 6, 2007, from http://www.apple.com/

Brain, M., & Wilson, T. V. (2007). *How WiFi works*. Retrieved November 4, 2007, from http://computer.howstuffworks.com/wireless-network1.htm

Budd, C. (2007). Using a Blackberry to support clinical practice. *Computers, Informatics, Nursing: CIN, 25*(5), 263–265.

Cellular-News. (2006, August 9). *PDA shipments reached record high in second quarter of 2006*. Retrieved November 22, 2008, from http://www.cellular-news.com/story/18733.php

Cornelius, F., & Gordon, M. G. (Eds.). (2007). *PDA connections: Mobile technology for health care professionals*. Philadelphia: Lippincott Williams & Wilkins.

Cuddy, C. (2006). How to serve content to PDA users on-the-go. *Computers in Libraries, 26*(4), 10.

Donnelly, G. F., & Rockstraw, L. (2003). *The personal digital assistant (PDA) – a tool for minimizing risk and error in nursing care*. Retrieved November 5, 2007, from http://www.nso.com/newsletters/advisor/2003_11/pda.php

Fox, M. K. (2007). *PDAs, handhelds and mobile technologies in libraries*. Retrieved February 7, 2008, from http://web.simmons.edu/~fox/pda/

Hodson Carlton, K., Dillard, N., Campbell, B. R., & Baker, N. (2007). Personal digital assistants in the classroom and clinical areas. *Computers, Informatics, Nursing: CIN, 25*(5), 253–258.

HPC: Factor. (2007, February 18). *The history of Windows CE*. Retrieved October 29, 2007, from http://www.hpcfactor.com/support/windowsce/

Layton, J., & Franklin, C. (2007). *How Bluetooth works*. Retrieved November 4, 2007, from http://electronics.howstuffworks.com/bluetooth1.htm

Lee, T. T. (2007). Patients' perceptions of nurses' bedside use of PDAs. *Computers, Informatics, Nursing: CIN, 25*(2), 106–111.

Maag, M. M. (2006). Nursing students' attitudes toward technology: A national study. *Nurse Educator, 31*(3), 112–118.

Medindia. (2007, October 15). *History of PDA*. Retrieved October 15, 2007, from http://www.medindia.net/pda/pda_history.htm

Microsoft. (2008). *Strong passwords: How to create and use them*. Retrieved February 7, 2008, from http://www.microsoft.com/protect/yourself/password/create.mspx

Miller, J., Shaw-Kokot, J. R., Arnold, M. S., Boggin, T., Crowell, K. E., Allegri, F., et al. (2005). A study of personal digital assistants to enhance undergraduate clinical nursing education. *The Journal of Nursing Education, 44*(1), 19–26.

Mitchell, B. (2007). *Wireless/Networking*. Retrieved November 5, 2007, from http://compnetworking.about.com/cs/wireless80211/g/bldef_wifi.htm

Skyscape. (n.d.). *Skyscape references in pockets of Drexel nursing students*. Retrieved November 5, 2007, from http://www.skyscape.com/group/Drexel_testimonial.pdf

Smith, C. M., & Pattillo, R. E. (2006). Technology. PDAs in the nursing curriculum: providing data for internal funding. *Nurse Educator, 31*(3), 101–102.

Thompson, M. J. (2007). 100 million sold [Electronic version]. *Macworld, 24*, 22–22. Retrieved October 30, 2007 from Business Source Complete Database.

W3C. (2006, June 27). *Mobile web best practices 1.0*. Retrieved November 8, 2007, from http://www.w3.org/TR/2006/CR-mobile-bp-20060627/

White, A., Allen, P., Goodwin, L., Breckinridge, D., Dowell, J., & Garvy, R. (2005). Infusing PDA technology into nursing education. *Nurse Educator, 30*(4), 150–154.

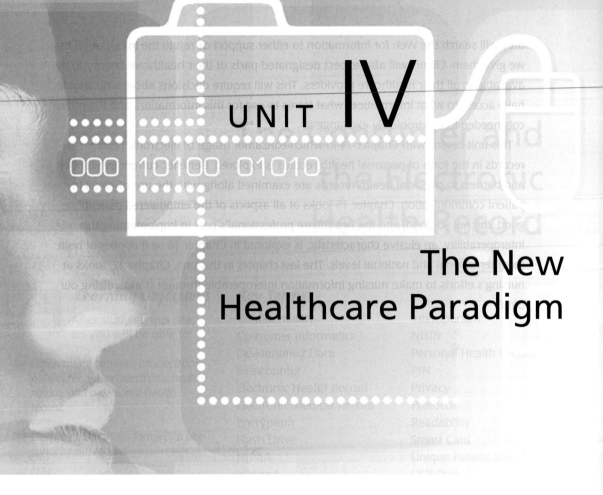

UNIT IV

000 10100 01010

The New Healthcare Paradigm

CHAPTER 14   The Consumer and the Electronic Health Record
CHAPTER 15   The Empowered Consumer
CHAPTER 16   Interoperability at the International and National Level
CHAPTER 17   Nursing Documentation: Is It Valuable?

An electronic health record for every American by 2014 was a goal set by President Bush in 2004 – a wonderful goal, but one with many required steps before it can be accomplished. These steps will involve both healthcare professionals and consumers. All of this is part of a new paradigm in healthcare in which consumers will change from patients to clients who make treatment decisions with healthcare professionals as they take more active responsibility for their care. As this paradigm slowly makes its perspective felt, professionals are finding that clients want reasons for treatments and that

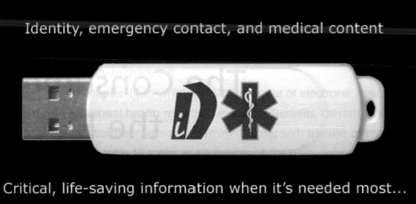

Figure 14-1 • Identification device. (Printed with permission of Identification Devices, LLC, Sandy, UT 84093; http://www.identificationdevices.net/)

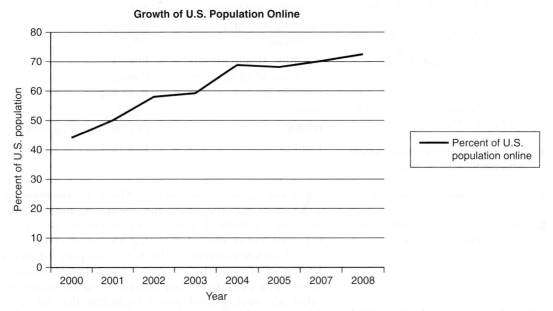

Figure 14-2 • Growth of U.S. population online. (Internet World Stats. (2007, April 12). *United States of America Internet usage and broadband usage report.* Retrieved August 29, 2007, from http://www.internetworldstats .com/am/us.htm)

are seeing a transformation of healthcare. The **Internet** is at the heart of this revolution. In less than a decade, the percentage of the U.S. population who are online has increased to over 70% (see Figure 14-2). Worldwide usage has also increased, with 15% of Asians and 48% of Europeans now online (Internet World Stats, 2008). With this trend, the pressure on healthcare providers to use the Internet for healthcare communication has increased. Additionally, consumers are starting to take more responsibility for their healthcare as the patient in the above scenario did when he purchased, entered data into, and wore the identification device. Further, as more and more "patients" use the Internet to learn about their conditions, you will see the relationship between patient and healthcare providers change and healthcare providers become more of an advisor while patients become clients or consumers.

Implementing the Promise of the Internet in Healthcare

Before the full promise of the Internet in healthcare becomes a reality, all healthcare records must be integrated. Many other countries are ahead of the United States in this endeavor, particularly those with a nationalized health service; however, none has yet reached the full potential. Many of the reasons for this, such as **privacy** issues and the development of a national network of healthcare records, are shared by all countries, although some, such as the Netherlands and the United Kingdom, are ahead of others.

In the United States, the National Health Information Network (**NHIN**)[1] is envisioned to serve this purpose. It is envisioned to be an electronic birth to death healthcare record that also provides consumer access. The development of the NHIN is dependent on each healthcare provider using electronic patient care records, these records being accessible by those designated by the patient anywhere in the United States, and patients having access to their healthcare records. Pieces of this will be built gradually, with full interconnectedness being the last step. In the past, there has been confusion regarding the terms to use for the three parts of this project. There is now agreement on the following terms (National Alliance for Health Information Technology, 2008), a diagram of which is seen in Figure 14-3. They will be used in this book.

▼ An **electronic medical record** (EMR) is a healthcare record created by healthcare providers or agencies such as a hospital.

[1] The NHIN will be addressed in Chapter 16.

▼ An **electronic health record** (EHR) is created when providers can access information from EMRs other than the one to which they belong. It is a longitudinal record of a patient's healthcare information (HIMSS Electronic Health Records Vendors Association, 2006) from all healthcare sources.
▼ A **personal health record** (PHR) is created when patients can communicate with their providers and document and create their own medical history (Clinfowiki, 2006).

The main difference between the terms "EMR" and "EHR" is the ability to exchange information interoperably.

There is overlap among these concepts; for example, some EMRs permit patients to view items in their records such as laboratory results. This is seen in Figure 14-3, where the client has access to an EMR from Dr. B's office, but this record is not yet part of an EHR.

ELECTRONIC MEDICAL RECORD

EMRs are the focus of most healthcare agencies today. They are owned and managed by the institution or provider that creates them. As healthcare agencies merge and form large corporations, these EMRs are often combined so that information from all member agencies and providers is accessible by those with the required authorization. Many agencies refer to their EMR as an EHR, but an electronic record that cannot interface with outside agencies is not a true EHR.[2]

ELECTRONIC HEALTH RECORD

When babies born in the United States are two months old, they probably have healthcare records in at least two places: the hospital where they were born and in the pediatrician's office. As the babies grow, the number and location of their healthcare records also grow.

[2] Electronic patient records will be discussed in Chapter 19.

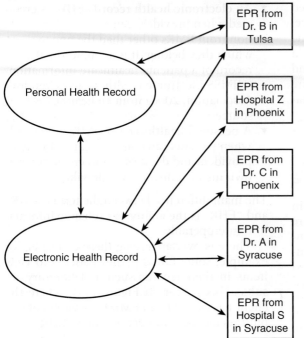

Figure 14-3 • Health record integration.

The current record system, whether paper or electronic, makes it difficult for individuals to have access to their healthcare records. Additionally, it handicaps healthcare providers by preventing them from having complete information about a person. Individuals who have not kept their own health records find it difficult to remember details. Try to remember what your last immunization was, where it was given, or if you have ever been immunized against a disease such as yellow fever. Even trying to remember all one's surgeries becomes difficult as one grows older, let alone being able to remember one's medical history. These problems can be life threatening in an emergency situation, as was seen in the aftermath of Hurricane Katrina. Paper records were either destroyed or inaccessible, making it impossible to obtain any past medical information or list of medications of people in need of care.

Under the EHR model, one's health information will be available from any location. This will make it easier for patients who visit multiple providers to supply each one with an up-to-date record, and the information available will usually be more than what a referring provider sends (Landro, 2000). It will also provide safer care in the advent of an emergency when regular records may not be available. With a record of all the prescriptions that a consumer has, adverse drug effects can be minimized. Additionally, so-called frequent fliers or those who use different sources to gain drugs will be identified and can be helped. Having healthcare data in an electronic format also means that **de-identified** data can be used in an aggregated form to assess patterns of disease, quickly identify potentially dangerous side effects of medications, and detect disease outbreaks. In a Markle Foundation study (Foundation, 2005), it was found that 72% of Americans are in favor of an EHR.

PERSONAL HEALTH RECORD

A PHR provides clients access to their healthcare information and may allow clients to enter data into their records. It will provide information from healthcare encounters along with information about the medications the client is taking, the results of various tests, and healthcare information designed for the consumer. At the present time, the term PHR may refer to a health record kept by the consumer, although it is hoped that this state is a temporary measure.

Consumers' access to their own health information is being gradually introduced into EMRs. Until just recently, a person's healthcare record, whether in a hospital or clinic, was regarded as the property of the agency providing the care. Patients were not allowed to see their records; in fact, in the not too distant past even providing patients with knowledge of their own temperature was regarded as improper. The Health Insurance Portability and Accountability Act (**HIPAA**) of 1996 changed this by mandating that patients be allowed to see their own healthcare records (Ross & Lin, 2003). Difficulties arise, however, because it was not stipulated how access must be provided (Halamka, Mandl, & Tang, 2008) and because in most cases pieces of a patient's medical history are scattered in many different locales.

Computerized PHRs today are in a state of evolution with no one agreeing on exactly what they are (Halamka et al., 2008). They range from Web pages on which clients can enter their own data to provider-hosted portals that allow client access to employer/payer to claim data. The one agreement is that they provide access to the consumers to healthcare information about the individual and enable them to manage their own information. To be a true PHR, however, consumers must be capable of managing and deciding how the information is accessed and used by National Alliance for Health Information Technology (2008, April 28). PHRs vary in their contents, scope, source of information, owner, location of the record, technical approach, and the identity of those who have access to the record (National Committee on Vital Health Statistics, 2006). The Markle Foundation's Connecting for Health in the final report of the personal health working group, in an effort to standardize efforts toward a PHR, offered an overall definition that closely resembles the PHR definition from the National Alliance for Health Information Technology (2008). The Markle Foundation defined a PHR as an electronic application that permits individuals to manage and share their health information as well as that of others (e.g., a child or spouse) for whom they are authorized (Markle Foundation Connecting for Health, 2003, p. 1379). It is person-centered and tracks and supports health activities from birth to death. There are at least five models of a computerized PHR.

▼ Patient owned and maintained. In this model, data is entered, maintained, and owned by the consumer.
▼ Portable, **interoperable** digital file such as **smart cards** (provider maintained) or a USB device (consumer maintained) such as the patient mentioned in the introduction had.
▼ Provider-owned and provider-maintained EMRs on the provider's server with limited access for consumers (Endsley, Kibbe, Linares, & Colorafi, 2006). Consumer access is mostly in the form of seeing test results, communicating with a provider, or both.
▼ A combination of provider and consumer access and data entry to the EMR. In this model, consumers and providers both contribute to the record (Simons, Mandl, & Kohane, 2005).
▼ A full PHR in which the preceding model is combined with a true EHR. Consumers will be able to limit what providers and others whom they designate can see. The record will be a two-way communication with providers, and the consumer will be able to enter data as needed.

As is to be expected during the building of the full PHR, none of these visions is pure, and there is often overlap between them. For example, the information on a smart card may be accessible to providers beyond the provider who originally created the card and, as with the EHR; another provider may be able to enter data. The first major step toward the goal of the full PHR is for all healthcare providers to have an EMR. This will be followed by merging healthcare information with other agencies into an EHR.

Allowing patient access and data entry will probably gradually be implemented first into EMRs and eventually into an EHR. As can be imagined, there are several barriers that must be overcome before the full PHR becomes a reality. Consumers are ready for PHRs. As part of their report, the Markle Foundation Connecting for Health Personal Health Working Group surveyed 1,246 online households to determine which elements of a PHR would be the most beneficial. One of the findings was that 71% would use it to help them understand their doctor's instructions (Markle Foundation Connecting for Health, 2003). Surprisingly, although data security is often seen by healthcare providers as a barrier to implementing PHRs, the majority of people in this survey believe that technology provides adequate protection and would not be reluctant to use PHR features. Interestingly, those who suffer from chronic illness, or are frequent healthcare users, are less concerned about privacy and security. People, however, do not want their PHR managed by their insurance company, their employer, or the government. Instead, they trust their doctor to host, manage, and access their PHR.

A Harris Interactive poll found that 42% of Americans keep some type of PHR, although only 13% keep them electronically. Forty percent of the 87% of those who do not keep their own EHRs think that it is highly likely that they will do so in the future (Harris Interactive Inc., 2004). In contrast to the Markle Foundation Study (Markle Foundation Connecting for Health, 2003), a Harris Poll found that for 68% of the respondents the biggest concern about electronic personal health records are privacy and security. Other concerns found in the Harris poll were worry about possible errors and that their information won't be available in an emergency, or that they won't keep their records up-to-date.

Benefits of PHRs

PHRs will further collaborative care, that is, care in which there is a partnership between the patient and their healthcare providers. When an individual's PHR is viewed together by both a healthcare provider and a consumer, instead of the healthcare provider giving orders, which the patient may or may not understand or accept, the healthcare provider can help the patient to understand his or her condition and work together with this individual to achieve an agreed-upon goal. Consumers can also collaborate in the creation and maintenance of the healthcare record.

Another benefit of PHRs is the ability to better manage one's disease treatment (Tang, Ash, Bates, Overhage, & Sands, 2006). For example, those suffering from a chronic disease will be able to track their disease together with their healthcare provider, which can lower the communication barrier between consumer and provider. A PHR will also permit the provider to link individualized information to the client, thus providing more personalized as well as higher-quality care. The improved communication that results will lead consumers to a better understanding of their healthcare responsibilities and disease management. A study done by the Dartmouth Cooperative Practice-Based Research Network (Wasson, Johnson, Benjamin, Phillips, & MacKenzie, 2006) studied the effects of various levels of collaborative care on chronic diseases. To judge the level of this care, they asked participants to evaluate the information given to them by their doctor, the explanation of the problem, along with the patient's confidence in their self-care ability. They found that when the provider and patient had a high exchange of information instead of a one-way flow, the patient's confidence in their self-care ability increased and outcomes improved.

Barriers to Implementation of PHRs

As can be imagined, there are several barriers that must be overcome before the full PHR becomes a reality. The technology to create a full PHR is here, but the agreements, **protocols**, and procedures are not.

Provider Reluctance and Responsibility. A PHR and EHR can threaten the autonomy of some healthcare providers who still want to practice in the traditional model (Tang et al., 2006). Despite the fact that patients can now get copies of their healthcare records, agencies and healthcare providers still see themselves as owners of this information, instead of guardians (Markle Foundation Connecting for Health, 2003). Healthcare practitioners have concerns about providing client access to information not designed for lay interpretation or that may contain information inappropriate to divulge to patients (Ross & Lin, 2003), such as psychiatric problems or diseases. Providers are also concerned about the effects on the patient, on the provider–client relationship, and on healthcare itself. There are also questions about a client's interest in reading and contributing to a healthcare record. Other concerns are that access to healthcare records may be used by the patient for litigious reasons. Also, there can be problems with client understanding of information in the records.

Some of the decisions that providers must make when implementing electronic client access to healthcare records include deciding which problems should be shared, whether or not to share the entire medication and allergy list, which laboratory and diagnostic tests should be shared, whether or not to share clinical notes, how to authenticate patient access, and whether minors should be allowed to access their records (Halamka et al., 2008). Some of the challenges that may become apparent as the building of the full EHR and PHR occurs are whether to provide a single PHR that works with all agencies, if data input from other agencies should be permitted to other agencies' record, how to integrate Web-based information with a PHR, allowing patients with specific diseases to connect with others with similar diseases, and how to permit clients to participate in clinical trials, pharmaceutical evaluation, and public health surveillance via their PHR.

Unique Patient Identifier. Besides an EMR, a full PHR requires that each citizen have a **unique patient identifier** for his or her healthcare information regardless of where it is stored.

Today individual providers have their own method of identifying EMRs. This despite the fact that the 1996 HIPAA required a unique patient identifier. The current situation of multiple identifiers for the same individual makes it impossible to relate patient information in any meaningful way (IEEE, 2004), a factor that raises administrative costs. However, because of the many privacy and security issues surrounding it, implementation was put on hold. One solution that has been endorsed by the Institute of Electrical and Electronic Engineers (IEEE, 2004), the Health Information Management Systems Society (HIMSS VPI Work Group, 2004), and the National Alliance for Health Information Technology (Pizzi, 2007) is a voluntary patient identifier. Under this proposal, individuals would decide whether or not they wished to have their healthcare records all identified by one identifier, which would be unique to that individual. The groups supporting this believe that a unique patient identifier will provide accuracy and safety when electronically exchanging medical information and wish the country to move forward on this.

Data Security. For consumers to feel comfortable with exchanges of their healthcare information, there must be assurances that their data will be protected from those without permission to access it. This will require not only that individual healthcare providers and agencies have state-of-the-art security but also that there are protocols that govern access to data.

Data Standards. Another barrier is the lack of standardization of data. It is necessary that all agencies involved in healthcare, including pharmacies, agree to record a defined set of data in a defined manner. That is, there must be decisions made about what information will be recorded and the protocols used to record and transmit it. Identification of this core set of data elements requires participation by representatives of all healthcare record users including consumers. There is also the problem of devising the actual terminology that will be used to record this data. Add to this the fact that these efforts need to be national and international in scope, and one begins to see the task that remains.[3]

Data Presentation. It is one thing to provide consumers with access to their healthcare data and it is another to present this in a useful, understandable manner. How will information be grouped? What should one screen present? This area is one of the primary focuses in the new field of **consumer informatics.** This area is also of concern for healthcare providers and often falls into the category of usability.

Consumers. There are also consumer changes that need to be considered. Patients need to start thinking of themselves as healthcare consumers with a responsibility to actively participate in their healthcare (Tang et al., 2006). We are only in the beginning stages of this transition. As you participate in these changes, you will find a need for re-education with some clients. Many were raised in an era in which one is a passive patient and therefore have developed security in placing responsibility for health with others. As consumers, people will need help in understanding new roles and responsibilities. One suggestion for helping the population make the transition is education starting in grade school about the responsibilities and use of PHRs (Tang et al., 2006).

Costs. Financing of EHRs and PHRs is another barrier. Although the U.S. government is starting to finance electronic records for some healthcare providers' offices, like so many informatics advances, the expectation is often that healthcare agencies and healthcare providers will pay for them. Yet, the majority of advantages accrue to payers and patients (Markle Foundation Connecting for Health, 2003). It is easy to say that electronic records will save money; these savings, however, generally come from the pocket of the healthcare agencies and healthcare providers who will lose business as patients do not require as many office visits,

laboratory tests, or hospitalizations. Thus, a method of financing healthcare that does not reward hospitalizations and procedures needs to be found. Managed care, theoretically, can offer this, but in many cases has had difficulties in implementation and patient acceptance. Incentives such as pay for performance, in which access to aggregated data is imperative for improving care, are an approach to motivating healthcare providers to find a business case for EMRs, EHRs, and PHRs.

Current PHRs in Use

Given the many barriers to creating EHRs, let alone a full PHR, along with the demand by consumers for a PHR, it is not surprising that consumers and providers have started on the road to a PHR. There are also some healthcare providers that permit client access to at least parts of their healthcare record.

Self-Created. One approach used by many consumers is to keep their own healthcare record. It may be on paper, or on their computer with or without special-purpose software. With this approach, the consumer needs to carry an updated print-out with them at all times if it is to be useful in an emergency. There are many fee-based Web services available that allow consumers to create their own Internet-based PHR; however, there are many variations in these services, especially in the data that the consumer records (Sittig, 2002). Some of these services permit healthcare providers, with permission of the record owner, to use a **personal identification number (PIN)** created by the consumer to interact with the records by phone, fax, or online. Less useful but helpful is the provision of a printed format that allows the consumer to take a hard copy to his or her physician. Those that only provide consumers with a view of their data have a limited value. Searching the Web with the term "personal health record" finds many of these commercial PHRs.

Potential users should always investigate the fine print in the privacy policy of the organization sponsoring a consumer-created and consumer-maintained PHR. A review

---

[3] Data standardization will be explored in Chapter 16.

requested by the Office of the National Coordinator for Health Information Technology about the privacy and security of online PHRs found that of the 30 privacy policies reviewed, none included more than 18 of the 31 criteria used in their review (Lecker et al., 2007). These criteria included such items as **readability** (of the privacy policy), details of how the information is shared, and definition of critical terms. It would also be wise to check the organization with the Better Business Bureau.

One of the difficulties with this model is the time-consuming task of entering data and deciding what data to enter. A Web-based record can be accessed by medical personnel if the patient is conscious and able to provide the Web site address and login and password. Currently, an online client healthcare record that delivers on its promises is still in its infancy. Kim and Johnson (2002) studied 11 online patient healthcare records identified through a Web search. They found that at a basic level these records provide Web-based access to personal medical information, but only a few provide the capacity for access to information in emergency situations. This situation exists, in spite of the fact that one of the touted benefits of an online personal healthcare record is to access to healthcare information in an emergency. There are also limitations that are a function of the prescribed data entry process such as requiring clients to select entries from a list or type an entry with very little explanation of what is wanted. Overall, they found that as they now exist, self-created and maintained patient healthcare records have limited functionality.

Another type of self-created PHR is one that plugs into USB ports on a computer such as the one that the patient in the introductory scenario had. They are affordable and small enough to carry on a key chain. Consumers plug them into their computer; fill in the labeled fields, and save the information. This information is then available to any emergency medical service (see Figure 14-1).

Smart Cards. Smart cards are devices that are created by providers for use by their patients.

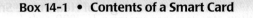

Box 14-1 • Contents of a Smart Card
A CPU for managing data
ROM to store the operating system
RAM for temporary storage

A smart card looks like a plastic credit card and, like a credit card, is embedded with information that can be read by a reader. In a smart card, however, the embedded data is on a computer chip that can not only be read but can also be written to with the appropriate computer system and access code. Functioning similarly to the central processing unit of a computer, smart cards contain RAM, ROM, and an operating system (see Box 14-1). They were first introduced in France to combat fraud in telecommunications and banking (Smart Card Alliance, 2003), and since then have found use in many industries including healthcare.

A smart healthcare card is defined by the International Standards Organization (ISO) as a card containing computer-readable data that is issued to a person or healthcare provider to facilitate providing healthcare (Barnhart, 2003). They are used by patients when making contact with the healthcare system for identification and to transmit information that will assist healthcare providers in their treatment. A healthcare smart card has four subsets of data: data necessary to operate the card including privacy protection, data unique to the consumer, administrative data such as insurance carrier, and clinical data. Access, however, is not automatic; users must provide a password, a PIN number, or both. These cards can also be designed to allow access by a biometric feature such as a thumbprint.

The first use of smart cards in healthcare was in France, and was instigated by insurance companies (Neame, 1997). Even today, smart health cards are more common in Europe and Asia than in the United States. However, their use in the United States is starting to grow. In their early years, smart cards were

rate of completion of the series of immunizations for children younger than two years (Dini, Linkins, & Sigafoos, 2001). Additionally, email has been found to improve the visitation rates for well-child visits.

Email communication with a healthcare provider avoids telephone tag. Waiting by the phone all day for a healthcare provider to return a call and having to use voice mail are frustrating for consumers. For providers, trying to return a phone call can be equally frustrating. Email can also be used for such things as sending patients' information or providing links to relevant information on the Web (Car & Sheikh, 2004). Patients can also use it to ask for further clarification after an office visit. Emails do not need to be transcribed; they can be printed and placed in a patient's record or, if the record is online, filed electronically. When properly implemented, email communication can result in time and cost savings.

Barriers to Email Communication With Providers

With more and more people using email, it may seem surprising that electronic communication with healthcare providers has not become more prevalent. Reasons that healthcare providers give for not instituting email are lack of time, lack of office staff, lack of interest in electronic communication, concerns about privacy and confidentiality (Gerstle, 2004), increased workloads (Baker, Rideout, Gertler, & Raube, 2005), reimbursement concerns, and potential malpractice liability (Harris Interactive Inc., 2002). These concerns are valid, but with some planning, they can be overcome.

Privacy of Email. Perhaps the biggest concern is privacy. Healthcare providers have a responsibility, both under HIPAA and ethically, to maintain confidentiality about their patients. They must be certain that the person requesting information is entitled to receive it, and that it is accurately transmitted and received (Gerstle, 2004). Additionally, in electronic communication, healthcare providers must be assured that the messages are not able to be intercepted by others. Most emails are not so

protected. However, email can be **encrypted** so that if intercepted by a third party it cannot be easily read (MacDonald, 2003).[4] Nothing, of course, is foolproof, and this includes mail and telephone calls. When a patient's voice mail message does not identify the person, there is no way of knowing if a wrong number has been reached.

In email, to assure that the email is going to the correct recipient, it is necessary to be certain that the correct email address is being used. If email is integrated with a person's EMR and messages sent from the record, the correct email address can be assured. Email needs to be both encrypted and sent with careful checking of the email address of the recipient. Without an EMR, protocols should be instituted to assure that the correct information is being sent to the correct patient. Just as paper information can be inadvertently slipped into the wrong envelope by harried office staff, so can information be emailed to the wrong patient. A suggested procedure is to use an address book with a previously tested address and carefully check the name in the address line.

Liability. Liability, although expressed as a concern, is not as big an issue as one might think. If one compares email liability with that for telephone calls, one finds that email is safer. Emails can be printed and filed in the patient's record, providing a written record of what was asked, as well as the answer. Healthcare providers, so familiar with telephone calls, may not realize that these calls expose them to liability, especially because they are so seldom documented (Sands, 2004). Policies that protect healthcare providers from liability with email communication can be seen in Box 14-3.

Workload. Increased workloads, especially without additional reimbursement, are another concern. One method of alleviating time demands for both client and provider is to develop structured forms accessible on a

---

[4] Encryption is discussed in Chapter 5.

Box 14-3 • Nationally Recommended Policies for Healthcare Providers' Use of Email

Print email communication and place in patients' chart.

Inform patients about privacy issues with respect to email.

When email messages become too lengthy, notify patients to come in to discuss or call them.

Establish a turnaround time for messages.

Request patients to put their names or identification numbers in the body of the message.

Send a new message to inform patient of completion of request.

Establish types of transaction.

Explain to patients that their message should be concise.

Remind patients when they do not adhere to [email] guidelines.

Develop archival and retrieval mechanisms.

Instruct patients to put the category of transaction in subject line of message (e.g., schedule an appointment, refill a prescription).

Configure an automatic reply to acknowledge receipt of patients' messages.

Request patients to use auto-reply features to acknowledge a clinician's message.

From Survey: Brooks, R. G., & Mencahemi, N. (2006). Physicians' use of email with patients: Factors influencing electronic communication and adherence to best practices. *Journal of Internet Medical Research, 8*(1) [Electronic Journal http://www.pubmedcentral.nih.gov/articlerender.fcgi?artid=1550692].

Web site that limit patient requests as well as facilitate a quick reply. For example, there can be forms for renewing a prescription, requesting an appointment, referrals, or follow-up communication with one's healthcare provider. Interestingly, where email communication has been instituted, an increased workload for healthcare providers has not materialized (MacDonald, 2003). For example, ConnectiCare found that online communication increased productivity by reducing administrative tasks. It has also been found that participating physicians were able to spend more time with patients because it is easier to integrate online communication than telephone calls into their daily work. Anecdotal

reports during a study of patient-physician emails found that physicians believed that Web messaging reduced their telephone calls and that they required less time than phone calls (Liederman, Lee, Baquero, & Seites, 2005). It was also reported that office visits triggered by emails are more efficient because the history is known.

IMPLEMENTING E-ENCOUNTERS

Clearly, the ability to perform many tasks electronically such as making an appointment will save patients and providers time (see Table 14-1). Instituting the reporting of tests online, however, requires careful planning. The first

---

TABLE 14-1 • Tasks Patients Would Like to Do Online

Task	Percentage of Clients Who Want
Ask questions with no visit	77
Make appointments	71
Get new prescriptions	71
See results of medical tests	70

Harris Interactive Inc. (2002, April 10). *Patient/Physician Online Communication: Many patients want it, would pay for it, and it would influence their choice of doctors and health plans.* Retrieved November 21, 2008, from http://www.harrisinteractive.com/news/newsletters/healthnews/HI_HealthCareNews2002Vol2_Iss08.pdf

hurdle may be winning over healthcare providers. Some may respond that "Patients can't handle this information" or fear that they will be deluged with "worried well" questions (Jirgis, 2007), factors that did not materialize at Vanderbilt University Hospital when they instituted email test results.

What to Post and When

Besides gaining buy-in from healthcare providers, decisions need to be made about what results will be posted and when. Having patients read online that they have cancer before the doctor has talked with them does not constitute good care. One organization solved this problem by organizing tests into three categories (Jirgis, 2007). Category one, routine laboratory tests such as complete blood counts and cholesterol levels, would be posted as soon as they were completed. Radiology tests, category two, would be posted after a week to provide time for the healthcare provider to contact the patient before results are seen. The third category included tests such as HIV, which are never posted online.

Email Contracts

Kane and Sands (1998) believe that email with clients should be characterized by a contractual relationship. They believe that before using email with a client, clinicians should negotiate several issues such as how long the turnaround time will be, whether the email will be triaged by the office staff or be sent directly to the provider, what content is permissible in the email, and what compensation, if any, the provider will require for email. Clients should also be instructed about permissible subjects for email, what content to place on a subject line, and to sign their full names to ensure accurate identification. Additionally, both patients and providers need to be aware that without encryption, their messages may be read by other than the intended parties. Some feel that the discussion of these points with a client should be recorded in the health record and would even commit these points to writing, with one copy given to the patient and another placed in the record.

Triaging Email Messages

Other planning that needs to occur is how to respond to and triage email messages. If Web form requests are used, they can be slotted to the correct box for attention. If email is used without a Web form, patients can be instructed to use given subject lines for various requests. It must be realized, however, that patients will not always adhere to this. In many ways, triaging email can follow methods used for telephone calls. It is important that a method be devised that assures a reply within a given time period and that this time period be communicated to the patient. If a patient sends an email and does not receive a reply within this time period, he or she will conclude that their provider is not serious about using email (Jirgis, 2007). When properly instituted, email communication with patients will save time now spent on the telephone by both the patient and the provider.

Who Pays?

Healthcare providers still need to be paid for the healthcare they deliver, whether through an office visit, through a telephone call, or electronically. Some considerations for payment are having either the payer or patient pay as for an office visit, or charge the patient an annual fee for these services (MacDonald, 2003). Given that patients have expressed a willingness to pay for email messaging (Harris Interactive Inc., 2002), any of these solutions may be feasible. Email messaging may be able to save money. One researcher has reported that supporting online patient–provider interaction could save up to $12 million in annual health costs (MacDonald, 2003). The question again becomes "Who should pay for a service that will benefit mostly patients and payers?"

HOME MONITORING

Although the technology for home monitoring is present, widespread use is slowed down because of financial hurdles and the rigid organization of healthcare (EurActiv, 2007). Home monitoring can prevent emergency hospital visits and decrease the number of office visits a client requires (eHealth News EU, 2007).[5] Home monitoring can also be designed to provide clients with recommended diet and lifestyle depending on the data submitted.

SUBSTITUTION FOR AN OFFICE VISIT

Using email instead of an office visit is a much more complex subject. Dartmouth-Hitchcock Clinic has instituted what they call "e-visiting" between a client and a provider with whom the client has a relationship (Wasson et al., 2006). An e-visit is set up by the client, who, using a secure Web site, requests the e-visit and provides an outline of the reason for the e-visit such as asking for advice, requesting a diagnosis, or therapy, tasks that previously required an office visit. The request is reviewed by a clinical person who brings it to the attention of the provider who determines if the reason meets the criteria for an e-visit. When the e-visit is complete, the provider enters information into the EMR and provides an ICD-9 code, which generates billing.

Summary

As the Internet and Web features are used more and more in healthcare, there will be a change in the relationship of the provider and client as client access to information previously held only by the practitioner increases. EMRs that provide healthcare records for only one provider will morph into EHRs that provide access to records from many different agencies from one access point. Subsequently, a PHR that permits and encourages client access to their healthcare information will emerge. Before this becomes a reality, there are many barriers that must be overcome including gaining provider compliance, a unique patient identifier, and a change in consumer behavior.

E-encounters, the exchange of information between healthcare provider and client, will become an expected mode of communication, one that nurses, particularly those involved in telephone consultations of private practice, will be involved. This will not happen without overcoming provider reluctance and planning that includes decisions such as what information to provide to clients and when. The final step of having an e-encounter substitute for an office visit will be sometime in the future for most agencies. Nevertheless, e-encounters and PHRs will become a normal part of healthcare delivery.

APPLICATIONS AND COMPETENCIES

1. Differentiate between an EMR, an EHR, and a PHR, as described in this chapter.
2. List the benefits of a PHR.
3. Find an online PHR by searching the Web and evaluate their privacy policy using the criteria on page 5 of the government report at http://www.hhs.gov/healthit/ahic/materials/01_07/ce/PrivacyReview.pdf. On the basis of this evaluation, make a recommendation to a client about whether to use this service.
4. Would you use a healthcare smart card? Why or why not?
5. Write a proposal for instituting email communication with clients in a specific practice such as obstetrics or cardiology.
6. Examine the pros and cons of a unique patient identifier.
7. Appraise the various methods of electronic communication with patients.

REFERENCES

Abrahamsen, C. (2004). Optimal patient safety a computer chip away? *Nursing Management, 35*(3), 47–48.

Alliance, S. C. (2006, February). *Smart card applications in the U.S. healthcare industry.* Retrieved November 21, 2008 from http://www.smartcardalliance.org/pages/publications-healthcare-industry

Baker, L., Rideout, J., Gertler, P., & Raube, K. (2005). Effect of an Internet-based system for doctor-patient communication on health care spending. *Journal of the American Medical Informatics Association, 12*(5), 530–536.

Barnhart, J. E. (2003). *The evolving standards for smart health cards.* Retrieved November 21, 2008, from http://www.icma.com/info/evolvingstds1204.html

[5] See Chapter 19 for more information about home monitoring.

California Health Care Foundation. (2001, November). E-encounters. *I-Health Reports*. Retrieved November 21, 2008, from http://www.chcf.org/documents/hospitals/EEncounters.pdf

Car, J., & Sheikh, A. (2004). E-mail consultations in health care: 1 – Scope and effectiveness [Electronic version at http://bmj.bmjjournals.com/cgi/content/full/329/7463/435]. *British Medical Journal, 329,* 435–438.

Center for Studying Health System Change. (2006, September). *Data Bulletin No. 32: Physicians slow to adopt patient email.* Retrieved November 21, 2008, from http://www.hschange.org/CONTENT/875/

Dini, E. F., Linkins, R. W., & Sigafoos, J. (2001). The impact of computer-generated messages on childhood immunization coverage. In R. Haux & C. Kulikoski (Eds.), *Yearbook of medical informatics: Digital libraries and medicine* (pp. 210–217). International Medical Informatics Association, Edmonton, AB Canada.

eHealth News EU. (2007, November 2). *St. Lucas Andreas Hospital to start home monitoring of cardiac patients.* Retrieved November 21, 2008, from http://www.ehealthnews.eu/content/view/805/26/

Endsley, S., Kibbe, D. C., Linares, A., & Colorafi, K. (2006, May). An introduction to personal health records. *Family Practice Management.* Retrieved November 21, 2008, from http://www.aafp.org/fpm/20060500/57anin.html

eHealth News EU. (2007, November 2). *St. Lucas Andreas Hospital to Start Home Monitoring of Cardiac Patients.* Retrieved November 21, 2008, from http://www.ehealthnews.eu/content/view/805/26/

EurActiv. (2007, December 6). *ICT networks prerequisite for healthcare at home.* Retrieved November 21, 2008, from http://www.euractiv.com/en/health/ict-networks-prerequisite-healthcare-home/article-168901

Foundation, M. (2005). *Attitudes of Americans regarding personal health records and nationwide electronic health information exchange.* Retrieved November 21, 2008, from http://www.phrconference.org/assets/research_release_101105.pdf

Gerstle, R. S. (2004). E-mail communication between pediatricians and their patients. *Pediatrics, 114*(1), 317–321.

Halamka, J. D., Mandl, K. D., & Tang, P. C. (2008). Early experiences with personal health records. *Journal of the American Medical Informatics Association, 15*(1), 1–7.

Harris Interactive Inc. (2002, April 10). *Patient/physician online communication: Many patients want it, would pay for it, and it would influence their choice of doctors and health plans.* Retrieved November 21, 2008, from http://www.harrisinteractive.com/news/newsletters/healthnews/HI_HealthCareNews2002Vol2_Iss08.pdf

Harris Interactive Inc. (2004, August 10). *Two in five adults keep personal or family records and almost everybody thinks it is a good idea.* Retrieved November 21, 2008, from http://www.harrisinteractive.com/news/newsletters/healthnews/HI_HealthCareNews2004Vol4_Iss13.pdf

HIMSS Electronic Health Records Vendors Association. (2006, October). *HIMSS EHRVA definitional model and application process.* Retrieved November 21, 2008, from http://www.himssehrva.org/docs/EHRVA_application.pdf

HIMSS VPI Work Group. (2004, February). *Voluntary patient identifier resolution.* Retrieved November 21, 2008, from http://www.himss.org/content/files/VPI_Resolution120920031.pdf

IEEE. (2004, June 17). *Voluntary health care identifier.* Retrieved November 21, 2008 from http://www.ieeeusa.org/policy/positions/healthcareidentifier.html

Internet World Stats. (2008, November 12). *Internet World Stats: Usage and Population Statistics.* Retrieved November 21, 2008, from http://www.internetworldstats.com/stats.htm

Jirgis, J. (2007, July 21). *Online patient access to test results and provider messaging: The technology is ready . . . Is the practice ready?* Paper presented at the 17th Annual Summer Institute in Nursing Informatics, Baltimore, MD.

Kane, B., & Sands, D. Z. (1998). Guidelines for the clinical use of electronic mail with patients. *Journal of the American Medical Informatics Association, 5*(1), 104–111.

Kim, M. J., & Johnson, K. B. (2002). Personal health records: Evaluation of functionality and utility. *Journal of the American Medical Association, 9*(2), 171–180.

Landro, L. (2000, May 26). Tools that can help you keep your own accurate medical files. *Wall Street Journal,* p. B2.

Lecker, R., Armijo, D., Chin, S., Christensen, J., Desper, J., Hong, A. et al. (2007, January 5). *Review of the personal health record (PHR) service provider market.* Retrieved November 21, 2008, from http://www.hhs.gov/healthit/ahic/materials/01_07/ce/PrivacyReview.pdf

Liederman, E. M., Lee, J. C., Baquero, V. H., & Seites, P. G. (2005). The impact of patient-physician web messaging on provider productivity. *Journal of Healthcare Informatics Management, 19*(2), 81–86.

MacDonald, K. (2003, November 18). *Online patient-provider communication tools: An overview.* Retrieved November 21, 2008, from http://www.chcf.org/documents/ihealth/PatientProviderCommunicationTools.pdf

Markle Foundation Connecting for Health. (2003, July 1). *Final report, Personal Health Working Group.* Retrieved November 21, 2008, from http://www.markle.org/downloadable_assets/final_phwg_report1.pdf

National Committee on Vital Health Statistics. (2006, February). *Personal health records and personal health record systems.* Retrieved November 21, 2008, from http://www.ncvhs.hhs.gov/0602nhiirpt.pdf

National Alliance for Health Information Technology. (2008, April 28). *Defining key health information technology terms.* Retrieved November 21, 2008, from http://www.hhs.gov/healthit/documents/m20080603/10_2_hit_terms.pdf

Neame, R. (1997). Smart cards – The key to trustworthy health information systems. *British Medical Journal, 314*(7080), 573–577.

Pizzi, R. (2007). *National Alliance for Health IT endorses voluntary patient identifiers.* Retrieved November 21, 2008, from http://www.healthcareitnews.com/story.cms?id=8305

Ross, S. E., & Lin, C. T. (2003). The effects of promoting patient access to medical records: A review. *Journal of the American Medical Informatics Association, 10*(2), 129–138.

Sands, D. Z. (2004). Help for physicians contemplating use of e-mail with patients. *Journal of the American Medical Informatics Association, 11*(4), 268–269.

Simons, W. W., Mandl, K. D., & Kohane, I. S. (2005). The PING personally controlled electronic medical record system: Technical architecture. *Journal of the American Medical Informatics Association, 12*(1), 47–54.

Sittig, D. F. (2002). Personal health records on the Internet: A snapshot of the pioneers at the end of the 20th century. *International Journal of Medical Informatics, 65*(1), 1–6.

Smart Card Alliance. (2003, September). *HIPAA compliance and smart cards: Solutions to privacy and security requirements.* Retrieved November 21, 2008, from http://www.smartcardalliance.org/pages/publications-hipaa-report

Smart Card Alliance. (2006, February). *Smart card applications in the U.S. healthcare industry.* Retrieved November 21, 2008, from http://www.smartcardalliance.org/newsletter/february_2006/feature_0206.html

Tang, P. C., Ash, J. S., Bates, D. W., Overhage, J. M., & Sands, D. Z. (2006). Personal health records: Definitions, benefits, and strategies for overcoming barriers to adoption. *Journal of the American Medical Informatics Association, 13*(2), 121–126.

Wasson, J. H., Johnson, D. J., Benjamin, R., Phillips, J., & MacKenzie, T. A. (2006). Patients report positive impacts of collaborative care. *Journal of Ambulatory Care Management, 29*(3), 199–206.

CHAPTER 15

The Empowered Consumer

Learning Objectives

After studying this chapter you will be able to:

1. Analyze the effect of consumer empowerment on healthcare.

2. Describe approaches to guiding clients to high-quality Web-based health information.

3. Analyze the effects of health literacy and health numeracy on patient care and teaching.

4. Demonstrate finding and evaluating a Web-based support group for a client with a specific condition.

5. Explore the potential for Web-based health education.

Key Terms

Accessibility	Health Numeracy
Alt Tag	HEDIS
Braille Reader	Image Map
Broadband	Navigation Bar
Consumer Informatics	NCQA
Decision Support	Patient Portal
Dial-up Connection	Plug-in
Electronic Mailing List	Screen Reader
Extranet	Support Group
Flash Animation	URL
Health Literacy	Usability

An imagined dialogue with Socrates in Chapter 13 of the book *Consumer-Driven Healthcare* asks why consumers who can intelligently purchase financial products, cars, and computers cannot do the same with healthcare (Hyde, 2004). The answer given was that they have never been allowed to. In the past, consumers did not have the knowledge that healthcare providers did, which resulted in a culture of paternalism. Patients were expected to accept what was prescribed disregarding cost and were labeled "noncompliant" if they did not. Additionally, there was an underlying assumption on the part of payers and consumers that all healthcare was equal, hence there was no concern about quality or cost.

Spearheaded by many large corporations, who formed the Leapfrog Group to study how they could work together to have an influence on the quality and affordability of healthcare (Leapfrog Group, 2007a), the movement to give consumers more control over how to spend their healthcare dollar is increasing. Much of this progress has been made possible through the use of the Internet and the World Wide Web (WWW). Consumers today can learn about the quality of care provided by many hospitals and find information about diseases that previously was only available to healthcare professionals. This move to consumerism in healthcare will permanently change the face of the healthcare industry (Singh, Hummel, & Walton, 2005). Healthcare providers will need to evolve from being care providers to health and wellness brokers, a role that fits naturally with nursing.

Consumer Informatics

The easy availability of information on the Internet, the push for more cost-effective healthcare, and the desire of many consumers to take more responsibility for their health (Centers for Medicare & Medicaid Services, 2007) has resulted in the development of the subspecialty in healthcare informatics of **consumer informatics**. Its goal is to improve the consumer decision-making processes and healthcare outcomes through the use of electronic information and communication (AMIA Consumer Health Informatics Working Group, 2007). This field is an applied science using concepts from communication, education, behavioral science, and social networking (Houston & Ehrenberger, 2001). It is designed to provide healthcare information to consumers, allow consumers to make informed decisions, promote healthy behaviors and information exchange, and social support to clients. Practitioners analyze consumer needs and information use, and develop ways to facilitate consumers in finding and using health information. They also evaluate the effectiveness of electronic health information and study how this affects public health and the consumer–healthcare provider relationship (Eysenbach, 2000; Lewis, 2007).

It is differentiated from healthcare informatics not by the technology, but by its focus on the consumer, rather than healthcare providers, as end user (Tetzlaff, 1997). The hope is that "intelligent informatics applications" will result in the healthcare information that reaches consumers creating a healthy balance between self-reliance and professional help (Eysenbach, 2000). It is related to all of healthcare informatics because full realization of its potential depends on the features and breadth of information systems. Consumer informatics applications may include interaction with healthcare providers, others may not. Examples include Web sites, information kiosks, blood pressure kiosks, and even personal health records.[1] Consumer informatics applications are part of the move to empower healthcare consumers.

Consumer Empowerment

The term *consumer empowerment* means that patients are provided with enough information so that they can make informed decisions. In other words, they can become consumers or clients, not patients. Patient empowerment got its start in a 1905 U.S. Supreme Court decision that established that patients have the right to know in advance what surgery is going to be performed (Millenseon, 2004). The case resulted from a physician who, believing that the patient would resist, performed a total hysterectomy on an epileptic patient without informing her beforehand. Although that was a beginning, it was another 50 years before a 1957 California Court of Appeals affirmed the right of patients to be told beforehand what procedure would be performed and what the possible adverse effects might be. Further court cases in the 1970s affirmed the rights of patients to be given this information in plain English. Despite this slow beginning we are seeing that today many consumers expect to receive understandable information about their health conditions and be full partners in their healthcare, not passive recipients (Kaplan & Brennan, 2001). They are also beginning to expect to be able to make intelligent decisions about healthcare on the basis of cost and quality.

---

[1] Personal health records are discussed in Chapter 14.

Consumer empowerment was advocated in the first report to the Secretary of Health and Human Services by Dr. Brailer, then National Coordinator for Health Information Technology. He supported the ability of consumers to select healthcare on the basis of their values and information (Brailer, 2004). Consumer empowerment has the ability to affect the rising rate of health plan costs by incorporating economic consequences for low-quality care. It can also improve healthcare by providing consumers with data such as the cost and quality of healthcare services along with information for self-diagnosis and referral to appropriate providers. At the same time, it can preserve the best elements of our present system of clinical support for those who suffer from acute illnesses, injuries, or chronic conditions.

ACCESSING QUALITY OF CARE INFORMATION

In an attempt to control healthcare costs, the U.S. Department of Health & Human Services (HHS) now requires hospitals to report quality indicators. Under the auspices of the Centers for Medicare & Medicaid Services (CMS) and the Hospital Quality Alliance (HQA), this information, which is updated quarterly, is posted on a Web page (Services, 2007). Visitors can see how often a given hospital provides recommended care for heart attack, heart failure, pneumonia, or surgery. The Leapfrog Group also rates hospitals, but they rate different things (Leapfrog Group, 2007b). They look at high-risk treatments for such things as abdominal aortic aneurysm repair, pancreatic resection, and bariatric surgery. They also rate intensive care units (ICUs) on the basis of the use of intensivists, or healthcare providers who have special training in critical care, and the use of computerized provider order entry systems (CPOE). Their site provides information and criteria to use in selecting a hospital as well as the dates that the information used for the rating was submitted. (On their page at http://www.leapfroggroup.org/cp it may be necessary to scroll to the right to see the dates!)

The Healthcare Effectiveness Data and Information Set (**HEDIS**) provides information to consumers and employers that allows them to compare the performance of health plans with other plans and to national or regional benchmarks. HEDIS measures performance in quality of care, access to care, and member satisfaction with the health plan and doctors. HEDIS is used by more than 90% of the U.S. healthcare plans. CMS requires that health maintenance organizations (HMOs) submit data to HEDIS if they provide HMO services for Medicare enrollees. This site was developed and is maintained by the National Committee for Quality Assurance (**NCQA**), which is a private nonprofit corporation dedicated to improving health quality (NCQA Organization, 2007).

Rating of hospitals is in the introductory stage and not yet perfect. Werner and Bradlow (2006) found that current performance measures predict only small differences in risk-adjusted mortality rates. The study authors recommend that more efforts be directed at developing measures more closely linked to patient outcomes. Like any database, what is collected to calculate the ratings determines the results. Even if not perfect, if consumers are to make good decisions about healthcare, providing even this level of information is needed. Expect to see this situation improve as more factors affecting the quality of care are teased out. In any quality study, nurses need to learn what data is being collected and how much of it reflects actual nursing care.

In 1998 the American Nurses Association (ANA) established the National Database of Nursing Quality Indicators™ (NDNQI) (Montalvo, 2007). The goal was to further the development of nursing knowledge "related to factors which influence the quality of nursing care" (Montalvo, 2007). Participation is voluntary, but currently there are over 1,100 U.S. agencies that contribute to the database. Results at this time are not available to consumers but only to participating agencies, but it is an excellent step toward helping nursing to further the quality of care. A primary area of study is the linkage between nurse staffing levels and patient outcomes.

HEALTH PORTALS

A portal is by definition any Web site that offers a wide array of resources and services such as email, forums, a search tool, and links to useful sites. It is the blending of many Internet tools into one useful service. Generally a portal is targeted at a specific population such as professionals in a discipline, healthcare consumers with a specific medical condition, those looking for either general or specific health information, or shoppers for specific products such as baby products.

Health portals are common; many are sponsored by governments. In Canada the government sponsors the Health Canada site (http://www.hc-sc.gc.ca/index_e.html), which has general health information as well as information specific to Canadians. Similar sites are provided by the Australian government (http://www.healthinsite.gov.au/) and the New Zealand government (http://www.nzhis.govt.nz/). The United States government sponsors the National Library of Medicine (http://www.nlm.nih.gov/), Medline Plus (http://www.nlm.nih.gov/medlineplus/), and Pub Med Home (http://www.ncbi.nlm.nih.gov/sites/entrez). Other governments also provide online health information; some of these sites are integrated with general information about the government.

PATIENT PORTALS

Patient portals take the portal concept one step further and individualize the portal using the patient's electronic health record. A patient portal may only offer one-way communication to a patient, but the information will be specific to that patient. An example would be an obstetric portal sponsored by an obstetric clinic that provided prenatal information targeted by the month or week of pregnancy of their patients. This type of personalization of information has been shown to be successful (Doupi & van der Lei, 2002), especially in the care of patients with chronic diseases such as diabetes and heart disease. Most of these systems also contain some type of **decision support** using computerized prompts (Dorr et al., 2007). Some patient portals provide email messaging features, and others provide patients access to their electronic medical record (EMR) (Weingart, Rind, Tofias, & Sands, 2006) similar to a personal health record (PHR), but without access to provider data outside the system. Using patient portals is one way of meeting the needs of clients who today expect more personal attention (Kaplan & Brennan, 2001). They desire the same services that the financial industry provides, namely personalized information that is targeted at them.

In the United Kingdom, NHS Direct (http://www.nhsdirect.nhs.uk/) provides a health portal that, although not tied to a consumer's patient record, provides answers to common questions, has a health encyclopedia, and a self-help decision support guide that helps consumers find out if their symptoms can be managed at home or if advice is needed from an NHS Direct nurse or whether to call an ambulance. This site also allows consumers to send a health inquiry to their healthcare provider and find a local health service. To accommodate the sight impaired, NHS Direct provides a free **screen reader**. Eysenbach (2000) predicted that the professionals who staff this service may evolve to "cyberlicensed professionals," or a healthcare provider who receives specialty education and whose practice is monitored for quality but whose practice is online. In the United States, specially trained nurses in hospitals provide some of these services.

Currently there are many nongovernmental groups that sponsor healthcare portals; some are commercial and some are nonprofit. Before recommending a site, or portal, to a client, it needs to be thoroughly evaluated. Because many portals depend on advertisements for support, special care needs to be taken to ensure that the information and links provided are bias free and complete.

THE DIGITAL DIVIDE

One of the criticisms often leveled against the growing importance of the Internet and Web as a means of dispersing information is that there is

necessarily the best practice (American Society of Anesthesiologists Task Force on Preoperative Fasting, 1999; Brady, Kinn, & Stuart, 2003; RCN Guideline for the multidisciplinary team, 2005).

Whatever your decision about the information, you will need to discuss it further with the client. If the information is from a reliable source and contradicts what you "know," you will need to acknowledge this. This may lead to you discovering that the client has unanswered questions, is scared, needs more understanding of the underlying disease, or just needs more information. In many cases, especially if the information is suspect, working with this client will take a great deal of patience and tact, but it is vitally important in providing care. More troubling can be the clients who have accessed information about their condition, do not discuss it with their healthcare provider, but use it in decisions regarding their treatment. Asking if a client has accessed information about his or her condition on the Web may start a conversation that leads to better understanding on both yours and the client's part.

CYBERCHONDRIACS

The searching by consumers for health information on the Web has led to a new term, "cyberchondriac." The term is a combination of the terms cyber and hypochondria to coin a word that tends to appear pejorative, or implying that a person is obsessive about illness. Researchers at Harris Interactive (2002) say that the term is not pejorative, but indicates a person who has concerns about health and searches for health information on the Web. They believe that this behavior is a positive sign. Although many worry that as the public gets more information from the Web, the healthcare provider–patient relationship will erode, these researchers believe just the opposite. In their 2002-posted survey they reported that 30% of the U.S. online population, 23% in France, 33% in Germany, and 17% in Japan found that online information influenced the discussions they had with their healthcare

provider in a positive manner. They also found that this information affected people's understanding of any health problems they had and improved their health management.

Unfortunately, there are many who imply that cyberchondriacs are those who think they have a given disease because their symptoms match those on an Internet health site (Word Spy, 2000). Although this is possible, it is no more likely that people who use the Web for health information will develop imaginary diseases than those who read about conditions in the popular literature or see health information on television. As a nurse you can influence how patients are affected by any information they have found (from any source) by answering clients' questions about this information and clarifying any misunderstandings. In these discussions always remember, that it is possible that a client may be accurate in self-diagnosis. More than one person has accurately diagnosed himself or herself from Web information.

INTERNET PHARMACIES

The high cost of drugs has forced many people to search for less expensive alternatives on the Web. There are lawful online pharmacies that require a prescription for any medication. However, there are also numerous pharmacies that bypass this practice and allow consumers to purchase medication without a prescription or consultation with a healthcare provider. Additionally, because their only interest is in making a sale, they may sell counterfeit or out-of-date medications, provide the wrong dosage, or sell medications that can create drug reactions. Furthermore, they do not warn purchasers of side effects or the appropriate method of taking a drug. To help your clients avoid the pitfalls of these suspect pharmacies, you should assess their sources for drugs and perhaps have the URL of a few legitimate online pharmacies to share (see Box 15-1). Warn your clients that any online site that does not require a prescription operates outside the law and may send questionable drugs.

Box 15-1 • When Considering Buying Health-Related Items Online

Be wary of extravagant claims about performance or treatment potential. Get all promises in writing and review them carefully before making a payment or signing a contract.

Read the fine print and all relevant Internet links. Fraudulent promoters sometimes bury the disclosures that they are wary of sharing by putting them in very small, fine print or in a location where you are unlikely to find them.

Look for a privacy policy. If you do not see one or if you do not understand it, seriously consider taking your interests elsewhere.

Be skeptical of any company or organization that does not state its name, street address, and telephone number. Web sites should have some form of feedback or contact information available. Check the site out with the local Better Business Bureau or consumer protection office.

Always consult a healthcare professional before altering any current treatment regimen or buying a "cure all" product that claims to treat a wide range of ailments or offers quick cures and easy solutions to serious illnesses.

Reproduced with permission from HIMSS from a White Paper: Marconi, J.E-Health. *Navigating the Internet for health information (Advocacy White Paper)*. Retrieved September 19, 2007, from http://www.himss.org/content/files/whitepapers/e-health.pdf

---

HEALTH LITERACY

The benefit that consumers will gain from all the information available today depends not only on its quality and availability, but also on the ability of the consumer to understand it. Referred to as **health literacy**, it is "the degree to which individuals have the capacity to obtain, process, and understand basic health information and services needed to make appropriate health decisions. It includes the ability to understand instructions on prescription drug bottles, appointment slips, medical education brochures, doctor's directions, consent forms, and the ability to negotiate complex healthcare systems. Health literacy is not simply the ability to read. It requires a complex group of reading, listening, analytical, and decision-making skills, and the ability to apply these skills to health situations" (Sullivan & Glassman, 2007). Health literacy is not static; it varies with context and setting and is not necessarily correlated with years of education or general reading ability. Today, especially in the developed world, health literacy is more important in determining health than the digital divide. It has been reported to be a greater predictor of health than age, income, employment status, level of education, or race (Health literacy: Report of the Council on Scientific Affairs, 1999). When working with clients, either face to face, by phone, or computer, or when designing educational materials, it is necessary to assess their health literacy (see Box 15-2).

HEALTH NUMERACY

Although much of the information that we provide clients is quantitative, for example, laboratory values, medication schedules, a growing body of knowledge demonstrates that clients are not able to fully comprehend or use this information (Ancker & Kaufman, 2007). Understanding a treatment, complying with a medication regime, or making decisions about a dosage of insulin on the basis of a glucosometer require not only health literacy, but also the ability to understand numbers in healthcare directions or information. Called **health numeracy**, it is the ability of a consumer to interpret and act on all numerical information, such as graphical and probabilistic information needed to make effective health decisions. (Golbeck, Ahlers-Schmidt, Paschal, & Dismuke, 2005). It involves the skills necessary to understand quantitative data, the ability to do basic calculations, make sense of numerical information, and enough statistical knowledge to compare knowledge presented with different scales, for

---

Box 15-2 • Skills Needed for Health Literacy

....

Skills Needed for Health Literacy

Patients are often faced with complex information and treatment decisions. Some of the specific tasks patients are required to carry out may include

- evaluating information for credibility and quality,
- analyzing relative risks and benefits,
- calculating dosages,
- interpreting test results, or
- locating health information.

In order to accomplish these tasks, individuals may need to be

- visually literate (able to understand graphs or other visual information),
- computer literate (able to operate a computer),
- information literate (able to obtain and apply relevant information), and

- numerically or computationally literate (able to calculate or reason numerically).

Oral language skills are important as well. Patients need to articulate their health concerns and describe their symptoms accurately. They need to ask pertinent questions, and they need to understand spoken medical advice or treatment directions. In an age of shared responsibility between physician and patient for healthcare, patients need strong decision-making skills. With the development of the Internet as a source of health information, health literacy may also include the ability to search the Internet and evaluate Web sites.

Reproduced from Sullivan, E., & Glassman, P. (2007, July 17). *Health literacy.* Retrieved September 20, 2007, from http://nnlm.gov/outreach/consumer/hlthlit.html

---

example, probability, proportion, and percent, and the ability to interpret graphs.

Even deciding the timing of medication dosages can be difficult without health numeracy skills, more so when several medications with different time schedules are involved. Lack of numeracy has been associated with poor outcomes in anticoagulation control and history of hospitalization in asthma (Ancker, Senathirajah, Kukafka, & Starren, 2006). This lack can also create difficulties when consumers have to calculate dosages as well as make it difficult for consumers to effectively use quantitative information to make health decisions and guide health behaviors. Studies have found that many consumers lack basic probability skills, making it difficult to decide the numerical probability of heads or tails in a coin toss, or to convert between percentages and whole numbers. Even determining which the larger risk is, 1%, 5%, or 10%, can be difficult. This lack will create difficulty in making informed healthcare decisions or in granting permission to be in a research study.

The ability to comprehend numerical information is greatly influenced by the presentation, whether in a questionnaire, document,

graphic, or medical device (Ancker et al., 2006). Some of these difficulties can be surmounted with a systematic design of information that takes these factors into consideration. For example, using stick figures to demonstrate 1 in 10 is usually clearer than using percentages or a graph. Although graphs appear to be an appealing alternative to using numbers, interpreting them often requires more effort and cognitive skills.[4]

HELPING CONSUMERS TO USE COMPUTERS

In your career, unless you work in an undeveloped country through the Peace Corp or missionary work, you will eventually find yourself both assisting consumers to find healthcare information and evaluating this information. Given that telemonitoring and computer support or education is becoming an accepted care protocol, you may be called on to help a client install or learn to use such a device. Box 15-3 lists some of the steps that are needed to accomplish this.

---

[4] See Chapter 9 for a more thorough discussion of graphs.

Box 15-3 • Installing a Technology Device in a Client's Home

Evaluate the technical skills of the new user.

Assess whether the physical skills needed to use the device are present.

Before visiting describe the physical needs of the device and ask the patient to select a location in the home.

Rehearse the installation steps so you are thoroughly comfortable with the skills.

Use a checklist to ensure a 100% installation.

Use everyday terms when teaching how to use the device. Explain any terms such as login, password, etc. before using them.

Explain how the device functions and any idiosyncrasies.

If there is a lag time between starting the device and it becoming functional, prepare the client.

If there are sounds such as one would find with a dial-up connection, describe and demonstrate.

Thoroughly teach the consumer how to use the device, including several return demonstrations.

Provide written instructions. As you teach you may want to revise these or highlight those where difficulties occur.

Have technical support available for follow-up instructions.

Adapted from Dauz, E., Moore, J., Smith, C. E., Puno, F., & Schaag, H. (2004). Installing comptuers in older adults' homes and teaching them to access a patient education Web site. *Computers, Informatics, Nursing: CIN, 22*(5), 266–272.

Internet Support Groups

Even in the earliest days of the Internet, clients sought online support, information, and decision support (Houston & Ehrenberger, 2001). The idea of **support groups**, however, is not new: They date back to the early 1900s as a method of working with persons suffering from psychological disorders (Klemm et al., 2003). Today, much of this support has migrated to the Internet. A 2005 survey by the Pew Internet Research Institute revealed that at least 36 million U.S. citizens were members of a support group (Ramie and Horrigan, 2005). Support groups may be a combination of the patient portals discussed above, a message board, email list, chat room, or any combination of these. Help given is similar to that in face-to-face groups.

Online support has been used in many areas including cancer support (Klemm & Wheeler, 2005), chronic illness (Cudney & Weinert, 2000; Weinert, Cudney, & Winters, 2005), Huntington's Disease (Coulson, Buchanan, & Aubeeluck, 2007), social support and health education (Hill & Weinert, 2004), caregivers (Brennan, 1994), breast cancer (Sharf, 1997;

Shaw et al., 2006), perinatal loss (DiMarco, M., & T, 2001), disability issues (Finn, 1999), menopause (Giordano, 1995), and alcoholism (Finfgeld, 2000). The GriefNet Support (http://www.griefnet.org/) offers support to persons suffering the loss of a loved one. Their discussion groups are varied and oriented to the type of loss. They include, but are not limited to, support groups for those affected by terrorist attacks, widows or widowers, parents who have lost children, children who have suffered a loss, and those who are grieving the loss of a pet. Many of their lists are moderated by trained counselors.

Support groups vary in sponsorship and the quality of the information. Some are sponsored by healthcare providers who will answer questions. Others are moderated; that is, nothing is posted that is not first vetted by the moderator. In groups sponsored by laypersons or organizations the moderator may or may not be healthcare providers. Most groups allow open discussion and permit members to answer each other's questions just as they do with listservs. Although there may be erroneous information posted, especially in non-moderated groups, often other members quickly correct the misinformation (Lewis,

2001). This, however, is a topic that needs research (Klemm et al., 2003).

For those groups that allow open discussion, membership is usually free and the discussion open for anyone to read, but one must join to post questions or replies. As a nurse you may want to find one or two such groups in your specialty so you can refer your patients to them. Before referring a patient, assess the group carefully. If referring a client to a group that is moderated, check the qualifications of the moderator. If the group is not moderated, look at the archives, and follow the list for a while before recommending it. You may even wish to join the group. A search by a Web search tool for the name of the disease or condition followed by "forum" or "support group" will yield many groups for that condition. For all support groups you should remind clients that the information they receive may be only an opinion; it may be an informed opinion, or it may not be (Martin & Youngren, 2000). If information posted is a new treatment, the client needs to do further research using qualified medical sites such as those sponsored by the government, or formal organizations whose reputation in the field is known. Just as with Web information, it may be necessary to teach clients how to evaluate information they find in these groups. Additionally, unless users are very familiar with the reputation of the site sponsor and the provider, they should be careful about giving their names, email addresses, and especially their credit card numbers.

MESSAGE CONTENT ANALYSES

Message content from support groups has been an object of study for several researchers.

Klemm, Reppert, & Visich (1998) analyzed messages from a colorectal cancer **electronic mailing list** and found many positives for this type of support. Members of this group exchanged information, gave and sought encouragement and support, related personal experiences, gave thanks, and provided humor and prayer for each other. Coulson and coworkers (2007) studied messages posted to a Huntington Disease support forum. They found

that informational and emotional support were the most frequent messages. Messages also often included teaching or referral to experts; those containing esteem support and tangible assistance were the least frequently posted, although they were not uncommon. Reminders that the group was available for support were also a common topic. These findings match the results of several other studies (Klemm et al., 2003; Klemm & Wheeler, 2005). Klemm (2008) analyzed messages from support groups for long-term cancer survivors and categorized them as focusing on information exchange, symptomatology, or frustration with healthcare providers. Results from studies of online groups are generally positive (Lewis, 1999; Lewis, Gundwardena, & El Saadawi, 2005).

ADVANTAGES FOR ONLINE SUPPORT GROUPS

There are many advantages to online groups over face-to-face groups. They are asynchronous, members can participate at any time of day or night, and membership is not restricted by time, geography, or space (Coulson et al., 2007). Messages to the group can be carefully thought out and edited before posting, which relieves participants from having to think on their feet, or having one or two people monopolize the conversation. Further, members come from diverse perspectives, which provides varied experiences, opinions, and information sources. Lastly, the provision of being anonymous, which many groups are, is helpful in discussing sensitive or potentially embarrassing situations. A drawback may be that the individual may be spending too much time online alone (Lewis, 2001) when the company of others is needed.

Provider-Sponsored Groups

It is not unusual for healthcare providers, particularly hospitals or healthcare organizations to provide online support for those for whom they provide care. These sites generally require passwords to enter, and sometimes specialized software. One of the earliest groups of this type was the ComputerLink project (Brennan, 1994). This service provided support to caregivers of those with Alzheimer's disease. Users could access the service at a time convenient to them and select from a variety of services. It was designed to link these individuals to each other and to a nurse moderator. Services were provided in three areas – communication, information, and decision support. Communication involved private email, a forum where members could post and read messages, and a question and answer session. The information module provided an electronic encyclopedia and over 200 indexed screens about selected illnesses, home care, and social services. In decision support, users were guided through an analysis process using their own words and preferences to making choices consistent with their values (Brennan, 1996).

Another example, although much different in scope, is the Comprehensive Health Enhancement Support System (CHESS). Instead of being designed for just one group, this service is a vendor-supported service, developed at the University of Wisconsin-Madison's Center for Health Systems Research and Analysis and provided to member organizations. Several major health organizations in the United States and Canada are using it. This product is provided to member healthcare agencies that can either use it as is or tailor it for their use. Using both computer-based and human support, the service is designed to help individuals cope with a health crisis or medical concern (What is Chess, 2006). Currently CHESS supports modules on breast cancer, HIV, prostate cancer, and heart disease with easily accessed, reliable, and organized health information in easily understood language. They also provide social support and decision-making and problem-solving tools. The service includes discussion groups, which are monitored by a nurse who is provided by the member agency (A.L. Salner, personal communication, October 1, 2007, CHESS). This person can provide expert advice or contact a physician for more help if needed. Participants must download and install the specialized software; then they use it in the privacy of their own home. If a potential user does not have a computer, it may be loaned one for a year. Research has demonstrated that CHESS has improved participants' quality of life, reduced demands on physician time, and sometimes, the cost of care. It has also been found that it can be used equally, although in different ways, by all people regardless of gender, income, age, or education. (See Box 15-4 for a description by a nurse of her experience with CHESS.)

Box 15-4 • One Nurse's Experience with CHESS

CHESS, for our breast cancer patients, was absolutely my best informatics experience. Our program was implemented in the early '90s, and many thought the older women would not participate because of the technology. They were wrong! We had age 40 to age 85 burning up the wires, which filled an obvious need. Any newly diagnosed breast cancer patient was eligible to join at no charge. We held fundraisers to defray costs of the technology and were able to purchase refurbished computers from local vendors at very low cost. The biggest problem then was to find space for the computer in patient homes.

The stories they shared were great and pretty intimate. We all got laughs when one woman, sunning herself after mastectomy, shared that she forgot she was bare chested (sans breast) and answered the door to the UPS guy who nearly fainted. I don't know how much of it was really true – but we all belly-laughed.

It was interesting that a lot of the activity occurred very late at night (I assume when their spouses and family were taken care of and asleep). Many developed intense support structures with the other patients as well as our designated CHESS nurse. At our annual "Celebrate Life" survivor event – many of them came to meet each other under the big tent in the cancer center parking lot.

I highly recommend programs like this that provide reliable information, support from those in the same situation, and access to healthcare providers when needed.

Deborah Ariosto, MS, RN, October 2007.

TABLE 15-1 • *Comparison of Some Methods of Web Page Creation*

Method	Advantage	Disadvantage
Office application program	Minimal knowledge required beyond use of the program itself	Creates "dirty code" that is difficult to maintain outside the application program used to create it. Often creates a very large file. May not provide needed flexibility
WSYWIG authoring tool	Fairly easy to use, but requires some learning Has many features such as methods to ensure that page designs are identical, spell check, and creating forms.	Some use nonstandard code that requires special software on the server
HTML editor	Provides good flexibility	Steep learning curve
Coding HTML	Provides good flexibility	Very steep learning curve

full-function screen readers are best for those who are visually limited. The bundled screen readers, however, can help a visually challenged person install a screen reader. Besides translating text to speech, some screen readers can send information to a **Braille reader**, a device that is placed near or under the keyboard. Users then use their fingers to "read" the information.

Screen readers have vastly improved from earlier times when they could not interpret tables; however consideration for alternatives to using the mouse, such as keyboard commands for navigation, are still necessary. Because screen readers cannot "read" a graphic, when graphics are used text alternatives (called **Alt tags**) should be used. The tag should either provide textual information that can be used by a screen reader in place of the illustration, or provide a link to a site that explains the illustration in text. If there are clickable spots on a graphic (known as an **image map**), make provisions for finding these links using a screen reader. **Navigation bars** or graphical bars across the top of a page that provide multiple choices also need alternative methods of access. Some sites provide this with a list of links for all these choices on the bottom of the page. Because this print is not intended for humans to read, it can be in a small font.

Color Blindness.   Color blindness, which affects 12% of males of European descent and about 0.5% of females, can interfere with reading a Web page, while the hearing disabled will miss any audio. Seizures can be caused in people with photosensitive epilepsy by blinking items on a Web page or quick changes from dark to light (Epilepsy Fact Sheet, 2008).

Usability

When health Web sites were evaluated by both **usability** experts and older adults they agreed on many problem areas such as difficulty finding drop-down menus, too much information on the screen, too small a font size, lack of instructions for playing video, and navigation problems (Nahm, Preece, Resnick, & Mills, 2004). To prevent these difficulties, it is imperative that a healthcare Web site be evaluated by other than the creators. When one designs a site, one is so familiar with its ins and outs that one tends to believe that everyone else is too. They are not! Thus, although healthcare providers can evaluate the Web content, it requires members of the intended audience to do thorough usability testing.

Some suggestions for making Web sites easier to understand are the use of adequate contrast between text and background, intuitive navigation, the avoidance of distracting features and the inclusion of users in the design phase. Designers should also gauge the health literacy and health numeracy skills of the intended audience. Additionally, content should be written clearly and simply in a language the user will understand. For example, medical terminology is appropriate when the audience is healthcare providers, but not with laypeople.

Summary

The field of consumer informatics has developed along with the empowerment of the healthcare consumer. Consumers now have access to information that was previously unavailable such as the quality of care provided by hospitals and disease conditions. As consumers use the Web more and more to find information, their relationship with healthcare providers will change. As this continues, greater attention will be paid to health literacy and health numeracy and how they affect the teaching of clients. Nurses will find themselves directing clients to high-quality Web sites and providing guidance in selecting support groups as another way to improve healthcare. Using patient portals healthcare agencies will provide more consumer education, some of it restricted to and individualized for their clients. These portals will also serve as a marketing device. Whether you ever design a Web site or part of a patient portal, you can still use the design principles as well as those in health literacy and health numeracy in evaluating the appropriateness of Web sites for clients and other educational materials. Helping clients to use computers, whether this involves installing a computer, referring clients to places where they can be taught basic computer skills, or providing help in finding and installing items to assist the physically challenged to use a computer will become more frequent nursing interventions.

APPLICATIONS AND COMPETENCIES

1. The fact that only slightly more than half the people who have found health information on the Web have discussed the information with their healthcare provider is somewhat disturbing (Cline & Haynes, 2001). Discuss the following statements.
   a. Patients are leery of discussing information with their healthcare providers versus just listening to advice.
   b. Patients are afraid to take a more participatory approach to their healthcare.
   c. Reluctance to discuss information found on the Web affects an individual's decision to follow the provider's treatment plan.
2. You are the nurse in a surgical center. A patient arrives with a printout of the complications of the surgery for which he or she is scheduled. Additionally, the information advocates alternative treatments. Discuss how you can work with this patient.
3. Find a high-quality Web-based support group for a client with a condition of your choosing and outline how you would teach the client about this site.
4. You are a nurse practitioner. The clinic where you are working wants to institute providing an online support group. What things would you want to consider?
5. Evaluate a Web-based health site.

REFERENCES

American Society of Anesthesiologists Task Force on Preoperative Fasting. (1999). Practice guidelines for preoperative fasting and the use of pharmacologic agents to reduce the risk of pulmonary aspiration: Application to healthy patients undergoing elective procedures [Electronic version]. *Anesthesiology, 90,* 896–905. Retrieved November 20, 2008 from http://www.asahq.org/publicationsAndServices/NPO.pdf

AMIA Consumer Health Informatics Working Group. (2007, July 12). *Mission statement.* Retrieved November 19, 2008, from http://www.amia.org/mbrcenter/wg/chi/

Ancker, J. S., & Kaufman, D. (2007). Rethinking health numeracy: A multidisciplinary literature review. *Journal of the American Medical Informatics Association, 14*(6), 713–721.

Ancker, J. S., Senathirajah, Y., Kukafka, R., & Starren, J. B. (2006). Design features of graphs in health risk communication: a systematic review. *Journal of the American Medical Informatics Association, 13*(6), 608–618.

Brady, M., Kinn, S., & Stuart, P. (2003, August 15). *Cochrane summary: Preoperative fasting for adults to prevent perioperative complications.* Retrieved November 19, 2008, from http://www.cochrane.org/reviews/en/ab004423.html

Brailer, D. J. (2004, July 21). *The decade of health information technology: Delivering consumer-centric and information-rich health care.* Retrieved November 20, 2008, from http://www.ihi.org/IHI/Topics/Improvement/ImprovementMethods/Literature/DecadeofHealth InformationTechnology.htm

Brennan, P. F. (1994). ComputerLink: An innovation in home care nursing. In S. Grobe & E. S. P. Pluyter-Wenting (Eds.), *Nursing informatics: An international overview for nursing in a technological era: Proceedings of the Fifth IMIA International Conference on Nursing Use of Computers and Information Science, San Antonio, TX, June 1994* (p. 407). Amsterdam, Netherlands: Elsevier.

Brennan, P. F. (1996). The future of clinical communication in an electronic environment. *Holistic Nursing Practice, 11*(1), 97–104.

Center for Personal Assistance Service. (2005). *US disability data table from the 2005 American community survey.* Retrieved November 19, 2008, from http://pascenter.org/state_based_stats/state_statistics_2005.php?state=us

Centers for Medicare & Medicaid Services. (2007, October 26). *Summary of responses to an industry RFI regarding a role for CMS with personal health records.* Retrieved November 19, 2008, from http://www.cms.hhs.gov/PerHealthRecords/Downloads/SummaryofPersonalHealthRecord.pdf

Cline, R. J. W., & Haynes, K. M. (2001). Consumer health seeking on the Internet: The state of the art. *Health Education Research, 16*(6), 671–692.

Coulson, N. S., Buchanan, H., & Aubeeluck, A. (2007). Social support in cyberspace: A content analysis of communication within a Huntington's disease online support group. *Patient Education and Counseling, 68*(2), 173–178.

Cudney, S. A., & Weinert, C. (2000). Computer-based support groups: Nursing in cyberspace. *Computers in Nursing, 18*(1), 35–43.

DiMarco, M. A., Menke, E. M., & McNamara, T. (2001). Evaluating a support group for perinatal loss. *MCN: American Journal of Maternal/Child Nursing, 26*(3), 135–140; 160–161.

Dorr, D., Bonner, L. M., Cohen, A. N., Shoai, R. S., Perrin, R., Chaney, E., et al. (2007). Informatics systems to promote improved care for chronic illness: A literature review. *Journal of the American Medical Informatics Association, 14*(2), 156–163.

Doupi, P., & van der Lei, J. (2002). Towards personalized Internet health information: The STEPPS architecture. *Medical Informatics and the Internet in Medicine, 27*(3), 139–151.

Epilepsy fact sheets photosensitive epilepsy. Retrieved November 20, 2008, from http://www.epilepsytoronto.org/photo.html

Eysenbach, G. (2000). Recent advances: Consumer health informatics [Electronic version]. *British Medical Journal, 320*(7251), 1713–1716. Retrieved November 19, 2008 from http://www.bmj.com/cgi/reprint/320/7251/1713

Eysenbach, G., & Kohler, C. (2002). How do consumers search for and appraise health information on the world wide web? Qualitative study using focus groups, usability tests, and in-depth interviews. *British Medical Journal, 324*(7337), 573–577.

Finfgeld, D. E. (2000). Resolving alcohol problems using an online self-help approach: Moderation management. *Journal of Psychosocial Nursing and Mental Health Services, 38*(2), 33–38; 48–49.

Finn, J. (1999). An exploration of helping processes in an online self-help group focusing on issues of disability. *Health and Social Work, 24*(3), 220–231.

Giordano, N. A. (1995). An investigation of the health concerns of the menopause discussion group on Internet. Columbia University Teachers College [Abstract]. *CINAHL.*

Golbeck, A. L., Ahlers-Schmidt, C. R., Paschal, A. M., & Dismuke, S. E. (2005). A definition and operational framework for health numeracy. *American Journal of Preventive Medicine, 29*(4), 375–376.

Harris Interactive. (2002, June 11). *4-Country survey finds most cyberchondriacs believe online healthcare information is trustworthy, easy to find and understand.* Retrieved November 20, 2008, from http://www.harrisinteractive.com/news/newsletters/healthnews/HI_HealthCareNews2002Vol2_Iss12.pdf

Harris Interactive. (2007, July 31). *Harris Poll shows number of "Cyberchondriacs" – adults who have ever gone online for health information– increases to an estimated 160 million nationwide.* Retrieved November 20, 2008, from http://www.harrisinteractive.com/harris_poll/index.asp?PID=792

Health literacy: Report of the Council on Scientific Affairs. (1999). Ad Hoc committee on health literacy for the council on scientific affairs, American Medical Association. *Journal of the American Medical Association, 281*(6), 442–557.

Hill, W. G., & Weinert, C. (2004). An evaluation of an online intervention to provide social support and health education. *Computers, Informatics, Nursing: CIN, 22*(5), 282–288.

Houston, T. K., & Ehrenberger, H. E. (2001). The potential of consumer health informatics. *Seminars in Oncology Nursing, 17*(1), 41–47.

Hyde, S. S. (2004). Dialogues with Socrates. In R. E. Herzlinger (Ed.), *Consumer-driven health care* (pp. 262–269). San Francisco, CA: Jossey-Bass.

Kaplan, B., & Brennan, P. F. (2001). Consumer informatics supporting patients as co-producers of quality. *Journal of the American Medical Informatics Association, 8*(4), 309–316.

Klemm, P. (2008). Late effects of treatment for long-term cancer survivors: Qualitative analysis of an online support group. *Computers, Informatics, Nursing: CIN, 26*(1), 49–58.

Klemm, P., Bunnell, D., Cullen, M., Soneji, R., Gibbons, P., & Holecek, A. (2003). Online cancer support groups: A review of the research literature. *Computers, Informatics, Nursing: CIN, 21*(3), 136–142.

Klemm, P., Reppert, K., & Visich, L. (1998). A nontraditional cancer support group. The Internet. *Computers in Nursing, 16*(1), 31–36.

Klemm, P., & Wheeler, E. (2005). Cancer caregivers online: Hope, emotional roller coasters, and physical/emotional/psychological responses. *Computers, Informatics, Nursing: CIN, 23*(1), 38–45.

Leapfrog Group. (2007a). *How & why Leapfrog started.* Retrieved November 19, 2007, from http://www.leapfroggroup.org/about_us/how_and_why

Leapfrog Group. (2007b). *Leapfrog hospital ratings.* Retrieved November 20, 2008, from http://www.leapfroggroup.org/cp

Lewis, D. (1999). Computer-based approaches to patient education: A Review of the Literature. *Journal of the American Medical Informatics Association, 6*(4), 272–282.

Lewis, D. (2007). Evolution of consumer health informatics. *Computers, Informatics, Nursing: CIN, 25*(6), 316.

Lewis, D., Gundwardena, S., & El Saadawi, G. (2005). Caring connection: Developing an internet resource for family caregivers of children with cancer. *Computers, Informatics, Nursing: CIN, 23*(5), 265–274.

Lorence, D. P., & Greenberg, L. (2006). The Zeitgeist of online health search: Implications for a consumer-centric health system. *Journal of General Internal Medicine, 21*(2), 134–139.

Martin, S. D., & Youngren, K. B. (2000). The virtual community: Helping patients use internet support groups. *Home Healthcare Nurse, 18*(5), 333–335.

McLeod, S. D. (1998). The quality of medical information on the Internet: A New Public Health Concern. *Archives of Ophthalmology, 116*(12), 1663–1665.

Millenseon, M. L. (2004). The role of providers. In R. E. Herzlinger (Ed.), *Consumer-driven health care* (pp. 549–560). San Francisco, CA: Jossey Bass.

Montalvo, I. (2007, September 30) The National Database of Nursing Quality Indicators™ (NDNQI®. *OJIN: The Online Journal of Issues in Nursing, 12*(3). http://www.nursingworld.org/MainMenuCategories/ANAMarketplace/ANAPeriodicals/OJIN/TableofContents/Volume122007/No122003Sept122030/NursingQualityIndicators.aspx

Nahm, E.-S., Preece, J., Resnick, B., & Mills, M. E. C. (2004). Usability of health Web sites for older adults. *Computers, Informatics, Nursing: CIN, 22*(6), 326–334.

NCQA Organization. (2007). *About NCQA.* Retrieved November 20, 2008, from http://web.ncqa.org/tabid/65/Default.aspx.

Nielsen, J. (1999). *Designing web usability.* Indianapolis, IN: New-Riders Publishing.

Ozdemir, Z. D., Akçura, M. T., & Altinkemer, K. (2006). Second opinions and online consultations. *Decision Support Systems, 42*, 1747–1758.

Pandolfini, C., & Bonati, M. (2002). Follow up of quality of public oriented health information on the world wide web: Systematic re-evaluation. *British Medical Journal, 324*(7337), 582–583.

Pew Internet Research Institute. (2005). *A decade of adoption: How the Internet has woven itself into American life.* Retrieved September 21, 2007, from http://www.pewinternet.org/pdfs/internet_status_2005.pdf

Prady, S. L., Norris, D., Lester, J. E., & Hoch, D. B. (2001). Expanding the guidelines for electronic communication with patients: Application to a specific tool. *Journal of the American Medical Informatics Association, 8*(4), 344–348.

Raimie, L., & Horrigan, J. (2005). (Pew Report) *Internet: The mainline streaming of online life.* Retrieved November 20, 2008, from http://www.pewinternet.org/pdfs/Internet_Status_2005.pdf

RCN Guideline for the multidisciplinary team. (2005, November). *Perioperative fasting in adults and children.* Retrieved November 20, 2008, from http://www.rcn.org.uk/publications/pdf/guidelines/PerioperativeFastingAdultsandChildren-002779.pdf

Services, U. S. D. H. a. H. (2007, July 27). *Hospital compare.* Retrieved November 20, 2008, from http://www.hospitalcompare.hhs.gov/

Sharf, B. F. (1997). Communicating breast cancer on-line: support and empowerment on the Internet. *Women & Health, 26*(1), 65–84.

Shaw, B. R., Hawkins, R., Arora, N., McTavish, F., Pingree, S., & Gustafson, D. H. (2006). An exploratory study of predictors of participation in a computer support group for women with breast cancer. *Computers, Informatics, Nursing: CIN, 24*(1), 18–27.

Singh, S. P., Hummel, J., & Walton, G. S. (2005). Consumer driven healthcare: Strategic, operational, and information technology implications for today's healthcare CIO. *Journal Healthcare Information Management, 19*(4), 49–54.

Sullivan, E., & Glassman, P. (2007, July 17). *Health literacy.* Retrieved November 20, 2008, from http://nnlm.gov/outreach/consumer/hlthlit.html

Tetzlaff, L. (1997). Consumer informatics in chronic illness. *Journal of the American Medical Informatics Association, 4*(4), 285–300.van Dijk, J. A. G. M. (2006). Digital divide research, achievements and shortcomings. *Poetics, 34*(4–5), 221–235.

Weinert, C., Cudney, S., & Winters, C. (2005). Social support in cyberspace. *Computers, Informatics, Nursing: CIN, 23*(1), 7–14.

Weingart, S. N., Rind, D., Tofias, Z., & Sands, D. Z. (2006). Who uses the patient internet portal? The PatientSite experience. *Journal of the American Medical Informatics Association, 13*(1), 91–95.

Werner, R. M., & Bradlow, E. T. (2006). Relationship between Medicare's hospital compare performance measures and mortality rates. *Journal of the American Medical Association, 296*(22), 2694–2702.

What is CHESS? (2006). Retrieved November 20, 2008, from https://chess.wisc.edu/chess/projects/about_chess.aspx

Word Spy. (2000, June 9). *Cyberchondriac.* Retrieved November 20, 2008, from http://www.wordspy.com/2000/06/cyberchondriac.html

Interoperability at the International and National Level

Learning Objectives

After studying this chapter you will be able to:

1. Define the three types of interoperability: technical, semantic, and process.

2. Describe a general pattern for developing standards.

3. Explain the need for standards.

4. Interpret the effects on nursing of standards at all levels of healthcare.

5. Identify organizations involved in setting standards at the international and national level.

Key Terms

Electronic Health Record

Electronic Medical Records

Granular

Health Information Exchange (HIE)

Interface Terminology

Interoperability

Mapping

Process Interoperability

Protocol

Reference Terminology

Reference Terminology Model

Regional Health Information Organization (RHIO)

Semantic Interoperability

Standards

Technical Interoperability

An individual who is unknowingly infected with a very contagious stage of a new type of flu walks into the international airport in Houston on his way to Seattle. While standing in the baggage check line, he starts up a conversation with the woman behind him, who will be in New Delhi in 24 hours. After checking his bag, he goes to the security line and there strikes up a conversation with a man who will be in San Diego in 4 hours. He is early for his plane, so he goes into one of the airport bars and starts talking to a woman who will be in Tokyo in 8 hours and then in Shanghai in 48 hours.

This is the world in which we live today. Jet travel makes all points on the globe vulnerable to any communicable disease. Thus, health is an international concern. To protect ourselves, it is necessary that countries be able to exchange information pertaining to contagious diseases with other countries, and within their own frontiers. This demands that healthcare systems be interoperable between communities, regionally and internationally. To achieve this goal, data transfer and reception must be interoperable.

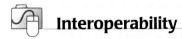

Interoperability

Simply stated, **interoperability** is the ability of two or more systems to pass information and to use the exchanged information. In healthcare, interoperability means that healthcare information systems can transmit and receive information within and across organizational boundaries to provide the delivery of optimum healthcare to individuals and communities (HIMSS, 2005). This can be achieved either by adhering to accepted interface and terminology **standards** or by using a third system that seamlessly integrates the two systems. An example of the first is the protocols that made the Internet possible plus the use of a standardized terminology. The use of an "rtf" file to "translate" a file from one word processor to another is similar to the second.

There are three different types of interoperability: technical (sometimes referred to as functional), semantic, and process. **Technical interoperability** refers to the transmission and reception of information so that it is useful (Gibbons et al., 2007). When systems are technically interoperable, they are able to receive usable data from a different system and send it to that system. This type of functionality enables data from a laboratory system to be exchanged with the pharmacy system. It also enables data from one healthcare provider to be exchanged with another.

Semantic interoperability takes this one step further. In semantic interoperability, not only is the information transmitted so that it is understandable, but at its highest level, messages exchanged by two computers can be automatically interpreted and acted on by the computers without human intervention. How effective semantic interoperability is depends on the interaction between algorithms, the data used in the message, and the terminology used to designate that data.

Process interoperability is a rather new concept that is intended to coordinate work processes. It has been referred to as workflow management and is related to integrating computer systems into work settings. It includes such considerations as a user-friendly system and effectiveness in actual use. Those of you who have had experience with healthcare systems that did not have interoperability are aware of the extra work and difficulties that this creates such as duplicate data entry and having to remember login and password for different systems.

Standards

Interoperability is not possible without standards. Imagine a situation in which each community sets its own time. In one city it would be 1:00 p.m., whereas in another 30 miles east it would be 1:30 p.m., and in still another 40 miles northwest it would be 12:30 p.m. This is more or less the situation that existed until the mid-19th century. Of course, then time was not so important and the population was not as mobile. When the railroads arrived, it became necessary to standardize the time. In the United States, the railroads set the first time zones, which eventually were adopted by state governments. As the industrial revolution progressed, it became necessary to have more and more standards if the economy was to prosper. Some of you may remember the Beta v. VHS videotape standards conflicts. This standard of course was decided in the market place. In healthcare, leaving standard setting to the market place has resulted in great inefficiencies.

A standard is an agreement to use a given protocol, term, or other criterion that has been formally approved by a nationally or internationally recognized professional trade association or governmental body. Standards are vital to communication as well as in other areas.

ISO has technical committees in many fields. The committee for health informatics is technical committee number 215 (TC 215). Each technical committee has working groups within it whose work is done by volunteers. Under TC 215, a working group of volunteers from many nations established a nursing **reference terminology model**. Known as ISO 18104:2003, some of the potential uses for this standard include facilitating the documentation of nursing problems (diagnosis) and actions (interventions) in electronic information systems, and the creation of nursing terminologies in a form that will make **mapping** (a form of matching concepts from one standardized terminology with those having similar meaning from another) among them easier. Box 16-2 explains ISO naming conventions.

INTERNATIONAL ELECTRICAL COMMISSION

The IEC creates and publishes international standards for all electrical-related technologies (IEC, 2008). These standards serve as the basis for national standards in international contracts. The objectives include efficiently meeting the goals of a global market, assessing and improving the quality of products covered by its standards, and contributing to the improvement of human health and safety. In the healthcare field, their standards include medical electrical equipment and magnetically induced currents in the human body.

ASTM INTERNATIONAL

Although ASTM International was originally created in 1898 as the American Society for Testing and Materials for the purpose of addressing the frequent rail breaks in the ever-growing railroad industry, it has become international (Wikipedia, n.d.). However, it still exerts a dominant influence among standards developers in the United States. Membership is by request, not by appointment or invitation, and anyone interested in its activities may join. Although there is no enforcement policy, in 1995, the United States passed the National Technology Transfer and

---

Box 16-2 • Naming Conventions in ISO

The name "International Standards Organization" is often incorrectly used instead of "International Organization for Standardization," possibly because the "acronym" for the organization is "ISO." The acronym is not a true acronym, but the word "ISO" derived from the Greek word "isos," which means equal. This name is used in all languages (international). If an acronym that represented the words "International Organization for Standardization" had been used as a basis for an acronym, there would be different acronyms in each language – not a standard!

Standards developed by ISO groups, or standards groups with whom they are collaborating, are named using first the acronyms of the organization involved in creating them, followed by a five-digit number indicating the number of the standard, and a four-digit number indicating the year in which they were published, and the title that describes the subject (Wikipedia). The title, however, is often omitted. For example, "ISO

18104:2003 Health informatics – Integration of a Reference Terminology Model for Nursing" is the full title of standard number 18104 that was developed in 2003. Often, however, it is just referred to as ISO 18104:2003.

Technical committees carry the prefix "TC." TC 215 refers to ISO's technical committee on health informatics.

When there is a subject that is still under development, but for which there is a possibility that in the future there may be a standard, a technical specification may be issued. In these cases, the prefix ISO/TS is used. The prefix ISO/TR indicates a technical report.

From International Standards Organization. (2006, September 29). *Discover ISO*. Retrieved November 20, 2008, from http://www.iso.org/iso/about/discover-iso_isos-name.htm; From Wikipedia. (2007, October 7). *International Organization for Standardization*. Retrieved November 20, 2008, from http://en.wikipedia.org/wiki/ISO

Advancement Act, which requires the federal government to comply with privately developed standards when possible. Other governments, both local and worldwide, also reference ASTM standards as well as corporations doing international business.

International Healthcare Standardization

Both the modern world with jet airplanes, which created a need for the quick dissemination of health data concerning disease outbreaks, and a new focus on healthcare outcomes have made the need for the collection of healthcare data more visible. Healthcare data collection is not new; the first healthcare data collections occurred in the 16th century in England. Known as the London Bills of Mortality, parish clerics recorded and published weekly the number of burials. These were used as an early warning system against the Bubonic Plague epidemics that decimated the European population several times in the 16th and 17th centuries. In 1570, baptisms were added to the statistics. Because the data was found to be valuable, in 1629 the London government took over responsibility for collecting this data. In the last half of the 17th century, John Gaunt used this data to make some insightful observations on the patterns of mortality (Chute, 2000). These efforts led to the modern concepts of epidemic and endemic disease patterns and the beginning of the disciplines of population-based epidemiology and the modern study of data terminologies and classifications.

INTERNATIONAL CLASSIFICATION OF DISEASE

Developing the standards needed to implement these efforts, however, was slow. It was 1900 before there was any agreement in medicine on standardizing even the causes of death. This standardization was the Bertillion Classification List of the Causes of Death, which had been presented by Jacques Bertillion in 1893 at the International Statistical Institute (ISI) in Chicago. It was accepted in 1900 and became the International Classification of Disease version 1 (ICD-1). At that time it was recommended that the classification be revised every 10 years to ensure that the system remained current with medical practice advances. The Mixed Commission, a group composed of representatives from the ISI and the Health Organization of the League of Nations, had responsibility for the updates through ICD-6, a version, which added morbidity and mortality conditions. The World Health Organization (WHO) took on this responsibility in 1948 and has published revisions ever since.

The ICD classification of codes, whose full name is the International Statistical Classification of Diseases and Related Health Problems, is a detailed listing of known diseases and injuries (Nation Master, 2005). It is used worldwide for mortality and morbidity statistics. Every known disease (or group of related diseases) is described, classified, and assigned a unique code. In the United States, the ICD codes are part of the standards required for use by the Health Insurance Portability and Accountability Act (HIPA).

The current version of ICD codes is ICD-10, but WHO has begun discussions and initiated the workgroup to address development of ICD-11. The United States, however, continues to use ICD-9 despite the fact that most of the rest of the world uses ICD-10 (Nation Master, 2005). The National Committee on Vital and Health Statistics (NCVHS) has forwarded several recommendations to the Office of the Secretary of Health and Human Services (HHS) to move to ICD-10. In August 2008, HHS proposed that by October 1, 2011, the United States adopt ICD-10. Because it will require reconfiguring many information systems, this change will be expensive; consequently the date will probably be pushed forward.

The ICD codes, which are now used worldwide for morbidity and mortality statistics, and in the United States for billing, were the first efforts to standardize healthcare data for both national and international use. Unless you are a nurse practitioner, it is unlikely that you will be asked to code a diagnosis, yet you need to be aware of these classifications. Although useful for statistical purposes, the ICD codes are not **granular** enough, that is, they do not capture enough data, to be used to document patient care in either **electronic medical records** (EMRs) or **electronic health records** (EHRs).

INTERNATIONAL CLASSIFICATION OF FUNCTIONING, DISABILITY AND HEALTH (ICF)

The International Classification of Functioning, Disability and Health (ICF) falls under the auspices of the WHO. The ICF codes are used to measure health and disability for both individuals and populations (World Health Organization, n.d.). These codes focus on the impact of disease on the human experience including social and environmental factors. They are relatively new, having been officially endorsed only at the Fifty-fourth World Health Assembly in 2001. The ICF classification acts to complement ICD-10 to provide information regarding functional status (Wikipedia, 2007). These codes are organized around body structure, functions, activities of living, and participation in life situations. They also contain information on severity and environmental factors. Although not intended as a measurement tool, these codes place emphasis on function rather than disease. They were designed to be relevant across all cultures, age groups, and genders making them useful with heterogeneous populations.

HEALTH LEVEL SEVEN

Although the Health Level Seven (HL7) organization is based in the United States in Ann Arbor, Michigan, and is accredited by ANSI, it is an international community of healthcare subject matter experts and information scientists (What is HL7?). Founded in 1987

(Wikipedia), it is an all-volunteer, not-for-profit organization that sets standards for functional and semantic interoperability for electronic healthcare data (Patterson, 2003). Its mission is "to create standards for the exchange, management and integration of electronic healthcare information" (HL7, n.d.).

The term "HL7" is derived from the position of these standards in the seven-level open systems interconnect (OSI) model. This model is a seven-layer model for implementing protocols that pass control from the bottom layer up the hierarchy to the top level (Webopedia, n.d.). The number seven in the name means that the standards being set are at the seventh, or the highest, messaging level of this model. At this level, the standards include those that address the terminology used, and at the functional level, identification of participants, electronic data exchange negotiations, and data exchange structuring. The lower six levels focus on the physical and logical connections between machines, systems, and applications. In very basic terms, HL7 standards are concerned with what data will be transmitted, for example, vital signs, demographic information, and so on, and what terminology and **protocols** will be used to transmit the data. There are many HL7 standards, each addressing a different portion of this process. The HL7 organization is very involved in setting standards for the EHR; several nurses are involved in these efforts.

DIGITAL IMAGING AND COMMUNICATIONS IN MEDICINE

Another standards development group that has ties to both national (National Electrical Manufacturers Association [NEMA]) and international groups (IEC) is the Digital Imaging and Communications in Medicine (DICOM) organization. DICOM sets and maintains standards that allow electrical transmission of digital images. Their work makes it possible to exchange medical digital images worldwide. Thus, if you have an MRI done in London, England, and your doctor is in Chicago, Illinois, using the DICOM standards, it is possible for him/her to see the image in Chicago just as if it had been done in his/her radiology department.

COMITÉ EUROPÉEN DE NORMALISATION

The European Committee for Standardization, or Comité Européen de Normalisation (CEN), is a collaboration of standards bodies in Europe. CEN has strong ties to the European Union politics, and common European legislation makes approved CEN standards national standards (Goossen, 2003). The standardization of healthcare informatics is the province of the CEN/Technical Committee 251. Several standards that are relevant to nursing have been developed including the PrENV 14032, health informatics systems of concepts for nursing. This standard focuses on the application of nursing terminology within electronic messages and healthcare information systems.

INTERNATIONAL HEALTH TERMINOLOGY STANDARDS DEVELOPMENT ORGANISATION (IHTSDO)

The International Health Terminology Standards Development Organisation (IHTSDO), a new standards development organization created in 2007, is the outgrowth of the joint development of the Systematized Nomenclature of Medicine – Clinical Terms (SNOMED CT) between the National Health Service (NHS) in the United Kingdom and the College of American Pathologists (CAP) in the United States (International Health Technology Standards Development Organisation, n.d.). Working with representatives of nine countries, this organization was created to promote more rapid development and worldwide adoption of standard clinical terminology for EMRs and EHRs.

They acquired SNOMED CT from the CAP and will maintain, further develop, and assure its quality. Coordination among these nations should "create new opportunities for international collaboration in research and public health, provide a better basis for making standard terminology available in developing countries, and align SNOMED CT with key international public health standards, including those produced by the World Health Organization" (SNOMED International, 2007). IHTSDO is incorporated as a not-for-profit commercial society in Denmark.

DEVELOPING STANDARDS

The work of the above standard setting organization groups is done by small groups of volunteers within the organization. Group members are experts in their field who become members of a working or technical group of an organization, which has been delegated to set a specific standard. Anyone (including you) who is an expert in an area, and has the time to devote to this endeavor, can be a member of a working or technical standard setting group. The first step in setting a standard is identification of a need. In the second step, the group, which has been designated to define the standard, must state in operational terms what the standard will accomplish and how it will do this. The third step is the longest, and one that will be returned to more than once. It involves a lengthy period of discussion, study of the literature, communication with those outside the group who will be affected by the standard, and possibly even research. Eventually, terms or specifications will be defined, which will be tested in the fourth step. If the number of parties who will be affected by the new standard is large, the proposed standard will be opened for public comment. If the comments indicate problems, the group will return to the third step to refine the standard. If the changes from the original are many, the new proposal will again be submitted for public comment. Eventually, members of the group will vote on the standard. If they vote in favor, it is submitted to the parent organization for endorsement. If accepted by the parent organization, it then becomes a standard with a prefix indicating the group that set the standard and a number specific to that standard. When updates are needed, steps three and four are repeated.

Billing Terminology Standardization

In the United States, over 20% of medical costs are in administration. Efforts to standardize government payments for hospital care were initiated in the 1980s with the diagnosis-related groups (DRGs) and modifications to the ICD codes. Following the lead of the government, many private insurers have also adopted them. Efforts to standardize billing for alternative healthcare such as nurse practitioners has led to the Alternative Billing Codes (ABCs).

ICD-CM

The ICD codes discussed above, although useful for certain statistical and billing purposes, present a one-dimensional view of disease because they focus only on etiology. To make the codes useful in billing, modifications were added. Currently in the United States, ICD-9-CM (clinical modifications) are used along with ICD-9-PCS for procedure codes (The Advanced Medical Technology Association, 2007) for billing purposes. There are efforts to make the base ICD codes for these modifications ICD-10.

DIAGNOSIS-RELATED GROUPS (DRGS)

The diagnosis-related groups, sometimes referred to as the "daily rate guide," or simply DRGs, is a standardized patient classification system developed in the early 1980s under the auspices of the former Health Care Financing Administration (HCFA), now called the Centers for Medicare and Medicaid Services (CMS). Originally intended as a review of the use of hospital resources, they have since become a system for prospective payment. Under this system, patients are categorized into groups for which studies have determined the average hospital resources patients in those groups consume. Hospitals are then paid based on the category into which a patient is classified. The criteria used for assigning categories include medical diagnosis, surgery,

complications, and usually age (Sermeus, Weber, Chu, Fischer, & Hunstein, 2006). Every patient is assigned a single DRG, a process that is done by a computer program called a "grouper" based on information from the uniform hospital discharge data set (UHDDS). More than one DRG system is in use beyond the main one used by CMS for Medicare patients. For example, the All Patient Refined – DRG (APR-DRG) is used to represent non-Medicare patients. Other countries, such as Australia, Belgium, Germany, France, the Netherlands, and Austria have developed their own DRG system based on the U.S. system. In some countries with nationalized health systems, these codes are used to determine hospital funding.

Although nursing is resource intensive, the DRGs do not do well in capturing this information. They tend to determine costs based predominantly on medical diagnoses and medical services consumption. It has been shown that adding nursing data to the DRG data can improve the DRG cost analysis by about 80%. One attempt to fix this was a project at Yale University (Doble, Curley, Hession-Laband, Marino, & Shaw, 2000). Using the APR-DRG, which has subclass ratings for severity of illness from 1 as minor to 4 as extreme, they sorted the DRGs into categories of high and not-high users of nursing resources. They used patient characteristics such as stability and complexity and added nursing competencies required to care for patients with a given DRG such as clinical judgment, collaboration, and systems. They then designated that DRG on a scale of 1 (low) to 6 (high) for nursing care requirements. This created a system that allowed nursing care to be articulated to payers in meaningful terms.

THE HEALTHCARE COMMON PROCEDURE CODING SYSTEM (HCPCS)

The Healthcare Common Procedure Coding System (HCPCS), established in 1978, "is a standardized coding system that is used primarily to identify products, supplies, and services not included in the CPT codes, such as ambulance services and durable medical equipment, prosthetics, orthotics, and supplies" (Centers for Medicare and Medicaid Services, 2008). It is intended to supplement the Current Procedural Terminology (CPT)® codes that were developed by the American Medical Association (AMA) in 1966. These are updated annually (American Medical Association, 2008).

ALTERNATIVE BILLING CODES

The ABC Coding Set or ABCs support electronic and paper claims processing for providers, healthcare payers, managed care organizations, and affiliated organizations. The system is intended for use in coding and support documentation for reimbursement by third parties for alternative medicine, nursing, and other nonmedical healthcare interventions. The codes are designed to fit into existing standard claim forms, software applications, and information management systems (ABC Coding Solutions). These codes permit accurate reimbursement for clinical nurse specialists, nurse midwives, nurse practitioners, licensed practical nurses, registered midwives, and registered nurses, and seven other healthcare specialists. Although not the typical terminology that the American Nurses Association (ANA) recognizes, these codes are one of the 13 standardized terminologies recognized by the ANA because they support nursing practice by providing a standardized method of billing for nurse practitioners.

U.S. Efforts Toward an Electronic Healthcare Record

The Institute of Medicine's Report "*To Err is Human*," resulted in the open realization that efforts toward improving the delivery of healthcare in the United States were needed. Creating electronic healthcare records has become one of the pillars of these endeavors.

OFFICE OF THE NATIONAL COORDINATOR FOR HEALTH INFORMATION TECHNOLOGY (ONC)

In May 2004, the president of the United States called for an EHR for Americans by 2014. To further this aim he established the position of National Coordinator for Health Information Technology (U.S. Department of Health and Human Services, 2007). This person heads the Office of the National Coordinator for Health Information Technology (ONC), which advices the Secretary of the U.S. Department of HHS on issues pertaining to the use of health information technology, and coordinates the health information technology policies and programs for HHS. Together with other executive branches, the ONC is responsible for developing, maintaining, and directing the implementation of the strategies for health information technology in both public and private healthcare sectors, and for providing advice to the Office of Management and Budget (OMB) about specific federal health information technology programs.

AMERICAN HEALTH INFORMATION COMMUNITY (AHIC)

The National Alliance for Health Information Technology (Alliance)

The American Health Information Community Successor (AHIC Successor) was originally known as the American Health Information Community (AHIC). As AHIC it was a federal advisory committee of public and private sector leaders representing a broad spectrum of healthcare stakeholders established to make recommendations to the Secretary on how to accelerate the development of interoperable EHRs (U.S. Department of Health and Human Services, 2007). In 2008, this group made the transition to a private/public partnership outside government and is now known as AHIC Successor. Besides members from the private sector, the Secretaries of HHS and Veterans Affairs serve as federal liaisons to the Board of Directors, and the National Coordinator for Health Information Technology is an ex officio federal liaison to the organization (AHIC Successor, 2008). The original AHIC delivered an initial set of four "breakthrough" recommendations to the Secretary of HHS in the areas of consumer empowerment, chronic care, EHRs, and biosurveillance. The new group will continue working toward national health information technology interoperability.

REGIONALIZATION EFFORTS

National Health Information Infrastructure (NHII)

The National Health Information Infrastructure (NHII) is the building block of the Nationwide Health Information Network (NHIN). This concept began to emerge in the United States about 20 years ago (Detmer, 2003). In 2000, NCVHS issued a report that stated the seven basic elements needed for the NHII (National Committee on Vital Health Statistics, 2001) (see Box 16-3). The NHII can be defined as an infrastructure for information and communication that connects users to each other, to information, and to analytical tools, all of which enable the management and generation of knowledge (Detmer, 2003). Clinical and public health information systems are the chief

building blocks of the NHII. They capture, store, organize, and present data about medical care and population health status that are crucial for routine work, problem solving, planning, and emergency response. It is envisioned that the NHII will strengthen the four pillars of healthcare: personal health management, healthcare delivery, public health, and research. It will enable national interoperability of all healthcare systems.

Nationwide Health Information Network (NHIN)

Achievement of the NHII will make the NHIN possible. This is envisioned as a network that allows health information to follow the consumer and be available for clinical decision making at any location (HHS). It will also support secondary use of healthcare information for the purpose of improving health of both individuals and communities. The NHIN is seen by the Office of the National Coordinator as a "network of networks," built out of state and regional health information exchanges (HIEs) and other networks to support the exchange of health information. Benefits that are envisioned from the NHIN are mentioned in Box 16-4. It will make possible a true EHR in which data

---

Box 16-3 • Basic Elements of the NHII

Values – The appropriate use of data, information, and knowledge in support of optimal health and quality of life for all Americans.

Practices and relationships – Facilitation of health information and knowledge flow both within and between healthcare organizations, community organizations, physicians, consumers, public health professionals, researchers, and policymakers.

Laws and regulations – A framework for how health-related businesses and individuals may use healthcare information, and for the reporting of information considered vital for public health.

Privacy – Legislation to specify the conditions under which personal health information may be collected, stored, and shared, as well as penalties for abuses.

Standards – For core data sets, classifications and terminologies, uniform identifiers, comparable methods for data collection and reporting, data access, disclosure and confidentiality, and data transmittal.

Technology – Network backbones such as the Internet, the World Wide Web, and other electronic communications that are interoperable.

Systems and applications – The ability for cross-system data exchange and enhancement of multimedia and geospatial capacities.

From National Committee on Vital Health Statistics. (2001, November 15). *A strategy for building the National Health Information Infrastructure.* Retrieved November 20, 2008, from http://aspe.hhs.gov/sp/NHII/Documents/NHIIReport2001/default.htm

---

Box 16-4 • Benefits of NHIN

- Standards-based, secure data exchange nationally.
- Improvements in the coordination of care information among hospitals, laboratories, physicians' offices, pharmacies, and other providers.
- The availability of appropriate information at the time and place of care.
- Secure and confidential consumers' health information.
- Consumers able to manage and control their PHRs and have access to their health information from EHRs and other sources.

- The reduction of risks from medical errors and the delivery of appropriate, evidence-based medical care.
- Lower healthcare costs resulting from correcting inefficiencies, preventing medical errors, and providing complete patient information at the point of care.
- A more effective marketplace, greater competition, and increased choice through accessibility to accurate information on healthcare costs, quality, and outcomes.

Based on HHS. *Nationwide Health Information Network (NHIN): Background*. Retrieved November 20, 2008, from http://www.hhs.gov/healthit/healthnetwork/background/

---

from many different sources is available from a given location.

Regional Health Information Organizations (RHIO) and Health Information Exchange(HIE)

The terms **Regional Health Information Organization** (RHIO – pronounced "Rio") and **Health Information Exchange** (HIE) have been used interchangeably (HIMSS, n.d.), although there are now definitions that differentiate them. The Alliance defines HIE as the electronic exchange of health-related information between organizations using agreed standards, protocols, and other criteria (National Alliance for Health Information Technology, 2008). A RHIO is an organization that governs the electronic exchange of health-related information among healthcare stakeholders within a geographic area. RHIOs are, as the name implies, regional, sometimes just a community, but they may also cover a large area that is not necessarily confined to state lines. The original concept dates to the 1990s when a few Community Health Information Networks were started (Overhage, Evans, & Marchibroda, 2005), but the idea then failed. How a RHIO is set up and funded and the services it provides differ with each RHIO.

RHIOs follow one of three models: a co-op model, the federated model, or a combination (hybrid) model (Gater, 2005). In the co-op model, the member hospitals have an overrid-

ing reason such as a need to share resources or to collaborate. In the federated model, strong health systems, which may or may not share their master patient index, join together, and share data from their electronic patient records. The hybrid model merges both models. Of the three, the federated model is the most technologically advanced.

There are currently quite a few RHIOs that are operational, with quite a few communities in the development process. Currently, one of the most successful is the Indiana Health Information Exchange, which was formed in 2005. It was an outgrowth of the 1996 Regenstrief Institute's Indiana Network for Patient Care, which shared data between hospital emergency departments (Solomon, 2007). Five hospital systems and many medical practices in the Indianapolis area were the first participants in the enlarged system, which was renamed the Indiana Network for Patient Care (INPC). These hospitals and medical practices share laboratory, pathology, radiology, EKG reports, and participate in public health reporting and clinical decision support.

Unfortunately, there are RHIOs that have failed. One difficulty is that they provide most of the benefits to patients and payers who do not pay for the RHIO, or pay a disproportionately small share (Conn, 2007). Some other difficulties include a lack of usability for healthcare providers and the unwillingness of participants to collaborate because of rivalries and mistrust. The same difficulties that caused the failure of the CHINs: issues about data ownership, inadequate buy-in, lack of trust, and a need for control (Overhage et al., 2005), and funding are also seen in failed RHIOs.

An early successful RHIO that failed was the Santa Barbara County Care Data Exchange, Inc. (SBCCDE), which was launched in 1998 with a grant from the California Healthcare Foundation (California Health Care Foundation, n.d.). It was a nonprofit, public utility designed to enable the sharing of patient health information between authorized users, including care givers and patients. It also provided access to laboratory results, radiology images and reports, clinical notes, and medications. Using a "peer-to-peer" network, when requested, a patient's information was collected from disparate sources. Despite its early success, SBCCDE folded in December 2006 (Miller & Miller, 2007). There were several reasons why it failed including the "lack of a compelling business case, distorted economic incentives, passive leadership among participants, vendor limitations and software delays, and due to a variety of factors, the venture's poor momentum and credibility" (Miller & Miller, p. 2).

It is important to realize that a RHIO is a business and must be structured and organized as such (Gater, 2005). Technology is the least important factor. Gaining collaboration between stakeholders for information sharing requires give and take, and trust. RHIOs cannot be pushed down from the national level, but must be built from local areas and gradually enlarged to include other communities or RHIOs. Before a RHIO can start, it is necessary to define what it will accomplish and then develop a strategy. Other tasks involve defining standards that all must follow and making technology decisions.

Beyond gaining collaboration, there remain many challenges for RHIOs. One of the biggest is determining who has a right to access information and how this will be controlled (Gater, 2005). There are technical barriers that include accuracy, security control, performance, scale, and nonstandardized data. Additionally, measures to ensure that information is matched with the correct patient must be developed, tested, and checked. This is complicated by the need to match patient information stored in different systems that may use a different name or identifier for the same patient and makes a very good case for a national unique patient identifier.

State Level Health Information Exchange Consensus Project (SLIECP)

The State Level Health Information Exchange Consensus Project (SLIECP) can be seen as an effort to facilitate the development of RHIOs. It is sponsored by the ONC and led by the American Health Information Management Association (AHIMA), Foundation of Research and Education (Foundation of Research and Education of American Health Information Management Association, 2007). SLIECP was established as part of the efforts to create the NHIN. The organizations that this project is designed to support are public-private collaborations that involve state governments in an effort to achieve statewide goals for quality and cost-effective healthcare. These statewide organizations are designed to be grassroots efforts, to encourage collaborative roles, bridge institutional and sector divides, build social capital, and foster statewide collaboration.

SYSTEM STANDARDIZATION EFFORTS

To make regional records possible, it is necessary for the data that goes into the records to be standardized and for systems used in these records to be interoperable. At the national level in the United States, there are many efforts underway to accomplish these efforts. Some are involved with standardizing EHR systems, others with terminology. The relationships between all of these groups and international groups varies from one group using the recommendations of another to a very few that are hierarchical. Most of the relationships involve such things as having a member of one organization take part in

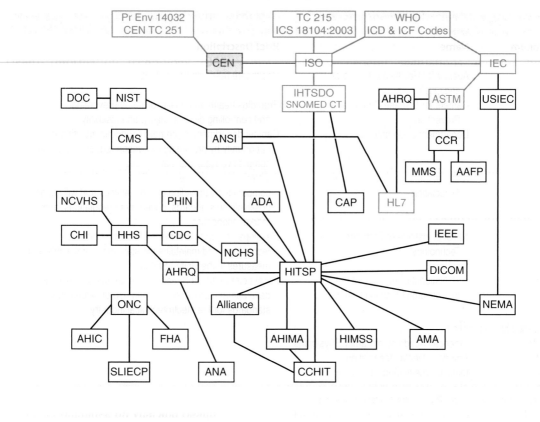

Figure 16-1 • Some relationships between standards organizations.

another, or other types of cooperative relationships. The diagram in Figure 16-1 is an attempt to show these relationships, which in some ways is more of a network, but there is no attempt to define the type of relationship. It looks confusing and it can be! What is important is that standards that will affect nursing are being promulgated. Table 16-1 describes the groups in the diagram that are not discussed in this chapter.

Health Information Technology Standards Panel (HITSP)

One of the groups that will have the most visible impact on nursing is the Health Information

Technology Standards Panel (HITSP). Like AHIC Successor, this is a cooperative partnership between the public and private sectors. They are responsible for designating standards that will be used in the structure and transmission of healthcare information; the standards that will affect how nursing and others document care, including the nursing and healthcare terminologies that will be acceptable. This multi-stakeholder, volunteer group operates under a contract administered by the ONC. HITSP was created in 2005 to reconcile the standards from various standards development organizations to enable the NHIN and health information interoperability (American

Although some of these express concepts particular to a specific discipline (those for nursing will be examined in the next chapter), there are many that are interdisciplinary. It is essential, however, for users to be able to find all the information related to a given concept in all machine-readable sources such as clinical records, databases, biomedical literature, and various directories of information sources. To meet this need, in 1986 the National Library of Medicine (NLM) began an ongoing effort to develop the Unified Medical Language System (UMLS). This project involves internal research and input not only by the NLM but also from the AMA, the ANA, and governmental agencies such as the Agency for Health Care Policy and Research (AHCPR) and the Institute of Medicine (Lindberg, 1995). The UMLS is intended to facilitate the retrieval of machine-readable biomedical information. It is not designed to be a terminology (Chen, Perl, Geller, & Cimino, 2007), but to map concepts from different terminologies so that related biomedical information can be located. The UMLS is intended as a **reference terminology**, not an **interface terminology**, or one that is used to enter data.

The UMLS contains 1.3 million concepts from more than 100 existing biomedical vocabularies and classifications and has grown to become the largest collection of medical terms (Chen et al., 2007). It includes concepts from all the currently ANA-recognized terminologies that support nursing practice. The UMLS concepts "are not optimized for particular applications, but can be applied [for finding information] in systems that perform a range of functions involving one or more types of information, e.g., patient records, scientific literature, guidelines, and public health data" (National Library of Medicine, 2006).

The UMLS consists of three different, but related, types of information: the Metathesaurus, Semantic Network, and the SPECIALIST Lexicon and Lexical Programs. The Metathesaurus is a large vocabulary database with information about health-related concepts, their names, and the linkages between them. The semantic network provides consistent categorization of the Metathesaurus concepts, including the categories that may be assigned to the concepts, and defines relationships between the semantic types. The SPECIALIST Lexicon provides information needed for the SPECIALIST Natural Language Processing System (NLP). It contains many biomedical terms along with the information needed by the SPECIALIST NLP. The future of the UMLS is envisioned to link information from EHRs with the biomedical literature.

Effect on Nursing and Patient Care

The decisions from the different HIT initiatives and the standards they set will affect nursing. These standards will be used in the EMR of the future and will determine what and how nurses document patient care. These decisions will determine the information that secondary analysis of the data will provide, which will determine national healthcare policy. Without nursing participation, the data will be unlikely to represent the contribution of nursing to patient care or provide national healthcare policy that is in the best interest of the patient/client.

Summary

Standards make commerce possible. From the light bulb you buy to the railroads, there are standards both nationally and internationally. The technology that is used to care for patients has also met standards. In information standards, healthcare is still in its infancy, particularly in electronic information standards. Currently there are many systems that are not interoperable with other systems. This situation prevents early identification of epidemics and serious drug side effects as well as contributing to errors in patient care.

Data input into computers will become the healthcare records of the future; if this data is to be useful, it must meet standards. Professional organizations at the international and national level, as well as governments have recognized this problem, and are working to overcome it. Healthcare, however, is very complex and composed of many different stakeholders and disciplines, which further complicates this problem. The standards that are developed and adopted will determine what is viewed as important in healthcare and will have a great effect on nursing and healthcare policy.

The information in a chapter of this sort, because it is tied to the politics of healthcare, is changeable. Every effort has been made to make this current at the time of its going to press.

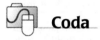

Coda

August, 2025.
The epidemic in the beginning of this chapter was avoided. Cooperation of the international community allowed data on the various outbreaks of flu to be collected at the time and place of origin and preventative measures be undertaken.

APPLICATIONS AND COMPETENCIES

1. In your own words, describe interoperability and its three subtypes.
2. Working with two or three others, arrive at some standards for something simple like entering a classroom or opening a book that could be interpreted by a computer.
3. Interview, in person or by email, a local person who is involved in a regional, national, or international standards setting group.
4. Using the Web, investigate further the activities of HITSP or CCHIT, or another of the standards setting groups. Employ the principles of evaluating Web sites for use seen in Chapter 11.
5. Describe the function of the Unified Medical Language System.

REFERENCES

ABC Coding Solutions. *What's in it for you.* Retrieved November 20, 2008, from http://www.alternativelink .com/ali/abc_codes/wiify.asp

AHIC Successor. (2008). Retrieved November 20, 2008, from http://www.ahicsuccessor.org/hhs/ahic.nsf/ index.htm

American Medical Association. (2008, November 13). *CPT® code information and education.* Retrieved November 20, 2008, from http://www.ama-assn.org/ ama/pub/category/3884.html

American National Standards Institute. (2006, November 1). *Standards panel delivers interoperability specifications to support Nationwide Health Information Network.* Retrieved November 20, 2008, from http://www.ansi.org/ news_publications/news_story.aspx?menuid=7& articleid=1361

California Health Care Foundation. (n.d.). *Santa Barbara County Care Data Exchange.* Retrieved November 20, 2008, from http://www.chcf.org/documents/ihealth/ SantaBarbaraFSWeb.pdf

Centers for Disease Control and Prevention. *National Electronic Disease Surveillance System.* Retrieved November 20, 2008, from http://www.cdc.gov/nedss/

Centers for Medicare and Medicaid Services. (2005, December 12). *OASIS overview.* Retrieved November 20, 2008, from http://www.cms.hhs.gov/OASIS/

Centers for Medicare and Medicaid Services. (2008, November 12). *HCPCS background information.* Retrieved November 20, 2008, from http://www .cms.hhs.gov/MedHCPCSGenInfo/

Chen, Y., Perl, Y., Geller, J., & Cimino, J. J. (2007). Analysis of a study of the users, uses, and future agenda of the UMLS. *Journal of the American Medical Informatics Association, 14*(2), 221–231.

Chute, C. G. (2000). Clinical classification and terminology: Some history and current observations [From a paper delivered in 1999 at AMIA 1999]. *Journal of the American Medical Informatics Association, 7*(3), 298–303.

Conn, J. (2007, August 30). RHIO experts talk problems, future of movement. *Modern Healthcare.* Retrieved November 20, 2008, from http://modernhealthcare.com/ apps/pbcs.dll/article?AID=/20070830/FREE/308290018

Health Information Technology. *Data & technical standards: Other standards activities.* Retrieved November 20, 2008, from http://www.hhs.gov/healthit/standards/other/

Detmer, D. E. (2003). Building the national health information infrastructure for personal health, health care services, public health, and research. *BMC Medical Informatics and Decision Making, 3*(1), 1–12 [Available at http://www.biomedcentral.com/1472-6947/1473/1471.pdf].

Doble, R. K., Curley, M. A. Q., Hession-Laband, E., Marino, B. L., & Shaw, S. M. (2000). Using the synergy model to link nursing care to diagnosis-related groups [Electronic version at http://www.certcorp.org/certcorp/certcorp.nsf/ edcfc72ba47aaa708825666b708820064bdcf/f708825660 cbf708110168a672488256904005dc672488256904002a 672488256904006?OpenDocument]. *Critical Care Nurse, 20*(3), 86–92.

Federal Health Architecture (FHA). (2006, August 29). Retrieved November 20, 2008, from http://www.hhs.gov/ fedhealtharch/index.html

Foundation of Research and Education of American Health Information Management Association. (2007, September 28). *State level health information exchange: Roles in ensuring governance and advancing interoperability.* Retrieved March 24 November 20, 2008, from http://www.slhie.org/Docs/FinalReportPart1.8.pdf

Gater, L. (2005, July 18). *The RHIO world.* Retrieved November 20, 2008, from http://www.fortherecordmag.com/archives/ftr_071805p16.shtml

Gibbons, P., Arzt, N., Burke-Beebe, S., Chute, C., Dickinson, G., Flewelling, T., et al. (2007, February 7). *Coming to terms: Scoping interoperability for health care.* Retrieved November 20, 2008, from http://www.hln.com/assets/pdf/Coming-to-Terms-February-2007.pdf

Goossen, W. T. F. (2003, June 25–28). *Standards, there are so many, which ones should we nurses choose?* Paper presented at the NI 2003 Post Congress Workshop, Mangaratiba, Rio de Janeiro, Brazil.

Health Information Technology. *Certification Commission for Healthcare Information Technology (CCHIT).* Retrieved November 20, 2008, from http://www.hhs.gov/healthit/certification/cchit/

Healthcare Standards Landscape. *Relationships with organizations for HITSP – Healthcare Information Technology Standards Panel (ANSI).* Retrieved March 24, 2008, from http://hcsl.sdct.nist.gov:8080/hcsl/index.html

HHS. *Nationwide Health Information Network (NHIN): Background.* Retrieved November 20, 2008, from http://www.hhs.gov/healthit/healthnetwork/background/

HIMSS. (2005, June 9). *Interoperability definition and background.* Retrieved November 20, from https://www.himss.org/content/files/interoperability_definition_background_060905.pdf

HIMSS. (2007). *What is HITSP?* Retrieved November 20, 2008, from http://www.himss.org/ASP/topics_hitsp.asp

HIMSS. (n.d.). *RHIO/HIE.* Retrieved November 20, 2008, from http://www.himss.org/ASP/topics_rhio.asp

HL7. (n.d.). *HL7 mission statement.* Retrieved November 20, 2008, from http://www.hl7.org/about/hl7mission.htm

IEC. (2008). *Mission and objectives.* Retrieved November 20, 2008, from http://www.iec.ch/about/mission-e.htm

International Health Technology Standards Development Organisation. (n.d.). *History.* Retrieved November 20, 2008, from http://www.ihtsdo.org/about-ihtsdo/history/I

International Organization for Standardization. (2008). *About ISO.* Retrieved November 20, 2008, from http://www.iso.ch/iso/en/aboutiso/introduction/index.html

Lindberg, D. A. B. (1995). The UMLS knowledge sources: Tools for building better user interfaces. In N. Lang (Ed.), *Nursing data systems: The emerging framework* (pp. 151–159). Washington, DC: American Nurses Publishing.

Miller, R. H., & Miller, B. S. (2007, August). *Santa Barbara County Care Data Exchange: Lessons learned.* Retrieved November 20, 2008, from http://www.chcf.org/documents/chronicdisease/SantaBarbaraLessonsLearned.pdf

Nation Master. (2005). *International statistical classification of diseases and related health problems.* Retrieved November 20, 2008, from http://www.nationmaster.com/encyclopedia/International-Statistical-Classification-of-Diseases-and-Related-Health-Problems

National Committee on Vital Health Statistics. (2001, November 15). *A strategy for building the National Health Information Infrastructure. Information for health.* Retrieved November 20, 2008, from http://aspe.hhs.gov/sp/NHII/Documents/NHIIReport2001/default.htm

National Library of Medicine. (2006, May 19). *About the UMLS Resources*®. Retrieved November 20, 2008, from http://www.nlm.nih.gov/research/umls/about_umls.html

Office of the National Coordinator for Health Information Technology. (2005, June 1). *Consolidated health informatics.* Retrieved November 20, 2008, from http://www.hhs.gov/healthit/chi.html

Overhage, J. M., Evans, L., & Marchibroda, J. (2005). Communities' readiness for health information exchange: The national landscape in 2004. *Journal of the American Medical Informatics Association, 12*(2), 107–112.

Patterson, G. (2003). *Health Level Seven (HL7).* Retrieved November 20, 2008, from http://healthinfo.med.dal.ca/HL7Intro/963/992/992.html

Public Health Information Network. (n.d.). *Detailed definition of PHIN.* Retrieved November 20, 2008, from http://www.cdc.gov/phin/about.html

Secretary of Health and Human Services. (2004, January 13). *Charter National Committee on Vital and Health Statistics.* Retrieved November 20, 2008, from http://www.ncvhs.hhs.gov/charter07.pdf

Sermeus, W., Weber, P., Chu, S., Fischer, W., & Hunstein, D. (2006). The DRG imperative: Overview and nursing impact. In C. Weaver, C. W. Delaney, P. Weber, & R. L. Carr (Eds.), *Nursing and informatics for the 21st century: An international look at practice, trends and the future* (pp. 231–245). Chicago, IL: Healthcare Information and Management Systems Society.

SNOMED International. (2007, January 15). *SNOMED International collaborating to create International Standards Development Organization.* Retrieved November 20, 2008, from http://www.snomed.org/news/documents/snomed_sdo.pdf

Solomon, M. R. (2007). Regional health information organizations: A vehicle for transforming health care delivery? *Journal of Medical Systems, 31*(1), 35–47.

The Advanced Medical Technology Association, AHIA, American Medical Informatics Association and Medical Devices Manufacturers Association. (2007, July 7). *Summary of joint position on adoption of ICD-10.* Retrieved November 20, 2008, from http://ahima.org/ICD10/Documents/MicrosoftWord-ICD-10StatementApproved7-18-2007.pdf

National Alliance for Health Information Technology. (2008, April 28). *Defining key health information technology terms.* Retrieved November 20, 2008, from http://www.hhs.gov/healthit/documents/m20080603/10_2_hit_terms.pdf

U.S. Department of Health and Human Services. (2007). *Health information technology initiative major accomplishments: 2004–2006.* Retrieved November 20, 2008, from http://www.hhs.gov/healthit/news/Accomplishments2006.html

Webopedia. (n.d.). *The 7 layers of the OSI model.* Retrieved November 20, 2008, from http://webopedia.internet.com/quick_ref/OSI_Layers.asp

What is HL7? Retrieved November 20, 2008, from http://www.hl7.org/about/

Wikipedia. *Health Level 7*. Retrieved November 20, 2008, from http://en.wikipedia.org/wiki/HL7

Wikipedia. (2007, September 23). *International Classification of Functioning, Disability and Health.* Retrieved November 20, 2008, from http://en.wikipedia.org/wiki/International_Classification_of_Functioning%2C_Disability_and_Health

Wikipedia. (n.d.). *ASTM International.* Retrieved November 20, 2008, from http://en.wikipedia.org/wiki/ASTM_International

World Health Organization. (n.d.). *International Classification of Functioning, Disability and Health (ICF).* Retrieved November 20, from http://www.who.int/classifications/icf/en/

CHAPTER 17

Nursing Documentation: Is It Valuable?

Learning Objectives

After studying this chapter you will be able to:

1. Compare the focus of documentation of patient care in an agency with the ways patient care data is used.

2. Define the concepts associated with standardized terminologies.

3. Describe the role of the American Nurses Association (ANA) in promoting standardized terminologies.

4. Compare and contrast the 12 current ANA-recognized standardized systems.

5. Analyze issues surrounding the use of nursing standardized terminologies.

6. List the benefits of using standardized terminologies.

7. Describe the function of the Unified Medical Language System.

Key Terms

Classification
Clinical Care Classification (CCC)
Committee for Nursing Practice Information Infrastructure (CNPII)
Department of Health and Human Services (DHHS)
Granularity
International Classification of Nursing Practice (ICNP)
Logical Observations: Identifiers, Names, Codes (LOINC)
Mapping
Minimum Data Set
NANDA, NIC, and NOC (NNN)
National Library of Medicine (NLM)
Nosology
North American Nursing Diagnosis Association (NANDA)

Nursing Information and Data Set Evaluation Center (NIDSEC)
Nursing Intervention Classification (NIC)
Nursing Minimum Data Set (NMDS)
Nursing Management Minimum Data Set (NMMDS)
Nursing Outcomes Classification (NOC)
Omaha System
Outcomes Potentially Sensitive to Nursing (OPSN)
Perioperative Nursing Data Set (PNDS)
Systematized Nomenclature of Medical Clinical Terms (SNOMED CT)
Taxonomy
Terminology List
Uniform Hospital Discharge Data Set (UHDDS)

While attending a special meeting of the ICN in Paris, I was naturally at once struck by the fact that the methods and the ways of regarding nursing problems were . . . as foreign to the various delegations as were the actual languages, and the thought occurred to me that . . . sooner or later we must put ourselves upon a common basis and work out what may be termed a "nursing Esperanto" which would in the course of time give us a universal nursing language. (Isabel Hampton Robb, 1909)

In polls, nursing is called one of the most trusted professions, but how does the public define the nursing activities that lead to this conclusion? How is nursing identified in healthcare planning? Occupational therapists, pharmacists, physical therapists, dieticians, and respiratory therapists, all can define their tasks. Nurses, however, perform many tasks in various roles, which makes it difficult to define what they do. Nationwide efforts to decrease healthcare costs have intensified the need for nursing to identify its contribution to healthcare outcomes (Larrabee, 2001).

Activities generally performed by nurses may be divided into three types: managerial, dependent or physician directed, and independent or autonomous (Bowles, 1997). Managerial and dependent activities are fairly well captured by most information systems. The third type of activity (e.g., autonomous tasks) is seldom captured. Without these data, the autonomous activities that nurses perform in patient care cannot be retrieved. This translates into a situation in which autonomous nursing activities are not recognized as having any value because they have not been identified as chargeable activities.

Nursing and Documentation

Although we conscientiously document care, nursing notes are often viewed as simply a means of communication between physicians and nurses, and hence of little use to either administration for billing or medicine for research. Before the age of litigation, nursing notes were often purged from patient records, leaving no lasting documentation of nursing contributions to healthcare, hence no way to retrieve this data (Bowker, Star, & Spasser, 1998). Although today nursing notes may be kept, nursing data is never included in patient discharge abstracts that are prepared by hospital medical records departments. These abstracts, which have no indication that nursing care is a part of hospital care, are used by different agencies for various funding and statistical purposes.

INVISIBILITY OF NURSING

In the absence of nursing data, too often nursing is measured by negative qualities, such as adverse events (Ozbolt, 2000). For example, when the government undertakes large studies that look at outcomes and their relationship to the nurse–patient ratio, they use **outcomes potentially sensitive to nursing** (OPSN) (Needleman, Buerhaus, Mattke, Stewart, & Zelevinsky, 2001). An **OPSN** is a medical diagnosis that is *thought* to measure the contributions of nurses in providing inpatient care. Some OPSNs are urinary tract infections, skin pressure ulcers, pneumonia, shock, upper gastrointestinal bleeding, and length of stay. Using OPSNs, a study done by the **Department of Health and Human Services** (DHHS) employing data from more than five million patient discharges from 799 hospitals in 11 states found that the more registered nurses, the fewer the adverse outcomes, that is, these complications did not occur as often. Additional studies have also demonstrated this as well as the fact that failure to rescue episodes increase as nurse staffing decreases beyond a certain level (Aiken, Clarke, Sloane, Sochalski, & Silber, 2002; "Hospital Death Rate," 2007; Needleman, Buerhaus, Mattke, Stewart, & Zelevinsky, 2002).

Although these studies identify that there is a relationship between nursing care and medically oriented outcomes, there is no explanation for what it is that nurses do that prevents bad outcomes. Additionally, OPSNs and failure to rescue describe only a small portion of nursing-sensitive outcomes. Such outcomes as the ability or inability of a client to perform unaided the activities of daily living, engage in wellness behaviors, practice safety measures, or control symptoms of a chronic condition such as pain management and fatigue (Oerman & Huber, 1999) are not part of these studies because of a lack of data. Yet failure to treat these conditions often results in higher healthcare costs. The lack of nursing data that demonstrate what it is that a registered nurse does that prevents adverse outcomes makes it impossible to determine the true value of nursing.

The roots of this problem lie in the "invisibility of nursing," a phenomenon identified in 1990 in an editorial in the *Journal of the American Medical Association* (Friedman, 1990). The editorial says that although nursing is critical to patient care, it has a low profile. Even administrators have trouble identifying nursing's contribution to patient care. Hansten and Washburn (1998) write about a chief executive officer in a hospital who says to his chief financial officer,

> To tell you the truth, George, I don't know what RNs do. Every time I've been on walking rounds in this hospital and asked nurses what they've done recently for our hospital's survival, some tell me I should already know, others struggle to come up with an answer, but can't explain. I know we need some RNs here, but I'm not sure why (p. 42).

There is no problem identifying what occupational therapists, pharmacists, physical therapists, dieticians, and respiratory therapists do – or in billing for what they do! Not only do administrators have difficulty in defining nursing, but on evenings and weekends nursing is often responsible for the tasks of other departments. Although the hospital may charge the patient for these non-nursing tasks done by nurses, the money rarely is credited to the nursing department. Instead it flows to either the hospital at large or the department responsible for the treatment during regular working hours. The absence of standardized data that can be coded and incorporated into electronic databases is behind these difficulties (Hansten & Washburn, 1998).

It is tempting to think that if one were to peruse nursing documentation it would be easy to obtain this data. There are several problems with this approach. One, retrieving information from paper records, which is where most nursing documentation is stored, is a labor-intensive, hence expensive, task. Also, much of it is in free text, which, although may be the most expressive form of communication, can also be incomplete. There is seldom a set format for documenting, and nurses are not consistent in either their documentation or the **terminology** they use. Even if the data is in an electronic information system, the terminology used to collect it is too often not standardized enough for it to be used for comparisons even within an agency, much less across different settings and geographical areas, and therefore unable to be used in healthcare planning databases. Present day nursing documentation is also lost to the purposes that Florence Nightingale envisioned. Nightingale saw documentation as a method for evaluating and enhancing patient care and furthering the profession. In its present state, nursing documentation is seldom used for either. Because it can't be easily identified, it is also not used for billing. Nursing care is a hidden charge, usually part of the room and board, but as was demonstrated earlier in the chapter, seldom bears any resemblance to the actual care provided.

DOCUMENTATION FOCI

Documentation can be classified as having two foci: 1) safe and quality patient care and 2) the secondary analysis that is used by the healthcare community. Nursing has for too long focused mainly on the first without realizing that healthcare data has many uses beyond the care of individual patients. Data is used institutionally for quality and infection control, and then designated data is aggregated and submitted regionally and nationally. Because patient records do not contain nursing data that identifies our cognitive and autonomous

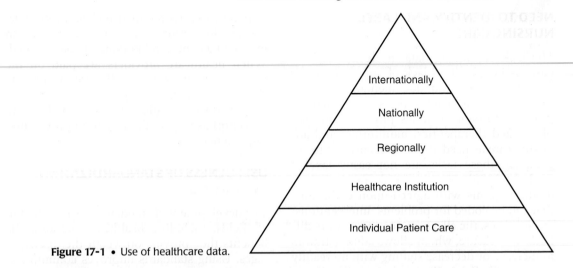

Figure 17-1 • Use of healthcare data.

TABLE 17-1 • *Comparison of Traditional Vs. Data-Driven Documentation*		
Outcomes Documentation		
Focus of data	**Traditional**	**Data-Driven**
Point of view	Lengthy, descriptive data to a specific patient-based objective	Structured data entry and focus using a computerized information system
Measurement of progress	Nurse estimates the optimal progress for a specific patient	Progress is indicated by the use of specified severity indicators
Terminology	Natural language used, which is often agency, or even unit, specific	Nursing observations are documented with standardized terminologies
Use of data	Outcomes are measured for only one individual	Outcome data is used for comparison across settings and populations

Adapted from Elfrink, Bakken, Coenen, McNeil, & Bickford C. J. (2001). Standardized nursing vocabularies: A foundation for quality care. *Seminars in Oncology Nursing, 17*(1), 18–23.

tasks, this data is lost as it moves upstream (see Figure 17-1). One consequence of this is that nursing data is not available for planning the use of healthcare resources.

Healthcare outcomes, which today have assumed great importance, are data dependent. To meet this need, it is necessary that the data be retrievable, comparable across settings, and measurable. Unfortunately, in nursing, the traditional ways of documenting do not lend themselves to any of these functions (Elfrink, Bakken, Coenen, & Bickford, 2001). Documentation is traditionally narrative text, often lengthy, and focused on a specific patient. The need for the use of documentation in determining the effect of interventions on outcomes that extend beyond an individual patient is not recognized.

Nursing documentation consists mainly of data such as medication administration, treatments, and other dependent nursing functions, that is, data about nursing tasks ordered by other disciplines. Because the information that might indicate nursing problems and guide interventions, or represent the cognitive component of nursing care, is rarely recorded, it is not part of a database. Lacking this data, nursing's contributions to patient welfare are never seen (Elfrink et al., 2001). See Table 17-1 for a comparison of traditional and data-driven documentation.

NEED TO IDENTIFY AND LABEL NURSING CARE

The lack of nursing data in electronic databases is not due to a lack of appreciation for nursing, or even our documentation, but to the difficulty in labeling the services that we provide. Nursing includes physical care, sophisticated therapeutics, monitoring, and adjusting care as needed; the skills needed to accomplish these tasks are not easily labeled (Ozbolt, 2000). Because we do not use standardized terms with agreed-upon definitions that can be coded for problems, interventions, or outcomes, the effects of nursing care are difficult to measure, which allows administrators to increase or decrease staffing with no readily apparent ill effects. We used to say that if you do not document it, you do not exist. Today, if your data are not in an electronic database in a way that they can be analyzed as secondary data, you do not count.

With the introduction of computerized information systems, the need for nursing to identify its data and to agree on the terminology to use for documentation has become of paramount concern. Given the push by various outside agencies for computerized information systems, there is only a small window to accomplish this if nursing is to be credited as a valuable asset in healthcare. The good news is that this work has been going on for over three decades. What is needed now is the realization of the importance of this work and the support of nurses and administrators to implement documentation systems that use standardized nursing terminologies. When nursing does not use standardized terminologies for documentation, their contribution to patient care does not allow for the multiple uses of healthcare data, placing the survival of the profession at risk (Sibbald, 1998).

Without standardized terms for the care that nurses give, a nursing information system (NIS) will not increase the visibility of nursing care. Our oral tradition of communication through shift report or written in a frequently modified Kardex needs to be updated for nursing to be represented in healthcare data. The pay-for-performance initiative provides an excellent chance for nursing to be counted. When healthcare providers are paid on the basis of outcomes, they will want all the data that can support quality care; standardizing nursing documentation of our data will add to this effort as well as allow us to improve nursing practice.

USEFULNESS OF STANDARDIZATION IN NURSING

The development of standards has occurred in all fields, including healthcare, because the benefits they provide outweigh the disadvantages. Using standards improves communication, facilitates research, and improves the ability to predict resource needs. Although we as nurses make sense of our nursing practice, we are very new at making explicit the value that is embedded in our clinical documentation (Clark & Lang, 1992). Despite almost 40 years of work, there is still a low visibility for the standardized nursing terminologies, which could uncover this value. Nurses, and even many involved in informatics, have little knowledge of our present standardized terminologies. This situation is worldwide, which results in several problems:

1. Nursing care is inadequately funded and billed (Goossen, 2000).
2. Nursing resources are inadequately planned and allocated.
3. The contribution of nursing to healthcare cannot be calculated.
4. It is very difficult to design decision support systems.

To quote Clark and Lang (1992), "If we cannot name it, we cannot control it, finance it, research it, or put it into public policy" (Clark & Lang, 1992, p. 128).

Goossen (2003) writes that there are five different types of standards in healthcare: to deliver quality patient care, to document and compare, to exchange information, for workflow, and to let technology work. The first type, standards for delivering quality care, tells nurses what to do; an example is a practice guideline. Standards for documenting and comparing involve terminology and **classifications**. The third type, exchanging information and developing electronic records, is concerned with interoperability. Workflow, the flow of information from one participant or machine for action, requires standards to prevent errors or omissions. In clinical care this is often the critical pathway. Standards that allow technology to work are also part of interoperability. In a good information system, these standards will all be integrated. This chapter concerns itself with standards for documenting and comparing nursing care, which encompasses **minimum data sets** and the nursing standardized terminologies.

Concepts Behind Standardized Terminologies

The science of developing a language or classification that adequately describes any healthcare discipline is very complex. It is part of a field called **nosology**, or the science of the classification of diagnostic terms. Developing a set of standardized terminologies involves much more than identifying and reaching consensus on the terminology. The terms must be part of a classification system or a logical arrangement of knowledge that is based on categories of concepts that are clearly stated and understandable to users. Moreover, the classification must be amenable to coding for use in a computerized system.

TAXONOMIES

A classification system is the final product that results from arranging the terms in **taxonomy**. A taxonomy is a way of organizing or classifying items that follow a set of rules and is focused on a given concept or philosophical base. That is, all items in the taxonomy have some features in common and are part of the group that forms the organizing concept. Members are further subdivided according to given features that are decided on by the developing entity. We are all familiar with taxonomies from our high school biology. They are pyramid shaped, and everything under a category is a type of the item above it (see Figure 17-2). The organizing concept, or axis, is vertebrates. The first level in Figure 17-2 contains fish and birds, each a vertebrate, but a different kind. The second level differentiates between different types of fish and birds, while the third level becomes even more specific, or granular. This type of taxonomy is known as monoaxial taxonomy, because it is organized around only one concept, in this example, vertebrates.

Taxonomies are often said to be either monoaxial or multiaxial. This refers to the organization of the taxonomy. In a monoaxial taxonomy, each item can have only one "parent," that is, it belongs to one category. Parents though, such as trout, in Figure 17-2, can have many children. In healthcare, a monoaxial taxonomy such as in Figure 17-2 is not always sufficient to describe the desired element. In these cases, a multiaxial taxonomy is created with users selecting words or phrases from

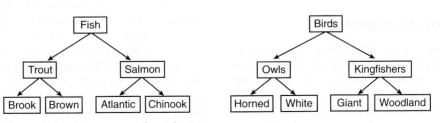

Figure 17-2 • A taxonomy of vertebrates.

TABLE 17-2 • *Comparison of Medical and Nursing Data*

68-Year-Old Female	
Medical Data	**Nursing Data**
Osteoporosis, mild	Physical injury, potentially because of: 1. Loose carpet edges 2. Bathtub without hand grips 3. Inadequate lighting in bedroom
Treatment: Calcium 500 mg three times a day Calcitonin – 200U intranasally in alternate nostrils daily	**Treatment:** Fix carpet edges Install hand grips in shower Use higher wattage bulb in ceiling fixture
Outcome: Fractured hip from fall	**Outcome:** Free from falls

- Where will the emphasis of planning be with just medical data?
- Where will the emphasis of planning be with just nursing data?
- Will the outcome of planning with both medical and nursing data yield a better outcome?

must be a named group who will be responsible for maintaining and revising the system.

In 1995, the **Nursing Information and Data Set Evaluation Center (NIDSEC)** was established by the ANA Board of Directors to evaluate the use of standardized terminologies in NISs by a vendor. Evaluation criteria include the use of the nomenclature, clinical content, clinical data repository (how the data is stored and retrieved), the general system characteristics, and a coding scheme that provides a unique identifier for each concept. The ANA encourages nursing system developers to have their information systems evaluated against these standards. When standardized terminologies are applied appropriately, nursing data is available for many uses, among them are the uncovering of knowledge embedded in clinical practice, developing decision support systems, and policy setting.

ANA-RECOGNIZED STANDARDIZATION EFFORTS

The ANA has recognized 13 standardization efforts pertinent to nursing. Two of these are minimum data sets, one, the ABC codes discussed in Chapter 16, consists of billing codes, and one, the Patient Care.

Data Set, has been retired. Of the remaining nine, all of which can be used in the interface mode, two are interdisciplinary and seven are nursing focused.

Minimum Data Sets

A **minimum data set** is a list of data elements with uniform definitions and categories that specify the minimum set of data that will meet the essential needs of multiple data users in a specific area. Thus, minimum data set requirements depend on how the data will be used. Most minimum data sets are designed to meet the needs of those who make policy. The data they contain is not, in most cases, sufficient to meet the needs of those who provide care. There are today many minimum data sets, each serving a different purpose. A minimum data set must meet the following criteria:

▼ The data must be useful to potential users, for example, legislators, healthcare professionals, administrators, or regulatory bodies.
▼ The items in the set must be readily collectable with reasonable accuracy.
▼ The items should not duplicate other available data.
▼ Confidentiality must not be violated.

Nursing Minimum Data Set (NMDS). The absence of nursing-sensitive data in the minimum data sets mandated in the United States for collection and used for healthcare planning was noted in the early 1970s by several nurse leaders. While discussing this among themselves at the 1977 Nursing Information Systems Conference, the idea for a **nursing minimum data set** (**NMDS**) originated (Werley, Ryan, & Zorn, 1995). The concept, however, was not quick to catch on – few nurses had much research background, and of those, few saw the value in everyday nursing data. Nevertheless, in 1985, Werley and Lang, with the sponsorship of the University of Wisconsin School of Nursing, Hospital Corporation of America, and IBM, invited 65 individuals to a conference to determine which items to include in an NMDS (Ozbolt, 1996). A postconference group refined the work of this conference and came up with the present set of 16 items (Table 17-3) in three categories: demographics, nursing care, and service elements. All but six of the items are already collected as part of the Uniform Minimum Health Data Set (UMHDS), which is not surprising, given that the NMDS was modeled after this data set. In the United States, the NMDS set designates the elements that need to be collected, but does not specify the terminology that is needed to collect this data.

The purposes of the NMDS are as follows:

▼ To make it possible to compare data from different clinical settings, populations, and geographical areas.
▼ To describe nursing care in various settings, including institutional and noninstitutional settings.
▼ To show or project trends regarding nursing care and resources needed for clients with various nursing diagnoses.
▼ To stimulate nursing research by providing links to data.
▼ To provide nursing data to influence clinical, administrative, and health policy decision making.

On the basis of the work done in the United States, many other countries have developed nursing minimum data sets, including Australia, Belgium, Japan, Switzerland, and Thailand (Mac Neela, Scott, Treacy, & Hy, 2006). Belgium has probably developed the concept the furthest, using their NMDS for

TABLE 17-3 • *Elements of the NMDS*		
Elements of the Nursing Minimum Data Set		
Nursing Care Elements	**Patient or Client Demographic Elements**	**Service Elements**
1. Nursing diagnosis*	5. Personal identification	10. Unique facility or service agency number
2. Nursing interventions*	6. Data of birth	11. Unique health record number of patient or client*
3. Nursing outcomes*	7. Sex	12. Unique number of principal registered nurse provider*
4. Intensity of nursing care*	8. Race and ethnicity	13. Episode admission or encounter date
	9. Residence	14. Discharge or termination date
		15. Disposition of patient or client
		16. Expected payer for most of this bill (anticipated financial guarantee for services)

Adapted from Leske, J. S., & Werley, H. H. (1992). Use of the nursing minimum data set. *Computers in Nursing 10*(6), 259–263.
*All items but these are in the Uniform Hospital Data Discharge Set

TABLE 17-4 ● *Some Non-Nursing Minimum Healthcare Data Sets*	
Data Set	**Acronym**
Minimum Data Set–Post Acute Care	MDS-PAC
Mental Health Minimum Data Set	MHMDS
Minimum Data Set (for Long-Term Care), Second version	MDS-2
Uniform Hospital Discharge Data Set	UHDDS
Uniform Ambulatory Care Data Set	UACDS

allocating nursing resources. At present there are efforts underway by the International Council of Nurses (ICN) and the nursing informatics working group of the International Medical Informatics Association (IMIA) to create an International Nursing Minimum Data Set (INMDS).

One difficulty that we have in nursing in the United States is differentiating the NMDS from the other minimum data sets seen in Table 17-4. In the United States, before the development of the NMDS, there were three patient-focused minimum data sets (Werley & Ryan, 1995). The **Uniform Hospital Discharge Data Set** (UHDDS), which was adopted in 1972 and is now mandated to be collected on all hospitalized Medicare patients, is one. The Long-Term Health Care Data Set and the Ambulatory Medical Care Minimum Data Set are the other two. Unlike the NMDS, these not only identify the data elements needed but also provide the terminology to use. Given the many health-related minimum data sets, it is not surprising that most people, nurses included, are not aware of the differences between the minimum data sets, nor of the fact that only the NMDS and the **Nursing Management Minimum Data Set** (NMMDS) contain nursing data that provide recognition of our cognitive work.

Nursing Management Minimum Data Set (NMMDS). When developed, the elements in the NMDS were identified as necessary for recognizing nursing care in the United States. Some nursing groups have found that more data

elements are needed for their purposes. The American Organization of Nurse Executives along with researchers from the University of Iowa have built on the NMDS and established an NMMDS that focuses on the nursing environment, nurse resources, and finances (Simpson, 1997).

Terminologies Developed by and for Nursing

Nursing is a very broad field encompassing many realms: hospital nursing, home health nursing, community nursing, office nursing, school nursing, occupational nursing, plus specialties within many of these areas. Thus, it is very difficult to find one standardized terminology that can meet the needs of all these groups. The result is that many have been developed and recognized by the ANA. There are also those in use locally, which, because they do not meet a universal standard, are not useful outside the agency. The seven active nursing terminologies collect either one or three of four of the nursing components in the NMDS. The element that is not captured by any of these seven is the intensity of nursing care.

The ANA-recognized standardized terminologies are discussed here in roughly the order in which ANA recognized them, with the exception of NANDA, which is discussed with **Nursing Intervention Classification** (NIC) and **Nursing Outcomes Classification** (NOC), because these are often used together. Each of these terminologies not only delineates terms and their definitions, for each term, but also classifies the terms to make it possible to study nursing at a more abstract level. It also makes it possible to link clinical data with the literature as well as provides decision support (Bakken, 2001).

Omaha System. The Omaha System is a research-based, comprehensive taxonomy that classifies and codes data elements for problems, interventions, and outcomes. It is designed to provide a consistent vocabulary for collecting, sorting, classifying, documenting, and analyzing data pertaining to individual patients, families, or communities. The Omaha

System was developed, tested, and revised through the efforts of public health and home care nurses in Omaha, Nebraska, and community health agencies in seven other geographical areas. Work started in 1970; four research grants were conducted between 1975 and 1993 and included 11 years of federal funding (Martin, 1999). From the beginning, the Omaha System was intended to provide a structure that was computer compatible. Because the Omaha System exists in the public domain and is not copyrighted, it is available for use without payment of a license fee. However, the terms and structure must be used as published and accompanied by a reliable source (Martin, 2005). Approximately 8,000 multidisciplinary practitioners, educators, and researchers use Omaha System point-of-care software nationally and internationally (The Omaha System, 2008). Current users are employed in home care, public health, school health, clinics, ambulatory care, long-term care/rehabilitation hospitals, and hospital-based and other case management sites. It is also used by nurse practitioners (Barton, Baramee, Sowers, & Robertson, 2003; Barton et al., 2003).

Clinical Care Classification (CCC). It was another standardized terminology that started with a community focus is the **Clinical Care Classification** (CCC). Until 2004, this was known as the Home HealthCare Classification (HHCC). The CCC was designed to be computerized, unlike many of the recognized terminologies. Like the Omaha System, the CCC includes within one system three of the nursing elements in the NMDS and provides codes for all. The CCC grew out of a project conducted at the Georgetown University School of Nursing under the leadership of Saba and colleagues in the late 1980s and early 1990s (Saba, 2002). The objective was to develop a method for assessing and classifying home health Medicare patients for purposes of predicting the resources that would be necessary in nursing and home health services. It has also proved useful for other disciplines such as social work, speech therapy, and physical and occupational therapy. Like the Omaha System, the CCC has been accepted by Health Information Technology Standards Panel (HITSP) as a nursing standard, and it too can be used free of charge.

North American Nursing Diagnosis Association (NANDA). What in 1982 became **NANDA** was initiated in the early 1970s by two nurses, Kristine Gebbie and Mary Ann Lavin (Gordon, 1998), who participated in a demonstration project requiring that patient data be computerized. They found themselves unable to comply because of the lack of any standards in the terminology used in nursing (Warren & Hoskins, 1995). This led them to call the first meeting of the National Conference Group for the Classification of Nursing Diagnoses in 1973. The conference objective was to identify terminologies that emphasized the unique role of the nurse. After two years of work, in 1975, the Second National Conference on Classification of Nursing Diagnoses proposed 37 nursing diagnoses to be used in classifying patient problems. Their first classification was simply an alphabetical list of the terms, but each had a definition, with an etiology and defining characteristics. As the list grew, a need for classifying the diagnoses beyond alphabetizing became obvious and a taxonomic vocabulary based on Gordon's 11 functional health patterns was created. Later the classification principle was changed to the nine human response patterns of exchanging, communicating, relating, valuing, choosing, moving, perceiving, knowing, and feeling.

The efforts by NANDA were one of the earliest attempts to define nursing terminology. Like the NMDS, it has become a building block for the nursing terminologies; the current nursing-created terminologies that capture more than one element use some form of a nursing diagnosis for labeling problems. NANDA 2 has progressed a long way from the first alphabetical list. It is now a multiaxial taxonomy using seven axes: the diagnostic concept, time, unit of care, age, potentiality (risk), descriptor, and topology (NANDA International, 2001). To create a diagnosis, users select terms from the axes necessary to express a patient-care concept. Every two years NANDA International meets to update and revise the terminology. There have been changes made to almost every NANDA International diagnosis to enable the defining characteristics, risk factors, and related factors to be coded, thus making each term more granular (Herdman, 2006). One of the criticisms of NANDA has been that the concepts are not unambiguous, a factor that has also been addressed.

Nursing Intervention Classification (NIC). As the work on the NMDS became more widely known, in 1987, researchers at the University of Iowa started work on NIC. This was an attempt to standardize the terminology used to describe nursing interventions for use with the NMDS. In 1990, they received a National Center for Nursing Research three-year grant and in 1993 a four-year grant (Bulechek, McCloskey, & Donahue, 1995) for development. Their work uncovered several interesting facets of nursing. In trying to identify nursing interventions from various sources such as textbooks, care planning guides, and NISs, they discovered that nursing actions are seen as discrete actions rather than as a part of a treatment for a specific condition (McCloskey & Bulechek, 1992). Additionally, the interventions listed for given conditions were not identical from one source to another and different terminologies were used for the same interventions. They also found confusion between what is an intervention, an assessment, or an evaluation activity. These difficulties are part of the problem nursing has in deciding which intervention works best with a given phenomenon. More revealing, they also found that interventions listed were often traditionally versus empirically based. Additionally, there was little record of the history of the decision making by nurses in choosing among interventions. At present, they have identified more than 500 interventions.

Nursing Outcomes Classification (NOC). A group at the University of Iowa also developed NOC, which is intended to be used with NANDA and NIC classifications as one large system to collect three of the four nursing care elements in the NMDS. Their efforts began in 1991, when a group of 43 nurses representing nursing education and service agencies began to identify and classify nursing-sensitive patient outcomes. For their purposes they defined outcomes as measurable, variable patient states or behaviors, including patient perceptions that result from nursing interventions (Johnson & Mass, 1992). Although the outcomes may be stated as goals, they are not intended as such. This group used current literature, research instruments, and information systems as the source for identifying the outcomes. Currently, there are over 300 research-based outcome labels that provide standardization of expected patient outcomes.

Unified NANDA, NIC, and NOC. Recognizing the need for NANDA, NIC, and NOC to work together, in August of 2001 an invitational conference was held to develop a first draft of a common taxonomic structure for these three classifications (McCloskey, Dochterman, & Jones, 2003). The structure, although somewhat different from those currently used in any of the three standardized terminologies, is not a radical change from any. There are 4 domains and 10 classes. The structure is in the public domain for use by any interested group. NANDA, NIC, and NOC are still separate terminologies and need to be licensed separately, but they are intended to work together. They are sometimes referred to as NNN. The NNN is not an ANA-recognized terminology, but rather the use in one system of three ANA-recognized terminologies: NANDA, NIC, and NOC.

A group that started at the University of Michigan, but is now housed at the University of Illinois, Chicago, developed a methodology for documenting using NANDA, NIC, and NOC, which is known as the Hands-on Automated Nursing Data System (HANDS). They developed a system that integrated the entering, storing, and retrieving of standardized NNN terms (Keenan et al., 2002).

The team included hardware and software experts, a database specialist, a standards specialist in HL7 and HIPAA (Health Information Portability and Accountability Act), nursing language experts, a statistician, nurse administrators, researchers, and clinicians. Developing the system revealed that there was a widespread misunderstanding by non-nurse team members about how to integrate standardized languages into documentation systems. Another lesson learned in this project was that the non-nurse members of the team had many misperceptions about the nature of nursing, believing it to be simple work. This led to difficulties in understanding the complexity needed for documentation of nursing practice. As they worked with the nursing team in this endeavor, these misperceptions were dispelled and the team came to understand the need to clearly represent what nurses do.

Perioperative Nursing Data Set (PNDS). The development of the **Perioperative Nursing Data Set (PNDS)** was started in 1993 by members of the American Operating Room Nurses association. The goal was to make visible to administrators, financial officers, and healthcare policy makers the patient problems that perioperative nurses manage (Baker, 2005; Beyea, 2000). The system encompasses the entire perioperative experience from preadmission to discharge using standardized elements for nursing diagnoses, interventions, and outcomes. It provides a framework for documentation for perioperative nurses (Kleinbeck, 2002).

International Classification of Nursing Practice (ICNP). The **International Classification of Nursing Practice (ICNP)** is an outgrowth of a failed attempt by the ANA to have the NANDA diagnoses included as part of ICD-10. They were turned down, not for poor content but because it was considered inappropriate to include work that had been developed within a single country in an international classification (Clark, 1998). This led the ANA to propose a resolution to the International Council of National Representatives in Seoul in 1989, which led to a project to develop the ICNP®.

Begun in 1990, the aims were to develop a standardized vocabulary and classification of nursing phenomena, nursing interventions, and nursing outcomes, which would be useful in both paper and electronic records. Its intention is to be part of a worldwide infrastructure that articulates ". . . nursing's contribution to health and health care globally" (International Council of Nurses, 2007) for the purpose of improving healthcare policy and patient care. It is also meant to establish a common language for nursing practice to enable communication among nurses and others, to describe nursing care in various settings, and to stimulate nursing research. Version 1 was released in 2005. Efforts now are underway to map the ANA-recognized nursing terminologies to ICNP as well as map ICNP to **Systematized Nomenclature of Medical Clinical Terms (SNOMED CT)**.

The ICNP encompasses nursing diagnoses that they term "nursing phenomena, nursing interventions, and nursing outcomes." In this multiaxial taxonomy, nursing phenomena and nursing outcomes use the same eight axes: focus of nursing care, judgment, frequency, duration, topology, body site, likelihood, and bearer. A nursing outcome is simply a new nursing diagnosis. The nursing interventions' taxonomy also has eight axes: activity, target, means, time, topology, location, routes, and beneficiary. To identify a nursing phenomenon, intervention, or outcome, a user selects terms from the axes. Terms from designated axes must be selected, others are optional. Because the number of terms that could be generated from such a system is large, currently catalogs, or a subset of nursing problems, interventions, and outcomes designed for a specialty, are being developed to facilitate data entry (Park, 2007).

Multidiscipline Standardized Terminologies

SNOMED® CT. The Systematized Nomenclature of Medical Clinical Terms–Reference Terminology (SNOMED-RT) was the first

preclude this. There is much knowledge that is currently concealed in nursing data that with the use of standardized terminologies could be uncovered. On the other hand, there are many gaps in the standardized terminologies for what is needed for documentation. In nursing, the standardized terminologies do, however, provide items of data that can be used in linking assessments, interventions, and outcomes as well as the literature, and making visible nursing's contributions to healthcare (Box 17-1).

One of the biggest difficulties in implementing a nursing terminology is not outside forces, but the culture of nursing. Nursing's religious and military history as well as the fact that nursing has been primarily a feminine occupation has contributed to our not voicing opinions or making our contributions known. Old customs of communicating to physicians with comments such as "The patient appears to be bleeding"

instead of stating it as a fact has also been a contributing factor. Fortunately, this type of communication is no longer as prevalent, but the mind-set behind it lingers along with our historical legacies. If we are to truly become valued for our contributions, we will need to take over responsibility for our nursing actions, visibly label them, and support one another in using the terminologies. Only nursing can accomplish this.

BENEFITS OF NURSING STANDARDIZED LANGUAGES

The benefits to patient care, nursing, and healthcare policy of using a nursing standardized terminology outweigh the drawbacks. Using a nursing terminology makes it possible to formalize nursing knowledge. This is important to improve communication between

---

Box 17-1 • Using a Standardized Terminology

In our public health nursing agency, we use the Omaha System, one of the ANA-recognized standardized nursing terminologies. Use of this standardized terminology has been very valuable from my perspective as both a field nurse and informatics consultant. The Omaha System has improved my ability to articulate the essence and the details of nursing care, in both my roles. Although it has taken patience and commitment for me to become proficient in "speaking the language," the results, in terms of strengthened patient care, have been well worth the effort. The learning task is made easier because the grammatical rules, syntax, concepts, and content are those of the nursing process: assessment, planning, intervention, and evaluation.

The terminology is fully integrated into my agency's computerized nursing information system (CNIS). On the basis of the terminology's foundation, powerful care plans have been created and are easily accessible at the point of care. They help me plan care and allow my charting to be more efficient and complete at the point of care. The care plans are easily customizable, allow me to address the unique needs of my patients, and

reflect the organization's policies and procedures. Because we are using a standardized terminology, we can engage in electronic exchange of information across the state. This has created opportunities to learn from and collaborate with my nursing colleagues in the delivery of highly diverse public health nursing services, from tuberculosis control to the prevention of childhood lead poisoning.

The standardized data generated by the terminology and stored in the CNIS enables quality assurance and improvement activities to be based on actual patient care data rather than data extracted from charting. The data are sufficiently atomic to generate meaningful information that enables me to describe to public health payers and partners the needs of patients, outcomes of nursing care, and the unique services that nurses provide in meeting the public's health needs.

Pamela Correll, RN, BSN, Nursing Informatics Consultant, Public Health Nursing Program, Maine Center for Disease Control and Prevention.

nurses, improve care, generate new nursing knowledge, educate nurses, and to gain the full benefits of an NIS (Goossen, 1996). Standardized languages also eliminate inconsistencies in investigating and documenting nursing practice, and allow the building of decision support systems for nursing.

Examples of the benefits from using a nursing standardized terminology can be found in Korea where a Korean version of the ICNP has been successfully used to populate the user interface (Park, 2007). Nursing interventions, when documented in this system, are billed, and the patient is charged for actual nursing care instead of an average for all patients. Another feature of this system is a printout of the nursing discharge record given to the patient as a record of his or her nursing care, a document that furnishes evidence that the nurse provides value. The system also provides decision support to clinicians by generating a list of possible interventions for a nursing problem. Some of the knowledge that has been unearthed in this system is the success of various interventions for pain and the outcomes of nursing interventions. Additionally, the quality and quantity of nursing documentation has increased. Interestingly, although the system keeps free text to a minimum, when free text is audited, the most frequent item found is "slept well."

As can be seen from the Korean example, data recorded using standardized terminologies will facilitate the examination of how nursing care contributes to patient outcomes. Because the terminology has exact definitions and is classified, it can be used in an aggregated format and hence will be available for export along with other nursing data, providing a more complete picture of needed resources as well as lending support to preventative care. An added benefit is that nursing ceases to be invisible. Although the dependent functions of nursing are important, they do not define nursing. The independent functions of nursing are equally, if not more, important in a healthcare system that is interested in cutting costs.

Perhaps the best benefit to nursing from standardized terminologies is the ability to study and reflect on our own practice. In the future, not only nurse managers but individual practitioners also should be able to retrieve de-identified date about their practice and study the outcomes of various interventions. The nurse should also be able to benchmark the data with averages for the unit as well as the agency. This can provide information to the nurse about areas she or he may wish to investigate more as well as areas where the information she or he has should be shared in presentations and writing. Clinical nurses have a wealth of knowledge that needs to be made part of the nursing literature.

Summary

Nursing data are elusive. To determine the benefits of nursing from healthcare data that are currently submitted to reporting agencies, it is necessary to use what are called OPSN. Most nursing documentation makes it difficult to find the nursing actions that produce these or other outcomes. Additionally, outcomes definitively sensitive to nursing are not easy to locate. Changing this requires that nursing identify the interventions, the nursing phenomenon to which they are directed, and the related outcomes. To make these available for research and policy planning, these items must be expressed using standardized nursing terminologies so that they can be entered into and retrieved from a computerized information system.

The science of the classification of diagnostic terms is known as nosology. Classifications are organized into taxonomies, which may be monoaxial or multiaxial. The classifying principle will depend on the purpose of the taxonomy. The granularity of a language determines the level of detail that a language will capture.

In the 1980s, the ANA recognized the need for nursing to standardize the data it uses in documentation. They have devised criteria for recognizing standardization efforts. Using these criteria, 13 different standardization efforts have been recognized, one of which has been retired. Two of these recognized systems are minimum data sets that designate the data elements that need to be collected, eight were created by and for nursing, and three are interdisciplinary. One of the main issues surrounding the use of standardized nursing terminologies has to do with the culture of nursing. Benefits from using standardized terminologies in nursing include the ability to develop nursing decision support systems, to discover the best interventions for phenomena that are part of the independent functions of nursing, to bill for actual nursing care, and to have nursing data present in a computerized information system. Many different standardized terminologies exist in healthcare in addition to nursing terminologies. Some of these were discussed in Chapter 16.

APPLICATIONS AND COMPETENCIES

1. List the uses of patient documentation in health planning. Compare these purposes with the documentation format used in a clinical area with which you are familiar. What conclusions can be drawn?
2. Match the data that you collect from a patient with potential uses beyond the care of an individual patient. Which of these data could be used to document:
   a. A nursing phenomenon that is part of the independent practice of nursing
   b. A nursing intervention directed to that phenomenon
   c. An outcome of this intervention
3. Investigate the many functions of the ISO at http://www.iso.org/iso/about.htm.
4. List organizations involved in standardization.
5. Describe the role of the ANA in the development of standardized terminologies.
6. Define the following terms:
   a. Taxonomy
   b. Axis
   c. Monoaxial
   d. Multiaxial
   e. Granular

f. Mapping
g. Minimum data set
7. Describe what is meant by a terminology used in the
   a. Interface mode
   b. Reference mode
8. Compare and contrast three of the 12 currently ANA-recognized language systems, one of which must include terms for nursing problems, interventions, and outcomes.
9. List the benefits of using standardized terminologies.

REFERENCES

Aiken, L. H., Clarke, S. P., Sloane, D. M., Sochalski, J., & Silber, J. H. (2002). Hospital nurse staffing and patient mortality, nurse burnout, and job dissatisfaction. *Journal of the American Medical Association, 288*, 1987–1993. [Electronic version available at http://www.premierinc .com/safety/topics/back_injury/downloads/R_04%20_ JamaRN.pdf]

Baker, J. D. (2005). Specialty nomenclature: A worthwhile challenge. *Gastroenterology Nursing, 28*(1), 52–55.

Bakken, S. (2001). An informatics infrastructure is essential for evidence-based practice. *Journal of the American Medical Association, 8*(3), 199–201.

Barton, A., Baramee, J., Sowers, D., & Robertson, K. J. (2003). Articulating the value-added dimension of NP care. *The Nurse Practitioner, 28*(12), 34–40.

Barton, A. J., Gilbert, L., Erickson, V., Baramee, J., Sowers, D., & Robertson, K. J. (2003). A guide to assist nurse practitioners with standardized nursing language. *Computers Informatics Nursing: CIN, 21*(3), 128–133.

Beyea, S. C. (2000). Standardized nursing vocabularies and the peri-operative nursing data set. *CIN Plus, 3*(2), 1, 5–6.

Bezon, B. J., Echevarria, K. H., & Smith, G. B. (1999). Nursing outcome indicator: Preventing falls for elderly people. *Outcomes Management for Nursing Practice, 3*(3), 132–137.

Bowker, G. C., Star, S., & Spasser, M. (1998). Classifying nursing work. *Online Journal of Issues in Nursing, 3*(2). [Electronic journal at http://www.nursingworld.org/ MainMenuCategories/ANAMarketplace/ANAPeriodicals/ OJIN/TableofContents/Vol31998/Vol31993No21998/ ClassifyingNursingWork.aspx]

Bowles, K. (1997). The barriers and benefits of nursing information systems. *Computers in Nursing, 15*(4), 191–196.

Bulechek, G. M., McCloskey, J. C., & Donahue, W. J. (1995). Nursing interventions classification (NIC): A language to describe nursing treatments. In N. M. Lang (Ed.), *An emerging framework: Data system advances for clinical nursing practice* (pp. 115–131). Washington, DC: American Nurses Association.

Clark, J. (1998). The international classification for nursing practice project. *Online Journal Nursing Informatics*. [Available at http://www.nursingworld.org/ojin/tpc7/tpc7_3.htm]

Clark, J., & Lang, N. (1992). Nursing's next advance: An international classification for nursing practice. *International Nursing Review, 39*, 109–112, 128.

Elfrink, V. L., Bakken, S., Coenen, A., & Bickford, C. J. (2001). Standardized nursing vocabularies: A foundation for quality care. *Seminars in Oncology Nursing, 17*(1), 18–23.

Friedman, E. (1990). Troubled past of "invisible" profession. *Journal of the American Medical Association, 264*(22), 2851–2857.

Goossen, W. T. F. (1996). Nursing information and processing: A framework and definition for systems analysis, design and evaluation. *International Journal of Biomedical Computing, 40*(3), 187–195.

Goossen, W. T. F. (2000). *Towards strategic use of nursing information in the Netherlands*. Gronigen, The Netherlands: University of Groningen.

Goossen, W. T. F. (2003, June 25–28). *Standards, there are so many, which ones should we nurses choose?* Paper presented at the NI 2003 Post Congress Workshop, Mangaratiba, Rio de Janeiro, Brazil.

Gordon, M. (1998). Nursing nomenclature and classification system development. *Online Journal of Issues in Nursing, 3*(2). [Electronic journal accessed at http://www.nursingworld.org/MainMenuCategories/ANAMarketplace/ANAPeriodicals/OJIN/TableofContents/Vol31998/Vol31993No21998/Nomenclatureand Classification.aspx]

Hampton Robb, I. (1909). *Report of the third regular meeting of the International Council of Nurses*. Geneva: ICN.

Hansten, R., & Washburn, M. J. (1998). Professional practice: Facts & impact. *American Journal of Nursing, 98*(3), 42–45.

Herdman, T. H. (2006). President's report. *International Journal of Nursing Terminologies and Classifications, 17*(3), 147–149.

Hospital death rate study reveals wide variations and stresses importance of registered nurses. (2007, January 15). *Medical News Today*. Retrieved November 22, from http://www.medicalnewstoday.com/articles/60785.php

International Council of Nurses. (2007). *Vision, Goals & Benefits of ICNP®*. Retrieved November 22, 2008 from http://www.icn.ch/icnp_ben.htm

International Health Terminology Standards Development Organisation. *SNOMED Clinical Terms® (SNOMED CT®) Core Content: January 2008 International Release*. Retrieved November 22, 2008, from http://www.cap.org/apps/docs/snomed/documents/january_2008_release.pdf

Johnson, M., & Mass, M. (Eds.) (1992). *Nursing outcomes classification (NOC)*. St. Louis: Mosby Year Book.

Keenan, G. M., Stocker, J. R., Geo-Thomas, A. T., Soparkar, N. R., Barkauskas, B. H., & Lee, L. L. (2002). The HANDS project: Studying and refining the automated collection of a cross-setting clinical data set. *Computers Informatics Nursing: CIN, 20*(3), 89–100.

Kleinbeck, S. V. M. (2002, March 1). Revising the perioperative nursing data set. (Clinical Innovations).

AORN Journal. Retrieved 2007, from http://www.encyclopedia.com/doc/1G1-84183558.html

Larrabee, J. H., Boldreghini, S., Elder-Sorrells, K., Turner, Z. M., Wender, R. G., Hart, J. M., et al. (2001). Evaluation of documentation before and after implementation of a nursing information system in an acute care hospital. *Computers Informatics Nursing: CIN, 19*(2), 56–95.

Lundberg, C., & Konicek, D. (2007, March). *Overview: SNOMED Clinical Terms® Nursing Working Group & Collaboration*. Retrieved November 22, 2008, from http://www.dsr.dk/dsr/upload/3/0/997/SNOMED_CAP_6.pdf

Mac Neela, P., Scott, P. A., Treacy, M. P., & Hy, A. (2006). Nursing minimum data sets: A conceptual analysis and review. *Nursing Inquiry, 13*(1), 44–51.

Martin, K. S. (1999). The Omaha system: Past, present and future. *Online Journal Nursing Informatics, 3*(1), 1–6. [Available at http://ojni.org/3_1/art1v3n1art.html]

Martin, K. S. (2005). *The Omaha system: A key to practice, documentation, and information management* (2nd ed.). St. Louis, MO: Elsevier.

Matney, S., Ozbolt, J. G., & Bakken, S. (2003). Update on logical observation identifier names and codes (LOINC). *Online Journal of Nursing Informatics, 7*(3), 1–8. Available at http://www.eaa-knowledge.com/ojni/ni/8_1/nurslangup.htm

McCloskey, J. C., & Bulechek, G. M. (1992). *Nursing interventions classifications (NIC)*. St. Louis, MO: Mosby Year Book.

McCloskey, J. C., Dochterman, J., & Jones, C. (2003). *Unifying nursing languages*. Washington, DC: American Nurses Association.

McDonald, C. J., Huff, S. M., Suico, J. G., Hill, G., Leavelle, D., Aller, R., et al. (2003). LOINC, a universal standard for identifying laboratory observations: A 5-year update. *Clinical Chemistry, 49*(4), 624–633. [Electronic version at http://www.clinchem.org/cgi/content/full/649/624/624]

NANDA International. (2001). *NANDA, nursing diagnoses: Definitions & classification 2001–2002* (4th ed.). Philadelphia: North American Diagnosis Association.

Needleman, J., Buerhaus, P., I., Mattke, S., Stewart, M., & Zelevinsky, K. (2001). *Nurse staffing and patient outcomes in hospitals (2001). Executive summary*. Retrieved October 17, 2007, from ftp://ftp.hrsa.gov/bhpr/nursing/staffstudy/staffexecsum.pdf

Needleman, J., Buerhaus, P., Mattke, S., Stewart, M., & Zelevinsky, K. (2002). Nurse-staffing levels and the quality of care in hospitals 10.1056/NEJMsa012247. *New England Journal of Medicine, 346*(22), 1715–1722. [Electronic version available at http://content.nejm.org/cgi/content/full/1346/1722/1715]

Oerman, M., & Huber, D. (1999). Patient outcomes: A measure of nursing's value. *American Journal of Nursing, 99*(9), 40–47.

Ozbolt, J. (2000). Terminology standards for nursing: Collaboration at the summit. *Journal of the American Medical Informatics Association, 7*(6), 517–522.

Ozbolt, J. G. (1996). From minimum data to maximum impact: Using clinical data to strengthen patient care. *Advanced Practice Nursing Quarterly, 1*(4), 62–69.

Park, H. -A. (2007, July 20). *International perspectives on nursing terminology and data standards*. Paper presented at the Summer Institute in Nursing Informatics 2007, Baltimore, MD.

Saba, V. (2002). Nursing classifications: Home Health Care Classification System (HHCC). *Online Journal of Issues in Nursing*. [Available at http://www.nursingworld.org/ MainMenuCategories/ANAMarketplace/ANAPeriodicals/ OJIN/TableofContents/Volume72002/No3Sept2002/ ArticlesPreviousTopic/HHCCAnOverview.aspx]

Sibbald, B. J. (1998). Canadian pioneer of nursing informatics. *The Canadian Nurse, 94*(4), 60, 59.

Simpson, R. (1997). Technology: Nursing the system, the nursing management minimum data set. *Nursing Management, 28*(6), 20–21.

The Omaha System. (2008, January 16). Retrieved November 22, 2008, from http://www.omahasystem.org/

Warren, J., & Hoskins, L. M. (1995). NANDA's nursing diagnosis taxonomy: A nursing database. In N. Lang (Ed.), *Nursing data systems: The emerging framework*. Washington, DC: American Nurses Publishing.

Werley, H. H., Ryan, P., & Zorn, C. R. (1995). The nursing minimum data set (NMDS): A framework for the organization of nursing language. In N. M. Lang (Ed.), *Nursing data systems: The emerging framework* (pp. 19–30). Washington, DC: American Nurses Publishing.

UNIT V

Healthcare Informatics

CHAPTER 18 The Informatics Discipline
CHAPTER 19 Basic Electronic Healthcare Information Systems
CHAPTER 20 Specialized Electronic Healthcare Information Systems
CHAPTER 21 Electronic Healthcare System Issues
CHAPTER 22 Carrying Healthcare to the Client

As this decade comes to a close and the next one unfolds, more changes in healthcare are bound to occur. Informatics is becoming more and more important in the quest for patient safety, a factor put into focus by the Institute of Medicine's reports. Other demands on this maturing field are created by requirements of third-party payers for data that provide outcomes for healthcare. These demands illustrate the reality of the interdisciplinary nature of healthcare; no single specialty can provide the needed data if these goals are to be met.

Chapter 18 starts this unit by exploring nursing informatics as a specialty and examining the multivaried roles in this specialty – a specialty in both nursing and health informatics – as well as the standards for roles within this specialty. Chapter 19 examines the basics of healthcare information systems with an overview of the process for system selection and implementation using the systems life cycle. Chapter 20 explores healthcare information systems as enterprise-wide systems designed to improve the quality and efficiency of patient care delivery. The advent of informatics opportunities is associated with new challenges. Chapter 21 discusses some of the unresolved issues associated with clinical information systems. Finally, Chapter 22 discusses some of the cutting-edge telehealth developments in which care is provided or monitored by healthcare professionals in another location.

CHAPTER 18

The Informatics Discipline

Learning Objectives

After studying this chapter you will be able to:

1. *Describe seven theories on which informatics relies.*

2. *Differentiate roles for informatics nurses and nursing informatics specialists.*

3. *Evaluate whether a specific nursing informatics educational program is appropriate for your career goals.*

4. *Analyze nursing informatics roles for all nurses.*

5. *Identify professional health informatics groups.*

Key Terms

Alliance for Nursing Informatics (ANI)
American Health Information Management Association (AHIMA)
American Medical Informatics Association (AMIA)
British Computer Society
Data
Driving Force
Early Adopter
Early Majority
European Federation for Medical Informatics (EFMI)
Healthcare Informatics
Healthcare Information Management Systems Society (HIMSS)
Informatics Nurse

Informatics Nurse Specialist
Information
Innovator
Input
International Medical Informatics Association (IMIA)
Knowledge
Laggard
Late Majority
Moving
Nursing Informatics
Nursing Informatics Working Group (NIWG)
Output
Refreezing
Restraining Force
Sociotechnical Theory
Throughput
Unfreezing
Wisdom

Introduction

Although the term "informatics"[1] is relatively new, the management of **information** started when the first caveman drew pictures to communicate and pass on **knowledge**. Society, however, has long since passed the time when pictures on a cave wall provided information. Although information is managed by persons and in a coordinated fashion in all disciplines, the term informatics has come to denote the use of a computer to manage healthcare information. **Healthcare informatics** is a broad multidisciplinary field with many different specialties such as **nursing informatics**, medical informatics, dental informatics, and pharmaceutical informatics. Generally, those who practice in their discipline's subspecialty are also licensed in their own profession such as nursing or dentistry. Health informatics is also broad enough to include subspecialties that are multidisciplinary, for example, social and consumer informatics. Despite all the subspecialties in healthcare informatics, a primary goal is interdisciplinary **data** management that facilitates holistic health and community health.

Nursing Informatics as a Specialty

Nursing is a subspecialty in informatics, with roles and tasks in both disciplines. The focus of **informatics nurses** varies with their job and specialty in healthcare, but the main focus of nursing informatics is in one of the following seven areas: 1) using data, information, and knowledge for patient care; 2) defining data in patient care; 3) acquiring and delivering patient care knowledge; 4) creating new tools for patient care from new technologies; 5) applying ergonomics to nurse–computer interfaces; 6) integrating systems; and 7) evaluating the effects of nursing systems (Pillar & Golumbic, 1993). Practice in each of these areas requires different knowledge and skills

---

[1] Definitions of informatics are in Chapter 1

on the part of the **informatics nurse specialist**. These areas can be matched with Warner's five categories of what people in medical informatics do: "1) signal processing, 2) database design, 3) decision making, 4) modeling and simulation, and 5) optimizing the interface between the human and the machine" (Warner, 1995, p. 207). These areas are compared in Table 18-1.

Ozbolt, Nahm, and Roberts (2007) state that those who enter the nursing informatics field with on-the-job training are informatics nurses and those with either a degree in nursing informatics or a postgraduate training are informatics nurse specialists. Despite her lack of a formal educational program, one would probably say that the first informatics nurse specialist was Florence Nightingale, given that the fundamental building block in informatics is data. Recognizing the value of data in effecting healthcare, she collected data and systematized record-keeping practices in Crimea (Audain, 1998). Using this data she developed the first version of the pie graph known as a "polar area diagram" to dramatize the need for reform to stop the needless deaths caused by the unsanitary conditions in military hospitals. With the advent of the computer, the use of data has become far easier and more widespread than it was in Ms. Nightingale's time. When decisions are based on the data available, collection and analysis of nursing data become very important. Without nursing data the value of nursing will continue to be hidden to those in policy-making positions. Through nursing informatics, the healthcare information systems that are being developed can include the nursing data needed to improve patient care and show the value that nurses add to healthcare.

One of the main objectives of nursing informatics in the clinical area is to integrate data from all areas pertinent to nursing care and present it in a manner that enables the clinical nurse to provide quality care. Many sources of information are needed for patient care. These were broadly classified into four areas by Corcoran-Perry and Graves (1990) who studied the information needs of practicing cardiovascular nurses as outlined in Table 18-2.

TABLE 18-1 • *Categories of Informatics Tasks*

Task	Warner's Description of Task	Nursing Informatics Areas of Focus from Pillar and Golumbic
Obtaining and processing data	Data must be obtained from diverse sources including, but not limited to, clinician input, diagnostic device, patient registration, insurance information, research, systematic reviews, practice guidelines	Acquiring patient care knowledge Integration of systems
Database design	Identification and definition of data needed and designing data storage so that it can be retrieved by others	Identifying and defining of data needed in patient care
Decision making	Restructuring of data and its presentation in a manner that facilitates decision making	Using data, information, and knowledge for patient care. Creating patient care knowledge
Modeling and simulation	Building of structural models that provide insight into the data. Purpose is to increase knowledge from the data	Creating new tools for patient care from new technologies Evaluating the effects of nursing systems
Optimizing the human interface	Improving the method that humans use to gain meaning from the output. Involves not only screen design and navigation, but also how the data is structured. Educating users	Applying ergonomics to nurse–computer interfaces

Adapted from Warner, H. (1995). Medical informatics: A real discipline? *Journal of the American Medical Informatics Association, 2*(4), 207–214; Pillar, B., & Golumbic, N. (Eds.). (1993). *Nursing informatics: Enhancing patient care.* Bethesda, MD: National Center for Nursing Research, U.S. Department of Health and Human Services.

TABLE 18-2 • *Sources of Information for Nursing Informatics*

Information Sources for Patient Care

Information about the patient	Documentation. History and physical, medications and laboratory reports, demographic information, and information about the patient's support system
Institutional information	Data of immediate concern such as tracking a piece of equipment or an individual as well as agency policies for admission criteria, release of information, and confidentiality of patient data. Information needed for external bodies, such as that needed for reporting to third-party payers, regulatory agencies, and policy-making bodies
Domain knowledge	Nursing knowledge as well as knowledge from related disciplines, literature, and clinical experiences
Procedural knowledge	Focuses on the procedures for performing tasks such as starting an intravenous line

Adapted from Corcoran-Perry, S., & Graves, J. R. (1990). Supplemental-information-seeking behavior of cardiovascular nurses. *Research in Nursing & Health, 13*(2), 119–127.

The overall goal in nursing informatics is to optimize information management and communication to improve individual healthcare and the health of populations (American Nurses Association, 2008).

In 1992 the American Nurses Association (ANA) recognized nursing informatics as a specialty with the first certification examination held in 1995. The prerequisites for writing the examination for certification include a bachelor's degree, an active registered nurse (RN) license, two years of practice as an RN, and 30 hours of continuing education in informatics within the last three years. The applicant must also meet one of the following three practice requirements: 1) 2,000 hours in informatics nursing within the last three years, 2) a minimum of 1,000 hours in informatics nursing in the last three years plus completion of a minimum of 12 hours of academic credit in informatics courses as part of a graduate level informatics nursing program, or 3) completion of a graduate program in nursing informatics containing a minimum of 200 hours of a faculty-supervised practicum in informatics (American Nurses Credentialing Center). Passing the examination provides certification for five years at which time the certification can be renewed if specified educational and practice requirements are fulfilled.

The ANA publishes the *Scope and Standards of Nursing Informatics,* now in its third edition. The publication outlines the characteristics of the specialty, defines the specialty, and describes how it differs from other health and nursing specialties (American Nurses Association, 2008). It also explains in detail the basic theories behind nursing informatics, presents a discussion of the sciences that provide a foundation for informatics, and discusses standardized nursing terminologies and the importance of interoperability. The publication is a necessary basic reference for anyone interested in the field.

Theories That Lend Support to Informatics

Although information has been managed in one way or another since the beginning of time, in the early 1900s as society became more complex, theories about managing information developed. Information theory itself is a mathematical theory about communication with the goal of finding the limits on reliably compressing, storing, and communicating data and is a branch of applied probability theory (Gray, 1991; Wikipedia, 2007). Informatics theory builds not just on information theory, but uses concepts from change theories, systems theory, chaos theory, cognitive theory, and sociotechnical theory.

NURSING INFORMATICS THEORY

Nursing informatics theory is concerned with the representation of nursing data, information, and knowledge to facilitate the management and communication of nursing information within the healthcare milieu. It focuses on nursing phenomena and provides a nursing perspective, clarifies nursing values and beliefs, produces new knowledge, and develops standardized nursing terminology for use in electronic records. Graves and Corcoran (1989), in their seminal article on nursing informatics, devised an information model for nursing informatics on the basis of Blum's taxonomy. This model identified data, information, and knowledge as the key components of nursing informatics. **Wisdom** was first added to this structure by Nelson and Joos (as cited in Joos, Whitman, Smith, & Nelson, 1992) shortly thereafter, but it was the 2008 ANA *Scope and Standards of Practice* that officially made this a part of the nursing informatics model.

Data

Data are discrete, objective facts that have not been interpreted (Clark, 2004) or are out of context; they are at the atomic level. Data are described objectively without interpretation. They are the building blocks of meaning, but lack context, hence are meaningless.

Information

Information is data that has some type of interpretation or structure; that is, it has a context. It is derived from combining different pieces of data (Clark, 2004). A set of data, such as vital signs when interpreted over a period of time is information.

Knowledge

Knowledge is a synthesis of information with relationships identified and formalized. It changes something or somebody by creating the setting for formulating possible effective actions, evaluating their effects, and deciding on the required action (Clark, 2004). For example, interpreting a set of vital signs over a period of time and deciding on an action based on this information combined with nursing knowledge and experience is an example of knowledge.

Wisdom

Wisdom is achieved through evaluating knowledge with reflection. It involves seeing patterns and metapatterns and using them in different ways (Clark, 2004) and knowing when and how to apply knowledge to a situation (American Nurses Association, 2008). For example, wisdom would be interpreting vital signs in a postsurgical patient as indicative of an infection and taking the appropriate action.

The Continuum

The above concepts are constructs, not absolutes, and are a continuum, or an analog process. The examples given are very simplified and are used to help you grasp the process of converting data into wisdom. Where something falls on the continuum depends on the person or situation. A nurse with 10 years of experience may possess a great deal of tacit knowledge. This is the knowledge that has been earned with experience and reflection, but the knowledge is so ingrained that it is difficult for the nurse to verbalize or acknowledge. Nonetheless this tacit knowledge provides a higher level of wisdom than that possessed by a new graduate. For a less experienced nurse, wisdom may be identical to knowledge in an experienced nurse.

The general idea of informatics theory is that the move from data to knowledge is a progressive process that follows a given path. As one moves up the continuum, each level

becomes more complex and requires more human intellect. In practice one finds that the lines between each of these entities are blurred and that the process is iterative. The processes of converting data into knowledge include capturing, sorting, organizing, storing, retrieving, and presenting the data to give it meaning and produce information.

Figure 18-1 is a simplification of this continuum, one that might apply to a nursing student or a new graduate. In this figure, data are combined to produce information, and information is combined to produce knowledge. As another example, the number 37 is a piece of datum. It is the smallest unit that can be processed. If we combine the number 37 with the datum that this is a Celsius temperature for a person, we now have some information. Combining this still further with the information that this is the normal body temperature, we have a small piece of knowledge. The individual adds wisdom by deciding on the action, if any, to take as a result of this knowledge.

SOCIOTECHNICAL THEORY AND SOCIAL INFORMATICS

Sociotechnical theory developed in the middle of the last century when it became evident that not all implementations of technology were increasing productivity. The overall focus is the impact of technology's implementation on an organization. To this end it focuses on the interactions of an organization between information management tools and techniques, and the knowledge, skills, attitudes, values, and needs of its employees, as well as the rewards and authority structures of the employer (Wade & Schneberger, 2005). Its precepts can increase the understanding of how information systems should be developed (Berg, Aarts, & van der Lei, 2003).

Introducing an information system is a social process that deeply affects an organization. Research based on sociotechnical theory is aimed at maximizing performance by designing or redesigning systems that fit the organizational system into which they are implanted. The sociotechnical point of view, which is the basis of social informatics, holds

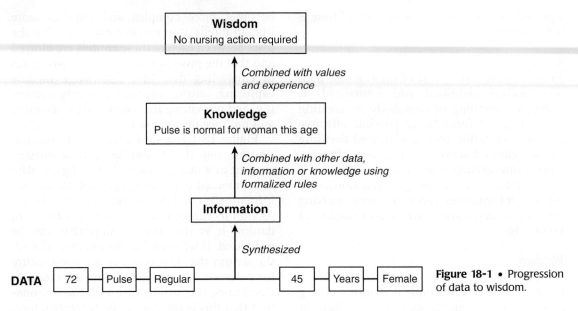

Figure 18-1 • Progression of data to wisdom.

that a good design is based on an understanding of how people work and the context of that work, not just technological considerations (Kling, 1999). The importance of social informatics is well evidenced by the failure of many information systems including the much publicized shutdown by Cedars-Lebanon Hospital in Los Angeles in early 2003 of their multi-million dollar computerized physician order entry. This system created a change that was seen as too radical by the physicians who believed that their interests were not sufficiently represented, the system was jammed down their throats, and that it was poorly designed (Chin, 2004).

CHANGE THEORIES

Instituting a change in documentation whether it is relatively simple such as a minor upgrade to a system, or major such as **moving** from a paper record to a completely paperless electronic system means change. "What will this mean to me?" is always uppermost in everyone's mind when faced with change. Whether affected individuals perceive the change as minor or major differs from individual to individual.

Change can be looked at in several ways. Rogers' Theory of Diffusion and Innovation looks at how change occurs in a society and in an individual. Lewin's Field Theory talks about stages in moving people and enterprises from a comfortable state before the change, through the discomfort of change, and finally back to a comfort with the change. Ignoring the psychosocial nature of changing information management is too often a one-way ticket to failure of the system.

Rogers' Diffusion of Innovation Theory

Rogers' theory, the diffusion of innovations, was first published in his book of the same name in 1962 (Rogers, 1983). This theory examines the pattern of acceptance that innovations follow as they spread across the population and the process of decision making that occurs in individuals when deciding whether to adopt an innovation. It was based on depression era rural research that studied how midwestern farmers adopted hardier corn. This theory is still timely in North America and developed countries with the same culture, but there is doubt if it applies to the areas of the world with different cultures.

Societal Changes. In looking at how innovations are accepted by the general population, Rogers divides people into five categories (Rogers, 1983). **Innovators**, the first category, readily adopt the innovation. They constitute a very small percentage, about 2.5% of the population (Anderson, 2001). These persons are often seen as disruptive by those who are averse to risk taking, and are not able to sell others on the innovation. This job is left to **early adopters**, the next category, who comprise 13.5% of the population. They are respectable opinion leaders who function as promoters of an innovation. The next group is the **early majority** (34%) who are averse to risks, but will make safe investments. The **late majority**, who make up another 34% of the adopters, need to be sure that the innovation is beneficial. They may adopt the innovation not because they see a use for it, but because of peer pressure. The last group, comprising 16%, is termed **laggards**. They are suspicious of innovations and change and are quite resistant. They see their resistance as a rationale and must be certain that the innovation will not fail before they can adopt it. This group, instead of being discounted, should be listened to. They may grasp weaknesses that others fail to see.

Individual Changes. In Rogers' theory, individuals go through five stages in deciding to adopt an innovation. Like all stage theories, progress is not uniform, and adopters can show behaviors from more than one stage at a time or revert completely to an earlier stage. The first stage is *knowledge of an innovation* in which the potential adopter gains an understanding of how the innovation operates (Rogers, 1983). This can occur either passively, through education or advertisements, or actively in response to a felt need. The second stage, *persuasion*, is based on the perception of the relative advantage of the innovation, compatibility with existing norms, and its observability. At this stage an individual forms an opinion about the innovation, negative, neutral, or positive. In the third stage, the individual uses his opinions to make a *decision*. A potential adopter may try the innovation or base an opinion on the experience and opinion of a respected peer who has tried the innovation. The individual then either decides to adopt or reject the innovation. If the decision is positive, the fourth stage, or *implementation*, follows. At this stage the adopter wants knowledge such as how to use the innovation and how to overcome problems with its use. *Confirmation*, or the fifth stage, may occur when reinforcement of the decision is sought. Conflicting information about the innovation may cause the adopter to reverse a decision.

Lewin's Field Theory

Rogers' theory identified the stages that individuals go through in making a change, whereas Lewin's field theory provides a guide to helping individuals achieve a positive decision in relation to an innovation. This theory holds that human behavior is related to both personal characteristics and the social milieu in which the individual exists (Clark, 2000). It focuses on the variables that need to be recognized and observed in a situation of change (Schein, 2004) and uses these variables to create a model of the stages that occur during change. Lewin divides these changes into three stages: **unfreezing**, **moving**, and **refreezing**. Ways of moving a group from the first to the last stage need to be part of a plan for implementation of a system.

Unfreezing. This stage is based on the idea that human behavior is supported by a balance of **driving** and **restraining forces** that creates an equilibrium. To institute change, the driving and restraining forces that are part of the maintenance of equilibrium in the organizational culture and individual have to be changed. To unfreeze, one must identify and change the balance so that the driving forces are stronger than the restraining forces. Driving forces can be involvement in the process, respect of one's opinion, and continuous communication during the process. Unfortunately restraining forces are harder to identify and treat because they are often personal psychological defenses or group norms embedded in the organizational or community culture (see Figure 18-2).

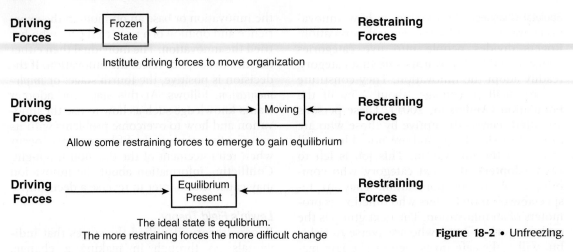

Figure 18-2 • Unfreezing.

Moving. In this stage the planned change is implemented. Its success depends on how situations were handled in the first stage. This is not a comfortable period. Anxieties are high, and if they are not successfully dealt with, the change may be unsuccessful. Additionally, it is important to recognize that in this stage movement may occur in the wrong direction. This is especially likely to happen if the new system has many problems, is not supported by administration, or has had no end user involvement. Thus it is important to have the support of administration in the planning process, involve users so that the system serves them instead of creating more work, thoroughly test the system before implementation for both bugs and usability, provide adequate training, and deal with any implementation problems immediately. In the Cedars-Lebanon case, the system created more work and resulted in a movement in the wrong direction despite a decree that all people must use the system (Bass, 2003). Decrees do not "move" people.

Refreezing. In this stage, equilibrium returns as the planned change becomes the norm and is surrounded by the usual driving and restraining forces. For this state to occur, individuals need to feel confident with the change and feel in control of the procedures involved in the new methods. A well-designed help system that can provide answers to frequent procedures as well as those that a user may use only occasionally will assist in this process, as will recognition by the organization of new skills. If too strongly reinforced, this stage can become a problem for the next change.

GENERAL SYSTEMS THEORY

General systems theory is a method of thinking about complex structures such as an information system or an organization. A simplified description of systems theory holds that any change in one part of a system will be reflected in other parts of the system. The original theory was introduced by von Bertalanffy in 1936 (Provost, n.d.). It was developed in part as a reaction against reductionism, or the reducing of phenomena to small parts, studying each, and ignoring the actions that each part creates in the other. In systems theory, the focus is on the interaction among the various parts of the system instead of regarding each individual part as standing alone. It is based on the premise that the whole is greater than the sum of its parts and is the basis for holistic nursing (Walonick).

To be part of a system, a phenomenon must be able to be isolated from its surrounding area for analysis, yet be part of the functioning of the whole system. Systems are described as being either open or closed. An open system continually exchanges information with the environment outside the system, while a closed system receives no **input** from the outside. This classification is more of a continuum than an absolute. Few, if any systems, are 100% closed or 100% open.

The objective of any system is to be in equilibrium, which is maintained by the correction forces from a feedback loop. Negative feedback results when there is a lack of something. The action it produces is to add the missing item to restore a variable to its state of equilibrium. Positive feedback results when there is too much of something. The action in positive feedback is to take away the excess. These two concepts can be confusing until one remembers that positive feedback results when the system finds too much of something and negative feedback when it finds something missing. Whether feedback is positive or negative is based on what the system finds, not its action.

The feedback loop operates using **input**, **throughput**, and **output**. Input involves adding information or matter to a system. Throughput is the processing, or evaluation of the input, that the system performs using the input information; output is the information or action that results from what the processing finds. This output may produce no action, or the action needed from either negative or positive feedback. A simple example would be inputting a patient's temperature into a computer system, the computer processing that data by combining it with the order that if this patient's temperature is more than 101°F, a specific medication should be given, and presenting the information to the nurse along with the action that needs to be taken. This is positive feedback – there was too much of something, body heat. The action it produced was to tell the nurse to give a medication. Another example is the physiological body processes that are governed by hormones as well as the entire human body.

You interact with systems all your life. Families, communities, and most inanimate objects are systems. The more complex the system, the more chaotic it is. A perfect example of a system is a computerized information system. Making a change in one area invariably affects other sections in ways that were never envisioned, which explains why it is often not a simple matter to make desired changes in systems. Adding an information system to a healthcare agency produces an even more complicated system. Systems theory provides a way of studying both the information system itself and its interaction with the environment. These interactions are also the focus of sociotechnical theory, but that theory would frame the problem in a different way.

CHAOS THEORY

Chaos theory was first encountered by a meteorologist, Edward Lorenz, in 1960 (Rae, n.d.), when attempting to predict the weather with a set of 12 equations. This theory is often associated with the so-called "butterfly effect," or the result on worldwide atmospheric conditions caused by the flapping of one butterfly's wings in the Amazon jungle. Yet, chaos theory has a true mathematical basis. The analogy comes from the small differences in the starting points of a butterfly flapping its wings, which produce different effects, and which over time produce changes. Chaos theory deals with the differences in outcomes depending on conditions at the starting point. For example, the conditions where an information system is first envisioned will affect the overall design.

Chaos theory, like general systems theory, addresses an entire structure without reducing it to the elemental parts. This makes it useful with complex systems such as information systems. The idea behind this theory is that what may appear to be chaotic actually has an order. It is based on the recognized fact that events and phenomena depend on initial conditions. Chaos theory is nonlinear. It allows us to question assumptions that we normally might reach using linear thought (Vincenzi, 1997). Seeing things reframed as a whole can stimulate new thinking and new approaches.

COGNITIVE SCIENCE

Cognitive science is gaining more importance in informatics. Basically, it is the study of the mind and intelligence (Thagard, 2004) and how this information can be applied. It is interdisciplinary and includes philosophy, psychology, artificial intelligence, neuroscience, linguistics, and anthropology and is a part of social informatics. It adds to informatics concepts that focus on how the brain perceives and interprets a screen (Turley, 1996). These factors are important in all aspects of information systems. When designing input screens, the screen locations where information is entered must be organized so as to facilitate data entry. Cognitive science is also a factor when presenting information; for example, characteristics such as color, font, and screen display affect clinical judgment because they are processed along with onscreen text and data. Additionally cognitive science addresses the amount of information that an individual can absorb and use constructively. Principles from these theories provide a guide to developing systems that allow users to concentrate on the task at hand, rather than requiring cognitive tasks to deal with the computer interface. Cognitive theory can also aid an informatics nurse specialist in understanding the information processing done by a nurse in decision making, thus facilitating the design of tools to support these processes (Staggers & Thompson, 2002).

USABILITY

Although usability has been a problem long before computers, this topic has become more visible with the advent of computer systems and the Web and is an integral part of informatics. It represents a multidimensional concept and involves users' evaluation of several measures, each one representative of their effectiveness in performing a task. It involves the ease of use, users' satisfaction that they have achieved their goals, and the aesthetics of the technology. It uses information from both the cognitive science and sociotechnical theories (see Box 18-1).

LEARNING THEORIES

Learning theories are important in informatics as well as in all nursing endeavors. Users must

---

Box 18-1 • The Five Goals of Usability

1. It is easy for users to accomplish basic tasks the first time they use the product.
2. Once learned, the design permits users to quickly and easily perform the needed tasks.
3. If it is not used for a period of time, it is easy to reestablish one's proficiency in using the product.
4. Users make very few errors, but any that they do make are easily remedied.
5. The design is pleasant to use.

From Peters, L. A. (2004, August). *Web site usability*. Retrieved March 26, 2008, from http://www.da.ks.gov/itab/was/usability.htm

---

be taught to use a system, and use of these theories can decrease the time for training as well as the time for learning.[2] See Table 18-3 for a summary of what the various theories contribute to informatics.

Roles for Informatics Nurse Specialists

As can be seen from the broad areas that informatics and its subspecialty nursing encompass, as well as the evolving nature of nursing informatics, the roles and areas in which informatics nurses work are many. Although the role they play may differ depending on the area, there is much overlap. You may find informatics nurses with only on-the-job training in many roles, but with the increase in complexity and expectations for systems, many of these roles are becoming limited to nursing informatics specialists. Informatics nurses may be systems educators, an information technology advocate, super user, system specialist, or clinical systems coordinator. Positions such as project director, director of clinical informatics, researcher,

---

[2] Learning theories are addressed in Chapter 23 about educational informatics.

TABLE 18-3 ● *Contributions of Theories to Informatics*	
Theory	**Contributions to Informatics**
Nursing informatics	Convert data into information and information to knowledge. Nurse adds wisdom
Sociotechnical theory and social informatics	Improve interaction between an information system and the organizational culture
Change	Increase the chance of success in implementing a system by attending to the reactions to the change
General systems	Contribute to the understanding of the complexity of an information system
Chaos	Improve the design of an information system
Cognitive science	Improve the ability of user to gain knowledge from an information system
Usability	Improve ease of use and satisfaction with an information system
Learning theory	Teach use of a system and design or select computer-aided instruction

product developer, policy developer, or entrepreneur are more apt to be filled by a nursing informatics specialist (see Table 18-4). Although job descriptions may vary from agency to agency, understanding the role of the informatics nurses in your area will help you to work with them to improve clinical systems.

Part of the job for all informatics nurses, regardless of their role or area of practice, is to interact with a variety of individuals at many different organizational levels, from anyone who uses the system to the chief executive officer (Heller & Romano, 1988). These interactions are important in gaining collaboration with clinicians, making decisions about how to interpret data, and obtaining administrative support for new practices. They also permit the informatics nurse to identify how information flows through an organization, assess for real and potential communication problems, and when necessary, devise alternative methods of communication. These are all areas where it is important for clinicians to provide information to the staff and administrators, who are, in effect, clients.

User liaison is an important role performed by informatics nurses. In this role, the nurse is the communications link between nurses and others involved in computer-related matters (Anderson, 1992; Hersher, 1985, 1995). Other job functions can be managing nursing

applications or chairing the nursing computer coordinating committee. Informatics nurses may also act as data systems managers for a specialty such as oncology.

Nursing informatics specialists working for either a healthcare agency or a vendor may be a project director for the installation of an information system. They may also be involved in product management or product definition. In this position the nurse may also be responsible for seeing that the product is updated. This involves being aware of new developments in the field as well as the current and future needs of clients.[3] Some nurse informatics specialists who work for vendors are involved in marketing. For marketing, skills in listening and anticipating needs, as well as the ability to identify the real decision maker, are necessary.

Some nursing informatics specialists act as consultants, either working independently or working for an organization. Consulting is a high-pressure field in which individuals often must make instant decisions based on personal knowledge and an analysis of only the known facts. This involves the role of a liaison and an expert. Many consulting jobs involve a

[3] When working in a role that involves working with system users, a client is not necessarily a person outside the agency, but an individual who needs the services that an informatics person can provide.

Box 18-2 • An Informatics Nurse Speaks (Continued)

you enter data and print reports to make sure the software does what it's supposed to do. This can take hours, days, or even weeks to complete.

Reports are the end result of information processing. When you buy software, you sometimes get standard reports (those that the majority of all users need) but you usually have to write custom reports. Users give me requests for reports that they would like to have. To create them I may be able to modify an existing report, or I may need to create a new one. This involves determining which file or files the information resides in, how the output of the report should look, what fields the report needs to include, what to name it so that the users will know which report to run, and perhaps which menu to put it on. Writing reports can take anywhere from a few minutes to several days, depending on the complexity, as well as the amount of time you can devote. (Remember all those interruptions!) Testing a report is also part of modifying or creating one. As the creator, I need to test it to be certain that it produces what the user wants. Then I need to have the user test it to see if the data and design meet his or her needs.

Another role of the informatics nurse is one of teacher. I develop the lesson plans and teaching materials to train the staff on the use of the computer systems. Training is done formally or informally, depending on the situation, and can take a few minutes to several days. In addition, I attend meetings, both in my department and with other departments. Many times, I am the leader of the meeting, which also involves putting together the agenda and handouts, and doing minutes. There are also user group and informatics organizations to which I belong.

A key element in this role is communication. When you are working in nursing informatics, you are providing help and support to end users: staff, managers, directors, and vice presidents, as well as the programmers/developers. (Very often, the programmer or developer is at your vendor's location and not in-house.) Nursing informatics is extremely dynamic, and I love the challenge. It offers me the opportunity to work with many different people, do many different things, and be creative. This role is never boring!

Judith Hornback, RN, BSN, MHSA
Informatics Nurse Specialist
Senior Consultant, RHI, Inc.
Highland, Indiana

---

alone, although helpful, is insufficient for a career in informatics. Computers are only a tool in informatics; information management is the focus. This knowledge cannot be gained without clinical experience.

To be a nursing informatics specialist requires a formal academic degree at the master's or doctoral level, or a formal post-master's or post-doctoral degree program leading to a certificate. All informatics careers require continuing education that is often obtained at professional conferences. The **American Medical Informatics Association (AMIA)**, **Healthcare Information Management Systems Society (HIMSS)**, and **American Health Information Management Association (AHIMA)** have large educational and research meetings including tutorials for novice practitioners. Additionally, some universities sponsor one- or two-week intensive informatics courses. Two annual conferences, one sponsored by Rutgers College of Nursing and the other by the University of Maryland School of Nursing, are excellent places for continuing education as is the annual conference of the American Nursing Informatics Association (ANIA) done in collaboration with the Capital Area Roundtable Informatics Nursing Group (CARING).

The nursing working group of AMIA classifies nursing informatics programs into four categories: 1) online courses, 2) graduate programs with a specialty in nursing informatics, 3) graduate and undergraduate programs with minors or majors in nursing informatics, and 4) individual courses in nursing informatics within graduate/undergraduate programs (AMIA Nursing Informatics Working Group, 2007). Their Web site provides links to a list of programs in each category. Online courses may be stand-alones that just provide continuing education, be part of a program that leads to a certificate in nursing informatics, or belong to a formal degree-granting program that may or may not be 100% online.

Many educational institutions have begun informatics programs. Given the many foci of informatics, it follows that each educational program will have a different focus. Some focus on applied informatics, others on informatics research. At present there are no accrediting bodies that examine informatics education. Thus there are many questions that prospective students need to ask of any program. Questions specific to an informatics program are listed in Box 18-3.

Informatics Missions for All Nurses

Informatics nurse specialists cannot work in a vacuum. The best systems are developed by collaboration between informatics nurse specialists and practicing clinicians. This avoids one of the common reasons for system failure: neglecting the expertise and needs of end users. To make this a productive relationship, practicing clinicians need to have a basic understanding of informatics (see Box 18-4). If a system is to truly assist the clinician in providing quality care, it is imperative that there be an understanding of the

---

Box 18-3 • Questions Specific to an Informatics Program

(In addition to those normally asked of any educational program)
1. What is the focus of the informatics program? For example:
   a. Clinical systems
   b. Knowledge generation/research
   c. Decision support
   d. Healthcare specialty
2. What types of jobs do graduates of the program obtain?
3. Who are the faculty in informatics?
   a. What is their informatics experience?

b. What are their qualifications to teach informatics?
c. What are there interests in informatics?
4. Is there a preceptorship or internship?
   a. If so, for how long?
   b. How are these assignments found?
5. How long has the program been operating?
6. What courses are currently available versus those being planned, but not yet offered?
7. If the program is online, how much on-campus time is required?

Box 18-4 • Some Informatics Facts for All Nurses

Data should be entered only once.
• One piece of data can be presented in many different ways and contexts.
• Data from monitors of physiological processes can be integrated into an electronic record.
• Computers can transform data by calculating either numbers or words.
• Computers require standardization of data if they are to permit learning from aggregated data.
• Decision support can be part of an informatics system.

• Output is only as good as input.
• Only a clinician understands how information flows through the clinical area, it is imperative that this information be communicated to informatics personnel.
• An information system will *not* solve organizational problems.
• Aggregated, unidentified data about patient care can, and should, be available to all practicing clinicians for the purpose of improving patient care.

role of data in not only providing but also tracking and trending individual patient care. As data is synthesized and converted to information and knowledge, all nurses need to use this information/knowledge wisely. Everyone needs to realize that a computer can only work with the data that it has. The principle "garbage in, garbage out" (GIGO) should have a corollary "data lacking, output defective" (DLOD). When evaluating output, whether research or from a computer, examine the data categories (fields) on which it was based.

There is often an unrealistic expectation that a new information system will solve all problems, some of which may be organizational problems. An information system is apt to magnify organizational problems such as poor communication between departments, lack of accountability, lack of administration support for the planned information system, etc. It is important to be able to separate organizational problems from informational system problems, and solve the former before the new system is implemented.

 Informatics Organizations

Health and healthcare concerns are worldwide, as is the interest in the use of informatics to improve healthcare.

MULTIDISCIPLINARY GROUPS

Given the interdisciplinary nature of informatics, it is to be expected that many of the formal organizations involve practitioners from all areas.

International Medical Informatics Association (IMIA)

The largest informatics group is the **International Medical Informatics Association** (**IMIA**), which was established in 1967 as TC4, a Technical Committee within the International Federation for Information Processing (IFIP). This group soon was renamed IMIA (International Medical Informatics Association). IMIA is a nonpolitical, international, scientific organization whose goals include promoting informatics in healthcare, promoting biomedical research, advancing international cooperation, stimulating informatics research and education, and exchanging information. Many countries belong to IMIA through national organizations such as the AMIA, which represents the United States, and the **European Federation for Medical Informatics** (**EFMI**), which represents Europe. The members have national meetings to focus on issues pertaining to their nation, which allow members to establish a national network where ideas can be shared, and provide a place to gain information for specific national problems. These organizations also provide journals and are a source of up-to-date information for their country. The members of IMIA also take part in MedINFO, a feature of IMIA, which is held every three years. A list of member countries' organizations is present on the IMIA Web page (http://www.imia.org/).

Healthcare Information and Management Systems Society (HIMSS)

Another international organization is HIMSS, which was founded in 1961, with offices in Chicago, Washington DC, Brussels, and other locations across the United States and Europe. HIMSS is a not-for-profit organization dedicated to promoting a better understanding of healthcare information and management systems. At present, HIMSS represents more than 20,000 individual healthcare professionals and more than 300 corporate members (Healthcare Information and Management Systems Society, 2007). In 2003 HIMSS formed a Nursing Informatics Community to provide support to the nursing role in informatics. HIMSS meets annually and publishes a quarterly journal and several guides to the field. They offer accreditation as a Certified Professional in Healthcare Information and Management Systems (CPHIMS).

American Health Information Management Association (AHIMA)

The American College of Surgeons formed AHIMA in 1928. This is mostly a North American group whose goal is the improvement of clinical records (American Health Information Management Association, 2007). Originally named the Association of Record Librarians of North America, the organization has had several name changes. Currently named AHIMA, this name was adopted to reflect today's situation in which clinical data has expanded beyond either a single hospital or provider. They offer credentialing programs in health information management, coding, and healthcare privacy and security.

NURSING INFORMATICS GROUPS

The multidisciplinary groups sometimes have smaller working groups, some of which are nursing focused. Since 1982 the IMIA nursing working group has sponsored an international nursing informatics conference every three years. The themes of these conferences provide a look into how the concerns of nursing informatics have broadened from a concern in 1982 with computers in nursing through integrating caring and technology in nursing, a realization of the impact of informatics on nursing knowledge, to the recognition of the importance of the consumer or human in healthcare (Table 18-5).

Working Groups of Larger Organizations

AMIA and EFMI both have nursing working groups. AMIA's nursing working group, the Nursing Informatics Working Group (NIWG), is responsible for promoting the integration of nursing informatics into the broader context of healthcare and influencing U.S. policy makers regarding the use of nursing information. EFMI's nursing working group was formed in 1988 to support European nurses and nursing informatics as well as to build informatics contact networks (Tallberg, 1994). Their Web page at http://www.helmholtz-muenchen.de/ibmi/efmi/ has a list of member nations.

British Computer Society Nursing Specialist Group. There are other professional informatics organizations that are primarily for nurses. A very active group is the British Computer Society Nursing Specialist Group, which is one of the five Health Informatics Specialist Groups of the **British Computer Society**. One of its aims is to disseminate information about current nursing informatics applications and to encourage the publication of research and development material in this area (British Computer Society, 2007). This is accomplished by interacting with other groups such as the Royal College of Nursing (RCM), the Clinical Professions and Health Visitor's Association (CPHVA/Amicus), and the NHS Connecting for Health's National Advisory Group for the National Programme.

Alliance for Nursing Informatics. In 2004, the **Alliance for Nursing Informatics (ANI)** was

---

TABLE 18-5 • *Themes and Locations of International Nursing Informatics Conferences*

Year	Title	Location
1982	The Impact of Computers on Nursing	London, United Kingdom
1985	Building Bridges to the Future	Calgary, Alberta; California, United States
1988	Where Caring and Technology Meet	Dublin, Ireland
1991	Nurses Managing Information in Health Care	Melbourne, Victoria, Australia
1994	An International Overview of Nursing in a Technological Era	San Antonio, Texas, United States
1997	The Impact of Nursing Knowledge on Healthcare Informatics	Stockholm, Sweden
2000	One Step Beyond: The Evolution of Technology and Nursing	Auckland, New Zealand
2003	E-health for All: Designing a Nursing Agenda for the Future	Rio de Janeiro, Brazil
2006	Consumer-Centered, Computer-Supported Care for Healthy People	Seoul, Korea
2009	Nursing Informatics – Connecting Health and Humans	Helsinki, Finland

formed to unite many of the local, smaller, nursing informatics groups. Membership is through membership in a nursing-focused informatics group, either a nursing working group or a local or national group. These groups still retain their dues, programs, publications, and organizational structures, but are united through ANI to create a unified voice for nursing informatics. Representatives of each of the organizational groups make up the governing directors group that guides the strategic goals and activities of ANI (Alliance for Nursing Informatics, n.d.). Their Web site (http://www.allianceni.org/) features links to all the member groups. Besides members of the nursing working groups of AMIA and HIMSS, other large member groups are CARING and ANIA.

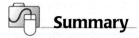 **Summary**

Nursing informatics is a subspecialty in both nursing and health informatics and is a relatively new field. Nursing informatics focuses on helping clinicians acquire and integrate patient care data from many sources. Concerns in this field have moved from hardware and healthcare applications to perspectives that embrace sociotechnical, change, general systems, cognitive science, usability, and chaos theories.

Within nursing informatics, there are many different areas of concentration and roles including project manager, systems manager, and independent contractor. Nursing informatics, however, is not solely the province of nursing informatics specialists; all nurses must be involved if successful information systems are to be developed and implemented. There are many areas where informatics nurses work, as well as many different job foci.

Many of the nurses working in informatics have learned on the job, but the trend today is for a more formal education in the field. Many different types of programs exist for those who wish to specialize in nursing informatics. They range from programs granting graduate degrees to continuing education offerings. There

is no accrediting body for education in this specialty as yet, and the wise prospective student should investigate any academic program before enrolling.

Health informatics organizations at the international and national level are mostly multidisciplinary. Besides nursing working groups in the multidisciplinary groups, there are organizations that focus only on nursing informatics interests.

APPLICATIONS AND COMPETENCIES

1. Using one episode in a recent clinical experience, describe how you mentally move data through information and knowledge to wisdom. Keep it small, such as giving a medication or assessing a patient for lung congestion.
   a. How did you evaluate and combine the different pieces of data?
   b. What was the outcome of this process?
   c. Reflect on how an information system could assist this process.
2. The theories supporting informatics come from many different areas.
   a. Using the sociotechnical theory make a plan to assess the readiness of an organization for either a new information system or an update to the current plan.
   b. In adopting a spreadsheet, in which category of Rogers' diffusion theory would you place yourself?
   c. Think of planning a change for an organization with which you are familiar. What are some of the restraining forces and the driving forces? How would you proceed?
   d. Think of some of the various organizations with which you are familiar. Where would you classify them on the open–closed continuum of systems theory?
   e. Relate the cognitive theory to the design of a Web page as discussed in Chapter 14.
3. Interview an informatics nurse to discover her/his responsibilities. Into which of the role(s) discussed in this chapter would you place this individual?
4. Using the Nursing Informatics Work Group from AMIA's Web page (http://www.amia.org/ni-wg/ni-wg-education), identify a formal educational

program in nursing informatics that would most interest you.

5. Investigate the activities of one of the informatics professional organizations. Some methods for accomplishing this include checking their home page, attending a meeting, or interviewing a member/officer in one of the groups.

REFERENCES

Alliance for Nursing Informatics. (n.d.). *About ANI.* Retrieved November 23, 2008, from http://www.allianceni.org/about.asp

American Health Information Management Association. (2007). *AHIMA history.* Retrieved November 23, 2008, from http://www.ahima.org/about/history.asp

American Nurses Association. (2008). *Nursing informatics: Scope and standards of practice.* American Nurses Association.

American Nurses Credentialing Center. *Informatics nurse certification.* Retrieved November 23, 2008, from http://www.nursecredentialing.org/Eligibility/InformaticsNurseEligibility.aspx

AMIA Nursing Informatics Working Group. (2007, July 12). *Categories of nursing informatics programs.* Retrieved November 23, 2008, from http://www.amia.org/ni-wg/ni-wg-education

Anderson, B. L. (1992). Nursing informatics: Career opportunities inside and out. *Computers in Nursing,* 10(4), 165–170.

Anderson, D. (2001, November 8). *Diffusion of innovation.* Retrieved November 23, 2008, from http://riccistreet.net/port80/charthouse/present/diffusion.htm

Audain, C. (1998). *Florence Nightingale.* Retrieved November 23, 2008, from http://www.agnesscott.edu/Lriddle/WOMEN/nitegale.htm

Bass, A. (2003, June 1). *Health-care IT: A big rollout bust.* Retrieved November 23, 2008, from http://www.radiologytoday.net/archive/rt_061305p18.shtml

Berg, M., Aarts, J., & van der Lei, J. (2003). ICT in health care: Sociotechnical approaches. *Methods of Informatics in Medicine,* 42(4), 297–301.

British Computer Society. (2007, August 1). *Health informatics (nursing) specialist group.* Retrieved November 23, 2008, from http://www.nursing.bcs.org/about.htm

Chin, T. (2004, February 17). *Doctors pull plug on paperless system.* Retrieved November 23, 2008, from http://www.ama-assn.org/amednews/2003/02/17/bil20217.htm

Clark, D. (2000, January 22). *Kurt Lewin.* Retrieved November 23, 2008, from http://www.nwlink.com/~donclark/hrd/history/lewin.html

Clark, D. (2004, May 2). *Understanding.* Retrieved November 23, 2008, from http://www.nwlink.com/~donclark/performance/understanding.html

Corcoran-Perry, S., & Graves, J. R. (1990). Supplemental-information-seeking behavior of cardiovascular nurses. *Research in Nursing & Health,* 13(2), 119–127.

Graves, J. R., & Cocoran, S. (1989). The study of nursing informatics. *Image: Journal of Nursing Scholarship,* 21, 227–231.

Gray, R. M. (1991). *Entropy and information theory* [Electronic version at http://ee.stanford.edu/~gray/it.html]. New York: Springer-Verlag.

Healthcare Information and Management Systems Society. (2007). *About HIMSS.* Retrieved November 23, 2008, from http://www.himss.org/asp/aboutHimssHome.asp

Heller, B. R., & Romano, C. A. (1988). Nursing informatics: The pathway to knowledge. *Nursing and Health Care,* 9(9), 483–484.

Hersher, B. S. (1985). The job search and information systems opportunities for nurses. In: D. Pocklington & J. Baron (Eds.), *The Nursing Clinics of North America,* 20, 585–603.

Hersher, B. S. (1995). Careers for nurses in healthcare information systems. In: M. J. Ball, K. J. Hannah, S. K. Newbold, & J. V. Douglas (Eds.), *Nursing Informatics: Where caring and technology meet* (2nd ed., pp. 77–83). New York: Springer-Verlag.

International Medical Informatics Association. *Welcome to IMIA.* Retrieved November 23, 2008, from http://www.imia.org/ about.lasso

Joos, I., Whitman, N. I., Smith, M. J., & Nelson, R. (1992). *Computer in Small Bytes.* New York: National League for Nursing Press.

Kling, R. (1999). What is social informatics and why does it matter? [Electronic version at http://www.dlib.org/dlib/january99/kling/01kling.html]. *D-Lib Magazine,* 5(1).

Ozbolt, J., Nahm, E.-S., & Roberts, D. (2007). How about a career in nursing informatics. *American Nurse Today,* 2(9), 34–36.

Pillar, B., & Golumbic, N. (Eds.). (1993). *Nursing informatics: Enhancing patient care.* Bethesda, MD: National Center for Nursing Research, U.S. Department of Health and Human Services.

Provost, W. J. (n.d.). *General systems theory.* Retrieved November 23, 2008, from http://www.n4bz.org/gst/gst1.htm

Rae, G. (n.d.). *Chaos theory: A brief introduction.* Retrieved November 23, 2008, from http://www.imho.com/grae/chaos/chaos.html

Rogers, E. (1983). *Diffusion of innovations.* New York: Free Press.

Schein, E. H. (2004). *Kurt Lewin's change theory in the field and in the classroom: Notes toward a model of managed learning.* Retrieved November 23, 2008, from http://www.a2zpsychology.com/articles/kurt_lewin's_change_theory.htm

Staggers, N., & Thompson, C. B. (2002). The evolution of definitions for nursing informatics: A critical analysis and revised definition. *Journal of the American Medical Informatics Association,* 9(3), 255–261.

Tallberg, M. (1994, January 9). *History of EFMI wg5 1988 to 1994.* Retrieved November 23, 2008, from http://www.nicecomputing.ch/nieurope/EFMI_aims_history.htm

Thagard, P. (2004, Summer). *The Stanford Encyclopedia of Philosophy* (Summer 2004 ed.). Retrieved November 23, 2008, from http://plato.stanford.edu/archives/sum2004/entries/cognitive-science/

Turley, J. (1996). Toward a model for nursing informatics. *Image: Journal of Nursing Scholarship, 29*(4), 309–313.

Vincenzi, A. E. (1997). Using chaos theory: The implications for nursing. *Journal of Advanced Nursing, 37*(5), 462–469.

Wade, M., & Schneberger, S. (2005, October 13). *Socio-technical theory*. Retrieved November 23, 2008, from http://www.istheory.yorku.ca/sociotechnicaltheory.htm

Walonick, D. S. *General systems theory*. Retrieved November 23, 2008, from http://www.survey-software-solutions .com/walonick/systems-theory.htm

Warner, H. (1995). Medical informatics: a real discipline? *Journal of the American Medical Informatics Association, 2*(4), 207–214.

Wikipedia. (2007, September 24). *Information theory*. Retrieved November 23, 2008, from http://en.wikipedia .org/wiki/Information_theory

Basic Electronic Healthcare Information Systems

Learning Objectives

After studying this chapter you will be able to:

1. Compare and contrast the electronic patient record with the electronic health record.

2. Discuss the importance of the clinical nurse's role in the selection of a clinical information system process.

3. Discuss the concept of workflow analysis as it relates to nursing care.

4. Compare the systems life cycle with the nursing process.

5. Discuss the role of the superuser in the systems life cycle.

Key Terms

Big-Bang Conversion
Bugs
Clinical Document
   Architecture (CDA)
Context-Sensitive Help
Contingency Plan
Continuity of Care
   Document (CCD)
Cost Benefit
Debugging
Electronic Health Record
   (EHR)
Electronic Medical Record
   (EMR)
Go-Live
Health Level 7 (HL7)
Initiating
Intranet

Needs Assessment
Phased Conversion
Pilot Conversion
Project Goal
Project Scope
Regression Testing
Request for Information
   (RFI)
Request for Proposal (RFP)
Return on Investment (ROI)
Rollback
Rollout
Scope Creep
Superuser
Systems Life Cycle
Test Scripts
Vanilla Product
Vaporware

Healthcare information systems (HIS) are a composite made up of all of the information management systems that serve an organization's needs. The complexity of HIS is largely *independent* of the size of the organization because healthcare provides a common core of patient care services. At the very minimum, most healthcare providers have electronic systems for billing patient care services. Facilities using advanced technologies have numerous systems that manage each and every service provided to the patient. This chapter will focus on a few basic components and processes common to HIS that are essential for all nurses to understand.

Every nurse needs to appreciate her individual role as it relates to HIS. As nurses we need to understand what systems can "do" to help efficiently manage information that relates to patient care. We must recognize how electronic documentation underpins the discovery of evidence-based practice for improved patient outcomes. We should expect HIS to support the nursing care delivery process and the documentation of care; HIS should *not* negatively impact our practice. That being said, we should not expect a technology solution to mimic the paper chart world. Adaption to electronic documentation requires a change in processes and workflow design. To effectively manage the change process, nursing leadership (Simpson, 2006, 2007) and clinical nurses must acquire technological competence and take an active role in the selection process and design for new systems. When participating in the system selection process, we should be able to talk with information technology specialists and vendor representatives using the appropriate terminology. Additionally, we must also understand the systems life cycle, the process for health information technology (HIT) system selection and implementation.

EMR, EHR, ePHR, and Their Relationships to Emerging Clinical Information Systems

The patient's health information is the forefront of clinical information systems. A brief review of the different types of patient records should help set the scene for emerging clinical information systems. The EMR (electronic medical record), EHR (electronic health record), and ePHR (electronic personal health record) are now being integrated into the design of clinical information systems.

The **EMR** is an electronic version of the traditional record used by the healthcare provider. It is a legal record that describes the care that a patient received during an encounter with the healthcare agency. The EMR is an electronic clinical data repository that uses a standardized healthcare vocabulary (Garets & Davis, 2006). The EMR comprises order entry, computerized provider order entry (CPOE), pharmacy, and other applications for clinical documentation. Instead of hospital visit information being located in one or more manila folders in medical records, the EMR is a searchable database. For example, providers could search for all admissions for treatment of congestive heart failure or all surgeries. A patient can have many EMRs – one at the health department for immunizations; one at each hospital where care has been provided; and one at each healthcare provider's office.

The value of EMRs has been challenged because there is no standard for recording data, which leads to data redundancy (repeated entries of the same information) and subsequent entry discrepancies. As an example, the hospital where the care was originally provided may have accurate dates for the admission or surgery; however, on readmission when asked about previous surgeries, the patient's memory of those dates or types of surgeries may vary from the actual information. Although the information belongs to the patient, the data in the EMR is owned by the healthcare provider. Except for a few very large healthcare organizations, the EMR data reside in virtual silos among all of the providers.

The **EHR** is a transportable subset of the EMR designed for use by healthcare organizations and physician practices, and other providers (HIMSS, n.d.). The EHR uses **Clinical Document Architecture** (CDA) data standards. CDA for common clinical document types was devised by **Health Level 7 (HL7)** to provide a common structure for clinical documents. The structure has three levels and provides the ability to send documents that have sufficient "code" in them to be machine readable and yet are also easily interpretable as a document by a human. This

---

Box 19-1 • Ways the EHR Can Address the Gaps in Clinical Knowledge

The EHR can address the gaps in knowledge in evidence and clinical practice by the following ways:

- Detecting information and knowledge from current records that can efficiently affect clinical outcomes
- Shortening the time from knowledge discovery to implementation
- Monitoring quality improvement outcomes that result from knowledge-driven changes in providers' practices

- Empowering the patient to become a partner in care with the healthcare provider(s)
- Providing real-world knowledge vs. controlled clinical trials about treatment effectiveness and outcomes

Adapted from Liang, L. (2007). The gap between evidence and practice. *Health Affairs, 26*(2), w119–w121.

---

can be achieved by the use of extensible markup language (XML) tags that designate what a piece of text is. For example, a first name will be tagged just like in HTML (see Figure 5-3 in Chapter 5 for an example of HTML tagging), as will other required fields. The tagged items can be automatically placed as data into an electronic record, while the document can be read by humans. This format is intended for use by any type of clinical document such as history and physical, a consult, a nursing document, or a discharge summary.

The new **Continuity of Care Document (CCD)** uses the CDA architecture to provide a "snapshot" of a patient's health information, including insurance information, medical diagnoses and problems, medications, and allergies (Kibbe, 2008), which is to be integrated with EHRs to provide the sharing of data with multiple providers. It is a result of the harmonization of the Continuity of Care Record developed jointly by the American Society for Testing and Materials (ASTM) International, Massachusetts Medical Society (MMS), Health Information and Management Systems Society (HIMSS), American Academy of Family Physicians (AAFP), and the American Academy of Pediatrics ASTM's with HL7's CDA specifications (Bazzoli, 2007a, 2007b). The CCD has defined what data is shared, and the CDA defines *how* data is shared with the EHR. In this manner the CDA will be used for other clinical documents that need sharing.

The terminology for an electronic record can be confusing because the terms EMR and EHR may be used as if the meanings are

identical. Not only can healthcare providers extract pertinent information from electronic records that would enhance the effectiveness of care, but the information also has the potential for use in quality and evidence-based care knowledge management. Both the EMR and EHR electronic clinical databases allow for healthcare providers to review and analyze changes over time. Liang (2007) forecasted five (see Box 19-1) potential solutions that the EHR can provide to fill gaps in knowledge between evidence and practice.

In the effort to improve patient care outcomes, there has been somewhat of a chaotic effort for healthcare providers to transition from a paper record to an electronic record. Without any "mental models" about how information can be extracted from electronic systems, the adoption process is tainted by "paper chart thinking" (Baron, 2007, p. 549). It will be several more years before universal standards for electronic records will be adopted and certified, although the process is under way. There is still inconsistent communication between those who are involved in the universal design of the electronic record, those attempting to implement it, and those who are considering implementation. Agencies that are adopting or want to adopt electronic documentation may not understand the advantages of an interconnected record and the importance of interoperability for sharing information pertinent to improvement of patient outcomes. In the ideal world, the EHR summary data is owned by the patient, has patient input, and is used by multiple healthcare organizations. The vision for EHRs

IMPROVED QUALITY

One of the most important benefits of the electronic record is improved patient care outcomes. In noncomputerized systems, test results can be easily lost or misplaced, requiring repeated testing. Ordered treatments can be overlooked or not documented. An electronic information system can improve the quality of care by preventing these all-too-common difficulties. When physicians enter orders into the system, transcription errors are eliminated. The electronic order can be compared with recommended dosages in the database, and the physician can be provided with information about the drug prescribed using clinical reminders (decision support system). When the order is integrated with the patient's information about the drugs that the patient is concurrently receiving, as well as drug allergies, drug mismatches can be better avoided. Clinical reminders can be generated to ensure that the patient is receiving the correct drug.

Healthcare Information Systems

Since the beginning of formalized healthcare, there have been HIS. As the complexity of healthcare has grown, so has the complexity of information. Patients see many providers and have records in many places. For several centuries, the paper record has proven its worth, but today's complex systems have outgrown the ability to be managed by paper.

STRENGTHS OF PAPER RECORDS

The wonderful thing about paper is that it is light and very transportable. The paper record can be used as soon as we find it and pick up a pen to write. We don't have to wait in line for a computer terminal, log in, click to drill down to menus, nor wait between windows opening. The paper record requires no electricity, no maintenance, and no downtime. In the paper chart world, we can chart very quickly.

A nursing student completing her senior internship in a hospital that used the paper record system stated that documenting on paper "made her think." When asked what she meant, she said that she was used to a computer documentation system that provided checkboxes and data entry screen prompts, which, she felt, guided her in electronic documentation. She said that when there was a blank nursing progress note, she had to "think" about *what to chart*. It was clear that she realized that without those prompts her entries might be incomplete.

WEAKNESSES OF PAPER RECORDS

Those of us who have used paper records can readily cite the inherent weaknesses. Unlike the electronic record, there is no backup system. Paper records can be easily damaged or destroyed. Parts of the paper record can be accidentally or, rarely, purposely destroyed. Part of the drudgery, particularly for night staff, includes stamping new forms and deleting duplicate updated patient information such as laboratory and x-ray reports. In the paper record world, it is very easy to stamp a chart form with the wrong stamp plate. Stamp machines are heavy and cumbersome and require maintenance. Filing copies of testing reports in paper records is very time consuming and prone to human error, such as misfiling a report.

Legibility is another criticism of the paper record. It is often very difficult to read handwriting of others. Script versions of certain terms have led to serious and sometime fatal medical errors. As a result, the National Coordinating Council for Medication Error Reporting and Prevention (MERP) (2008) and the Joint Commission (2001) made recommendations to stop using certain dangerous abbreviations. The Joint Commission issued a Sentinel Event Alert on the use of dangerous abbreviations in 2001, and healthcare agencies have worked fervently ever since to correct the problems. For example, the abbreviation for cubic centimeter (cc) was being misinterpreted as *units*, every day (q.d.) was being misinterpreted as four times per day (q.i.d.), and morphine sulfate (MSO_4) was being misinterpreted as magnesium sulfate ($MgSO_4$).

Trending data in the paper record world is tedious and prone to error. The user has to graph vital signs data and draw connecting lines to portray a trend on a vital signs flow sheet. Information such as intake and output (I&O) is initially charted on a clipboard in the patient's room and then transferred to the paper record at the end of the shift. If the patient got behind or ahead of his or her fluid volume needs, it usually is not discovered until the nurse charts the date – when it is too late to make an efficient correction. Totaling the I&O for complex care patients can be extremely time consuming and prone to error. A calculator is often required to add and subtract numbers for an I&O total. All of this is avoided with an EMR; the data can be entered as it is generated, and the total is automatically calculated. Further, it can provide an up-to-date record for the physician who wants this information before the end of the shift.

Paper records for patients who require a lengthy hospital stay can become very large, heavy, and difficult to store on a nursing unit. Retrieving old records for a new admission is often challenging. It isn't unusual for paper records to be misfiled, so there may be a significant time delay before the paper record is delivered to the nursing unit. Finding information for a patient with multiple readmissions is often overwhelming and may require searches through stacks of manila folders.

THE NEED FOR AN ELECTRONIC PATIENT RECORD

Why is there a need for an electronic patient record? As clearly outlined in the IOM reports, it is to make patient care safer (Committee on Quality of Health Care in America & Institute of Medicine, 2001; Committee on the Work Environment for Nurses and Patient Safety, 2004; Institute of Medicine, 1999). The paper record and the associated information silos are not good enough anymore. The need for an electronic record is recognized worldwide, not just in the United States.

WORKFLOW REDESIGN

The need for workflow redesign when making a change from the paper record to an electronic documentation system cannot be emphasized enough. In contrast to the paper record environment where forms were often designed for the care providers, the electronic system focuses on the patient with collaborative information sharing patient data among the care providers. This means that workflow redesign has to consider the patient, the work done by all of the care providers, and organizational needs, not just nursing needs. All participants in the design and implementation process must carefully listen to users' perceptions about the impact of a system implementation, recognize barriers to change, and identify strategies to work through the barriers (Lee, 2007). "Applying automation, even the newer, more sophisticated solutions, without focused, intentional process redesign can increase the very complexities intended to be streamlined" (Ball, Weaver, & Kiel, 2004, p. 454).

One approach for workflow redesign is to use the same method as we do for patient problems: identify the purpose, goals and expected outcomes (Schulman, Kuperman, Kharbanda, & Kaushal, 2007). The workflow redesign should be orchestrated by a multidisciplinary committee, which first identifies what an automated system is expected to accomplish. The committee should also establish broad goals and maintain compliance with standard setting organization requirements and rules and laws of regulatory agencies. The design of an efficient workflow process must include documentation of patient care, creation of reports, electronic prescribing of medications, and CPOE.

Workflow redesign is not for the faint of heart. It requires a tremendous amount of work and collaboration between the various discipline members. Without that communication, the work could easily be compared to the Chinese parable about the blind men and the elephant. According to the parable, each blind man touched a different part of the elephant and came away believing that the part he

Flow Chart Symbols and Their Meaning Using the Systems Life Cycle

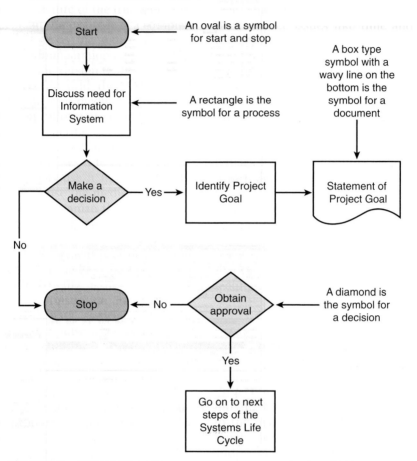

Figure 19-2 • Systems life cycle.

the use of terminology across an organization, healthcare agencies often provide glossaries and templates for users. One example is the Duke University Web site at http://www .oit.duke.edu/enterprise/lifecycle/index.html, which includes a glossary, templates, and flow charts (Duke Office of Information Technology, n.d.).

Initiating
Every system begins with an idea. In the **initiating** phase, the project goals and needs (requirements) are identified and analyzed. This first phase is a critical step. Many system implementation failures can be attributed to a poor needs assessment. All system stakeholders must be a part of this process, not just the information systems personnel. A **stakeholder** is anyone who has something to gain or lose from a project (Nuseibeh & Easterbrook, 2000). Examples of stakeholders include the healthcare agency's top executives, nursing executives, financial personnel, and any other personnel who may need to use the system.

Project Goals and Scope. The first task in initiating the process is to identify the project goal. The **project goal** is a succinct statement that

---

Box 19-2 • Example of Project Goal Statements

- Implement computerized patient order entry CPOE by 12/1/12. Implement computerized documentation in the ED by 4/1/11.

---

describes the project. Goals should be specific and measurable. Instead of using the term *project goal,* some references use the term *project definition* (see Box 19-2).

The next task is to define the **project scope,** which refers to all of the elements that are entailed in the project. For example, a project scope may address the implementation of an electronic documentation in the ED, or it may entail deployment of electronic documentation throughout the entire hospital. **Scope creep** is a term that describes unanticipated growth of the project. It can develop because of "we don't miss what we never had" situations. Once the users understand that a database or new system can manage information more effectively, they often specify new requirements, causing the scope of the project to creep (get larger). The problem with scope creep is that time and resources add up to money. Scope creep can cause project budget overruns.

Project Requirements. Every project involves risks; they should always be carefully explored and never be minimized. Risks are all of those things that could interfere with the success of the project. They include personnel, finances, equipment, interoperability issues, training, security, and time issues.

The **needs assessment** is identification of the expectations or requirements of the system. In this part of the cycle, data and information pertinent to the project goal and scope are put together and translated to the needs for the system. The team identifies what features are essential to the new system and which features would be nice to have. At this point, a team member may go back to the clinicians and ask them to differentiate their needs from their wants. Some teams use a rating scale to deter-

mine the necessity of a feature, with patient safety features being given a higher priority.

The assessment is comparable to a brainstorming session. Questions that should be addressed include the following:

▼ Why do we want an information system?
▼ What do we want the system to do?
  ▼ Communicate with another department?
  ▼ Generate alerts?
  ▼ Record information in the patient record?
  ▼ Print reports?
▼ Of all of the system "wants," which are essential needs and which are nice to have?

As a comparison, think about the needs assessment process when purchasing a vehicle. Considerations for making a purchase would include the amount of money you have to spend. You also would want to consider the expected number of passengers and when and why you want to use the vehicle. Gas consumption may be another consideration – whether there is a cost benefit in purchasing a hybrid. Service should be important. You would want to consider the reputation and reliability of the service department, the cost of oil changes, and routine maintenance. In the process of making a purchase decision, the buyer usually reads news reports, compares auto manufacturers, vehicle types, and auto dealers. Likewise, all of the factors considered for the purchase of a vehicle should be taken into consideration when selecting an information system: the reason for the purchase, what we want the system to accomplish, and the alternatives available. When reviewing the alternatives, decision makers must consider which alternatives best meet their requirements, the experiences of other users, and the type and reliability of service. This detailed analysis is done to determine the **return on investment** (ROI)[3] and cost benefit. ROI[3] is the cost savings that are realized. **Cost benefit** is "an analysis of the cost effectiveness or different alternatives in order to see whether the benefits outweigh the costs" (WordWeb Online, 2008).

---

[3] ROI is discussed in greater detail in Chapter 21.

The needs assessment for a HIS is similar to a vehicle purchase. All participants in the needs assessment process must do their homework. A list of possible vendor products should be determined. This is often done using word of mouth, reading news reports, reading journal article reports, and listserv communication. A **request for information** (RFI) with a summary of the information is sent to vendors. Information from the return of the RFI is used to determine which vendors should be considered. Vendor products should be compared using a tool such as a matrix. In doing so, participants need to learn the information technology terminology. The time and quality of a needs assessment can make or break the success of system implementation. A **request for proposal** (RFP) is a detailed document sent to potential vendors asking them to submit information on how their product will meet the user's needs. The document should be a list that can be answered with using yes, yes with customization, yes with future releases, and no (Hunt et al., 2004). A well-written RFP will allow the users to compare products effectively. It has three parts – one that describes the method and deadline for responses; one that describes the organization; and one with a listing of details of expectations such as requirements, training, and support.

HIS project requirements refer to needs, such as

- schedule, design, and budget constraints;
- the number of system users;
- the department(s) that will use the system;
- the type of application, for example, desktop application or enterprise application;
- where the software and data will reside;
- how and where the data is backed up;
- requirements for system redundancy (if one system fails, another system takes over seamlessly); and
- the type and availability of system support.

PLANNING

Planning is the second step in the systems life cycle. This critical phase requires detailed assessment of the current processes including workflow analyses, timelines, and the implied changes of the new processes. Effective planning can breed trust and confidence among the users and team members (Hunt et al., 2004).

Analysis of Workflow

Workflow analyses are critical components of the planning phase. A workflow analysis analyzes and depicts how work is accomplished. Each nursing task has a distinct workflow. It is important to analyze workflow in the paper record system (or legacy electronic system), and then project work might best be accomplished using the new electronic system. As an example, consider the workflow

- that begins with a physician's medication order and ends with medication administration of digoxin,
- that begins with administering intravenous (IV) Lasix and ends with documentation of the drug, and
- that begins with checking a blood glucose level, subsequently administering a combination of NPH and regular insulin, and ends with documentation of the procedures.

The process for "who" does what, when, and how differs for each example. The "it depends" has to be considered. In the first example, it depends on how the physician's order was written. Was it written by the physician or was it a verbal or phone order? If the order was written on the paper chart, was the order transcribed by a medical secretary or a nurse?

An effective way to visualize what happens is to diagram the activity. Diagramming can be done using drawing tools in any program that includes the use of drawing shapes such as OpenOffice.org Draw, MS PowerPoint®, or specialized software, such as MS Visio®. A process flow diagram uses special symbols to convey a certain meaning. As an example, the oval shape is used to convey the start and stop processes, the rectangle shape indicates a process, and the diamond shape indicates a decision (see Figure 19-3).

Systems Life Cycle

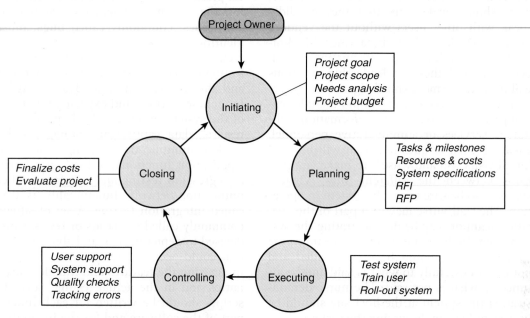

Figure 19-3 • Flow chart diagram symbol meanings.

Selecting a System

Selecting a system is one of the most daunting decisions for the stakeholder committee members. Healthcare organization enterprise solutions have the potential of improving or disrupting the complex care delivery process and are significant financial investments that range from thousands of dollars to millions of dollars. The risks of making a mistake can be mitigated with the use of a structured process, effective risk and needs analyses, and careful product investigation.

The selection member participants must educate themselves to be able to make an informed decision. Participants should investigate pertinent literature. Journals with comprehensive pertinent articles include *Computers, Informatics, Nursing: CIN, JAMIA: Journal of the American Medical Informatics Association, The Journal of Healthcare Information Management,* and the *International Journal of Medical Informatics.*

Nursing participants should consider membership in nursing informatics professional or-

ganization and stay abreast of common issues and concerns using informatics listservs. Nurses should network with other system users and attend professional informatics education sessions, such as HIMSS and American Medical Informatics Association (AMIA). Listening to the experiences of others without a vendor present can uncover important issues, both good and bad.

It is important for the selection committee not to be overly dependent on the vendor's advice. Vendors are in the business of making money, and they are trained to market their product to make sales. They have been known to minimize system weaknesses. Be cautious about vendors' promises of upcoming new features or product releases. Broken promises of computer system products are known as vaporware. The selection committee members should also make site visits to interview others. Before selecting sites to visit, it is important to talk with several agencies and listen to both good and bad features. No system is perfect, and the success of a system may have as much to do with the agency as the vendor. Although the visits are often arranged by the vendors, users should make sure that they candidly speak with other users without the vendor's presence. During a site visit, talking with clinical users as well as with information system personnel and those in leadership positions will provide the most knowledge.

The site visitation team should include several potential users, not just information technology services or administrative personnel. Creating a list of questions that will be used for all visits will allow users to make comparisons between the different sites. Visitors should also be sure to see the system in operation. The staff nurse may be a part of the visitation team or may be demonstrating the system from the host site. In either position, the selection team should be open-minded and both listen carefully to what is said and be attuned to what is not said. The nurse demonstrating the system at the host site should be honest and fair in discussing the system.

System Design and Testing

Once the system is selected, the next step is to customize the system design so that it is compatible with the user requirements. Typically, the vendor will provide the user with a standard product, sometimes known as a **vanilla product.** It is similar to the standard desktop PC that the buyer can customize with additional features such as additional memory or an extra monitor. Just as in the customization of a desktop PC, extra features come at an additional fee.

During the system design phase, system documentation must be developed. It is an important feature started in the planning phase and continued with each change made in the system. Some vendors provide "canned" or standardized data entry objects and output boxes, while others allow unlimited customization by the customer. The decision to build-your-own or take-what-you-get should be made in the very early stages of the vendor selection and discovery process. The need for up-to-date and complete system documentation that flows with the user processes cannot be overemphasized.

The testing phase is just one of many critical phases that must be addressed intently before the system is implemented. System errors and issues, commonly called **bugs,** must be identified and addressed. The process of correcting the errors is called **debugging.** The testing of the new system is ongoing, during and after the system build. The testing needs to include features and expected functionality of the system, hardware, backups, downtime, restarts, data capture and storage, and network communication, among other factors. Application functionality is often referred to as **regression testing** and interface, and communication/network functionality is usually called **integration testing.** A set of situations commonly called scenarios or **test scripts** are devised to depict normal and abnormal events that could occur. Clinicians may be involved in devising the features and functionality scenarios and in the actual testing. Several test scripts should be written for each functional part of the software and for the integration of data across interfaces to ensure consistent quality of output. A test script may not catch everything that doesn't work as expected, but each time a new issue is discovered, it should be added to the set of scripts. Over the years, a collection of test scripts can become extremely accurate and reduce the issues discovered during implementation. This will improve user acceptance of the system or changes to an existing system and the user's trust and confidence in the Information Services (IT) department. The trust and confidence for IT is imperative for moving the institution forward with an electronic information system.

System **superusers** are identified to assist in the system build and testing. Superusers should be clinical nurses and staff who are recruited from each of the areas where the system will be deployed. Superusers can help sell the other clinicians and assist in later implementation and training. They are invaluable to the success of the implementation phase. The participation of end users in initial testing provides the design team with valuable developmental information. Observer users during testing highlight training needs. Many times, something that is considered intuitive by the design team may prove confusing for the user.

Training

The need for basic computer training that is uncovered in the needs assessment phase should be met before training for the actual system occurs. Computer literacy issues can be dealt with in separate learning sessions and target only those who need to know instead of planning training with the lowest common denominator of learner in mind. User training is another essential step leading to a successful **go-live** or **rollout**. Both terms refer to the implementation of a new system. The training sessions should use effective pedagogical teaching/learning theory and methods[4]. It should be done within a few weeks of the system implementation for "just-in-time" learning. If completed too early, without reinforcement, the learning will be forgotten.

Training should be done with the user needs in mind. Many facilities use superusers to assist with the training sessions. A needs assessment may be helpful to identify training resources. Analysis of needs can assist the training developers to create modules that meet the needs of novices to expert computer users. It can also be helpful to identify availability of the staff. Training should also include instructions on how to obtain help for the system. An ideal system will contain **context-sensitive help**, or help that is modified on the basis of where in the system help was accessed. Providing online tutorials and video clips on the computer can also assist clinicians to successfully use the system.

During training sessions, end users should take responsibility for learning to use the new system by asking questions and providing feedback on the functionality and features for the system to best serve their needs. Training activities should be viewed as multipurpose activities. The trainer not only teaches intended users how to use a system but also makes determinations about specific support

that will be required during the rollout. During the training sessions, security and data accuracy must be addressed. By discussing these issues in the context of system use, the user responsibilities related to security become more meaningful.

A common training mistake is to simply show the user where system features are located and explain how they are used. A better approach is to develop several scenarios or simulation case studies that the clinician experiences on a daily basis so that the user can apply learning. After a brief introduction to the system, the user is allowed to work through the learning modules. Some agencies develop self-learning modules and place them on the nursing unit PCs and use them in addition to classroom training.

Another mistake is to provide too much information in a single training period. Rather than planning a four- to five-hour class, it is better to break the training session down into shorter one- to two-hour classes. Learning to use a new computer system can be overwhelming to many. After a short period of time, the mind can become absolutely saturated, evident by restlessness and inattention of the learners.

IMPLEMENTATION

The implementation or **go-live** is a significant milestone. Many agencies build the momentum to that milestone with preparatory "count down the days . . ." presentations, memos, and posters. The implementation team may choose to order t-shirts – one color for the trainers and superusers and another for the staff. The celebration often includes a media release to the local newspapers. The implementation is yet another key phase in the systems life cycle. It needs to be carefully planned and implemented. If not done well, the users might be tempted to bypass essential features that were put in place to make patients safer.

Success of the go-live is dependent on the support system. Adequate system and user support are crucial. It may be necessary to schedule additional staff for the first few days

---

[4] Information about teaching/learning theory is in Chapter 23.

beginning with the physicians order in either the paper record environment or with that of an electronic information system.

5. Compare the systems life cycle with the nursing process. How are they alike or different?

6. Discuss how the role of the nurse clinician superuser is helpful in the design and implementation of life cycles.

7. Create a lesson plan to use when implementing a clinical documentation system on a nursing unit. Be sure to incorporate concepts of change theory and teaching learning theories.

REFERENCES

American Nurse Association. (2008). *Nursing informatics: Scope and standards of practice.* Washington, D.C.: American Nurses Association.

Ball, M. J., Weaver, C., & Kiel, J. M. (Eds.). (2004). *Healthcare information management systems: Cases, strategies, and solutions* (3rd ed.). New York: Springer-Verlag.

Baron, R. J. (2007). Improving patient care. Quality improvement with an electronic health record: Achievable, but not automatic. *Annals of Internal Medicine, 147*(8), 549–552.

Bazzoli, F. (2007a, February 14). Continuity of care document is approved by HL7, endorsed by HITSP [Electronic version]. *Healthcare IT News.* Retrieved February 28, 2008, from http://www.healthcareitnews.com/story.cms?id=6408

Bazzoli, F. (2007b, March 1). Continuity of care standards reach milestone [Electronic version]. *Healthcare IT News.* Retrieved March 12, 2008, from http://www.healthcareitnews.com/story.cms?id=6615

Business Wire. (2008, February 11). *Homer Memorial Hospital selects HMS to provide information technology infrastructure.* Retrieved November 23, 2008, from http://www.reuters.com/article/pressRelease/idUS162438+11-Feb-2008+BW20080211

Committee on Quality of Health Care in America, & Institute of Medicine. (2001). *Crossing the quality chasm: A new health system for the 21st century.* Retrieved November 23, 2008, from http://books.nap.edu/catalog.php?record_id=10027#toc

Committee on the Work Environment for Nurses and Patient Safety. (2004). *Keeping patients safe: Transforming the work environment for nurses.* Retrieved November 23, 2008, from http://books.nap.edu/catalog.php?record_id=10851#toc

Duke Office of Information Technology. (n.d.). *Systems life cycle.* Retrieved November 23, 2008, from http://www.oit.duke.edu/enterprise/lifecycle/index.html

Garets, D., & Davis, M. (2006, January 26). *Electronic medical records vs. electronic health records: Yes, there is a difference.* Retrieved November 23, 2008, from http://www.himssanalytics.org/docs/WP_EMR_EHR.pdf

Hayes, H. B. (2008). Virginia makes two grants for innovative uses of health IT [Electronic version]. *Government Health IT, 2008.* Retrieved November 23, 2008 from http://www.govhealthit.com/online/news/350201-1.html

Health Information and Management Systems Society. (n.d.). *EHR: Electronic health record.* Retrieved November 23, 2008, from http://www.himss.org/ASP/topics_ehr.asp

Hunt, E., Sproat, S. B., & Kitzmiller, R. (2004). *The nursing informatics implementation guide.* New York: Springer-Verlag.

Institute of Medicine. (1999). *To err is human: Building a safer health system.* Washington, D.C.: National Academies Press.

Institute of Medicine, & National Academy of Sciences. (2001). *Crossing the quality chasm: A new health system for the 21st century.* Washington, D.C.: National Academies Press.

Kibbe, D. C. (2008). *Unofficial FAQs about the ASTM CCR standard.* Retrieved November 22, 2008, from http://www.centerforhit.org/x1750.xml

Lee, T. T. (2007). Nurses' experiences using a nursing information system: Early stage of technology implementation. *Computers, Informatics, Nursing: CIN, 25*(5), 294–300.

Liang, L. (2007). The gap between evidence and practice. *Health Affairs, 26*(2), w119–w121.

Medication Errors Reporting Program (2008). *About medication errors: Dangerous abbreviations.* Retrieved November 22, 2008, from http://www.nccmerp.org/dangerousAbbrev.html

Nuseibeh, B., & Easterbrook, S. (2000). *Requirements engineering: A roadmap.* Retrieved November 22, 2008, from http://www.doc.ic.ac.uk/~ban/pubs/sotar.re.pdf

Schulman, J., Kuperman, G. J., Kharbanda, A., & Kaushal, R. (2007). Discovering how to think about a hospital patient information system by struggling to evaluate it: A committee's journal. *Journal of the American Medical Informatics Association, 14*(5), 537–541.

Simpson, R. L. (2006). Evidence-based practice: How nursing administration makes it happen. *Nursing Administration Quarterly, 30*(3), 291–294.

Simpson, R. L. (2007). The politics of information technology. *Nursing Administration Quarterly, 31*(4), 354–358.

Staggers, N., Kobus, D., & Brown, C. (2007). Nurses' evaluations of a novel design for an electronic medication administration record. *Computers, Informatics, Nursing: CIN, 25*(2), 67–75.

The Joint Commission. (2001). *Medication errors related to potentially dangerous abbreviations.* Retrieved November 23, 2008, from http://www.jointcommission.org/SentinelEvents/SentinelEventAlert/sea_23.htm

WordWeb Online. (2008). *Dictionary and thesaurus.* Retrieved November 23, 2008, from http://www.wordwebonline.com/en/COSTBENEFITANALYSIS

Specialized Electronic Healthcare Information Systems

Learning Objectives

After studying this chapter you will be able to:

1. Discuss the potential impact of quality measures for use of health information technology (HIT) on patient care.

2. Discuss the pros and cons for use of best-of-breed versus integrated HIT solutions.

3. Identify two quality measures that would benefit the nurse who has a voice in selection of an electronic clinical system.

4. Describe the advantages for integration of data from pharmacy, laboratory, and radiology information systems with the electronic patient record.

5. Explain why the Leapfrog Group recommends the use of computerized provider order entry (CPOE).

6. Discuss the factors that impact the management of patient flow in hospitals.

7. Identify at least three factors that would promote the adoption of clinical information systems (CISs) by nurses.

Key Terms

Active RFID
Aggregated Data
Best of Breed
Certification Commission for Healthcare Information Technology (CCHIT)
Clinical Decision Support System (CDSS)
Clinical Documentation
Closed-Loop Safe Medication Administration
Electronic Medication Administration Record (eMAR)
Enterprise

Health Information Technology (HIT)
Integrated Interface
Mission Critical
Passive RFID
Physician Quality Report Initiative (PQRI)
Picture Archiving and Communication System (PACS)
Positive Patient Identifier (PPID)
Radio Frequency Identifier (RFID)

The healthcare industry uses a variety of information systems to support and communicate for the delivery of patient care and to manage business operations. Healthcare information systems (HIS) comprise applications that track patients and manage financial data associated with the staff payroll and billing for services rendered and patient care services including nursing, including pharmacy, radiology, and laboratory services. In a well-designed system, there is an interface between systems to support the sharing of data so that the data does not have to be reentered. An **interface** allows for sharing of data

linked to this basic information. Laboratory results find their way to the appropriate provider or care area on the basis of the important information contained in this portion of the information system. It is important, therefore, that the data in this system should be updated and verified on a regular basis.

FINANCIAL SYSTEMS

Financial systems are another distinct application in the HIS. They are considered by some as the second backbone of the system because they track financial interactions and provide the fiscal reporting necessary to manage an institution. Financial systems are **mission critical**, which means that the services are vital to the existence of the organization. A few functions of financial systems are to assure a higher collection rate from payers, to expedite payments for accounts receivable, to minimize third-party payer denials of care, and to prevent underpayment for care.

The problem that many healthcare organizations are facing today is how to get their legacy financial system to communicate with the clinical information system (CIS). Some of the systems in use date back several decades and are not able to meet the demands of regulators and consumers (Conn, 2007). To avoid building costly interfaces at the institutional level, some healthcare organizations choose to purchase enterprise systems that include financial systems, but it is an expensive proposition that costs in the hundreds of millions dollar range. The integration of the two systems is necessary for efficient billing and to allow for process improvement analysis.

Healthcare agencies recognize the challenges of being able to stay in business and meeting the requirements of regulators and payers. Besides the billing and reimbursement from third-party payers, consumers want to know their out-of-pocket expenses prior to checking into the hospital. Hospitals want to be able to bill Medicare without being accused of fraud. Fraud accusations, true or not, are in the news daily. As an example, in 2008 three New Jersey hospitals were accused of inflating charges to increase Medicare reimbursement. Two of three hospitals filed for Chapter 11 bankruptcies. In the same year, a Louisiana hospital settled with the Department of Justice for "knowingly" allowing a physician perform unnecessary procedures between 1999 and 2004 (FierceHealthcare, 2008). Between 1997 and 2007, Medicare received $11 billion from fines and settlements related to fraud (FierceHealthcare, 2007).

Clinical Information Systems

Clinical information systems (CISs) are a conglomerate of integrated and interoperable information systems and technologies that provide information about patient care. The core information systems are the ancillaries: laboratory, radiology, and pharmacy. The clinical documentation system is built using data from the core ancillary systems. Other components of the CIS are the CPOE, the **electronic medication administration record (eMar)**, and **positive patient identifier (PPID)** systems, such as the bar-coded medication administration system.

CIS vendors, like other software companies, continuously work to improve the quality of their products. They make the improvements available as version releases and as major upgrades. Major upgrades are usually associated with a fee and may also require equipment upgrades. Major software upgrades could also introduce new software bugs. For these reasons and others, healthcare institutions may choose not to make software changes. On the other hand, nurses who are critical of a certain CIS need to be aware that their concerns may be related to the version of software, not the manufacturer.

ANCILLARY SYSTEMS

The laboratory and radiology systems provide a means of storing and viewing clinical testing and diagnostic patient information. Laboratory systems, one of the earliest clinical systems, have been in use by small and large hospitals for several decades. Laboratory systems integrate data from all of the standard laboratory departments including hematology, chemistry, microbiology, blood bank, and pathology. Radiology systems integrate data from patient diagnostic and therapeutic services, including the **picture archiving and communication system** (**PACS**). PACS allows for digital versions of all of the diagnostic images, such as x-rays and magnetic resonance images (MRIs), to be stored in the electronic patient record. The pharmacy system provides a means for stocking and recording medications dispensed by the pharmacy. The three ancillary information systems provide a foundation for other clinical systems.

CLINICAL DOCUMENTATION

Clinical documentation applications are available in various formats. A good documentation system, whether for nursing or another discipline, is part of the clinical workflow and provides communication of real-time information. Clinical documentation software is designed using rules so that when assessment data with abnormal values, such as a pulse rate or blood pressure, is entered, the abnormal values stand out because they are displayed in a different color (see Figure 20-1). These systems remove the need to go find the paper chart and allow all who use the electronic chart to access information whenever and wherever it is needed.

Screens can be designed to support assessment documentation by listing systems, or practitioners can be alerted by the system with a pop-up box to complete or verify essential information, such as allergies. Numerical laboratory data, such as a white blood count (CBC), hemoglobin (Hgb), and platelet count, can be displayed in a graph format to visual trends (see Figure 20-2). In a well-planned documentation system, there is little need for entry of free text, although the ability to do so should be there for the occasional time when there is no place to document the information and a comment is necessary. When these

systems work well, it is because the healthcare professionals who use the system were involved in planning, design, implementation, and evaluation of the system.

Nursing information systems sometimes use the nursing process approach with nursing diagnoses as the organizing framework. When properly designed, data collection supports clinical workflow instead of being distracting. It should provide flexibility in both data entry and in viewing data necessary for patient care. Additionally, it should provide easy access to reference information such as policies and procedures as well as online literature.

Clinical documentation systems should provide for retrieval of data used in long-range planning and research. Use of clinical data by practicing nurses can be facilitated by easy availability of **aggregated data**. Aggregated data is a collection of data that is useful to see a big picture. It can be useful in determining best practices, evidence-based care, and form the basis for decision support systems.

COMPUTERIZED PROVIDER ORDER ENTRY

The CPOE system allows a clinician to place an order by simply selecting a patient and the needed service from a computer screen. The letter "P" in CPOE can mean physician; however, this textbook uses P to refer to all care providers who write orders, including physician's assistants and nurse practitioners. The use of CPOE is the number one recommendation made by the Leapfrog Group to improve patient safety and quality (Leapfrog Group, 2008a). The advocacy group promotes safety, quality, and affordability of healthcare (Leapfrog Group, 2008b). Results of their research study indicate that CPOE has the potential benefit of saving approximately 567,298 serious medication errors (Birkmeyer & Dimick, 2004).

When a provider writes an order using CPOE, the order is immediately sent to the appropriate department. This saves time, and it also prevents transcription errors. Additionally, order entry systems facilitate the capture of financial information for restocking and billing

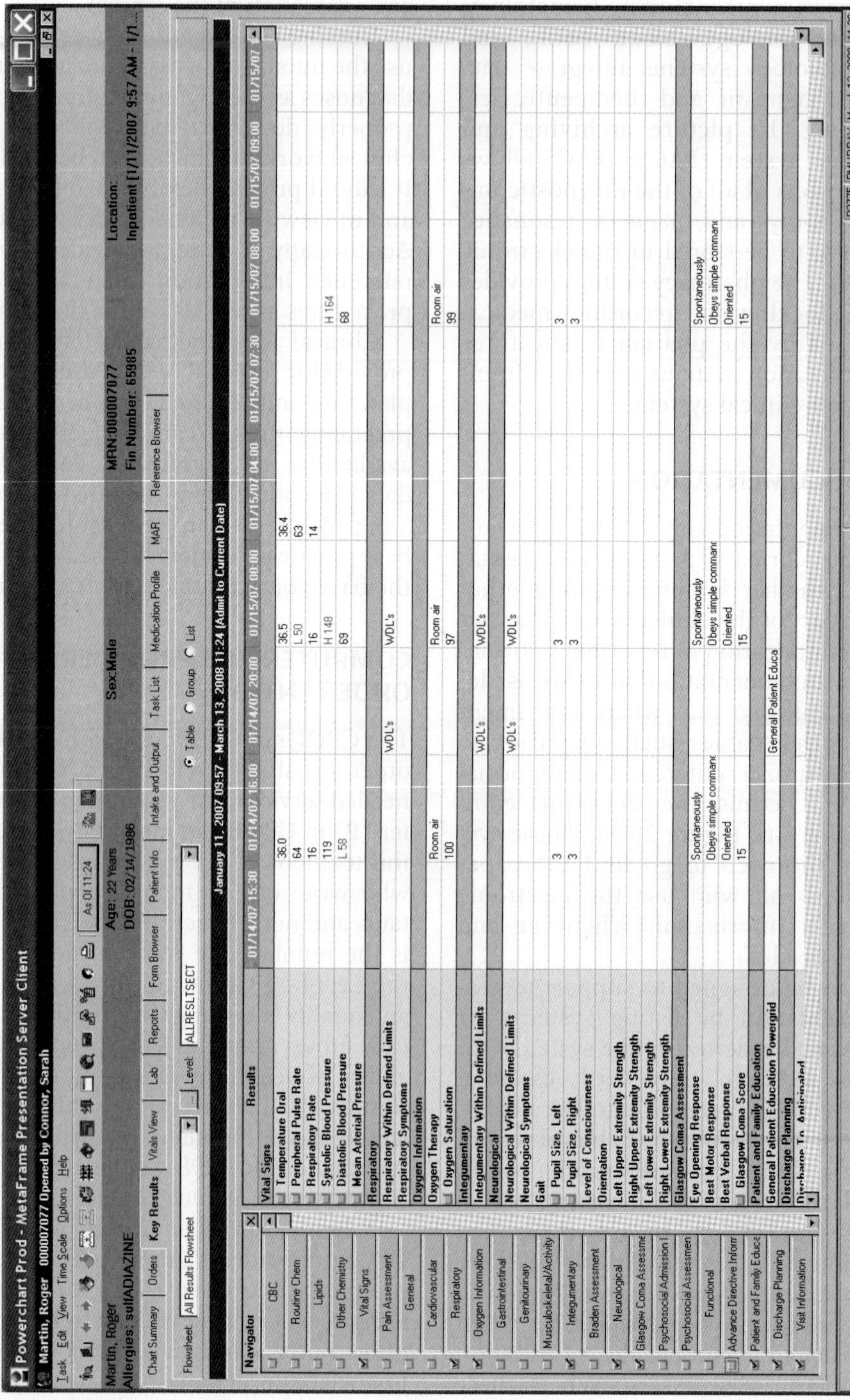

Figure 20-1 • Clinical assessment data display with abnormal values. (Used with permission from Cerner Corporation.)

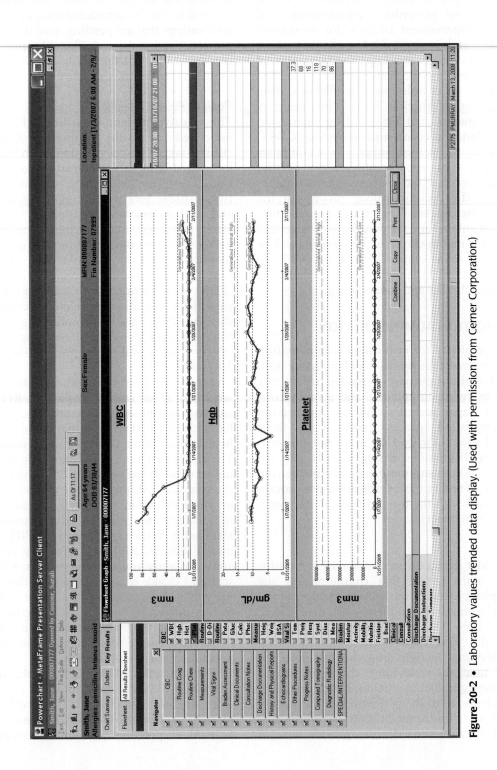

Figure 20-2 • Laboratory values trended data display. (Used with permission from Cerner Corporation.)

purposes. The advantages attributed to CPOE are electronic prescribing (e-prescribing) and quality improvement (Agency for Healthcare Research and Quality, n.d.). Use of e-prescribing can reduce errors and improve the quality of care because the medication order is checked against a set of rules such as allergies, drug dosage, administration routes, frequency of administration, and drug-to-drug interaction using **clinical decision support system (CDSS)** information. Decision support is a computer application that uses a complex system of rules to analyze data and presents information to support the decision-making process of the knowledge worker. That is, if a medication order is entered and the dosage exceeds normal limits for that medication, the provider will be given this information. The system should also provide information about any potential drug incompatibilities and patient allergies.

MEDICATION ADMINISTRATION

The use of HIT for medication administration is a process that works hand in hand with CPOE with the purpose of making patient care safer by reducing potential and actual errors. In the paper record world, the medication administration process resided in three record silos – the doctor's order, the pharmacist's verification/dispensing records, and the nurse's administration/paper documentation record. In reality, it is a medication-use process addressed with the use of the eMar (Hagland, 2006, September).

eMar

The eMar discussed in Chapter 19 is a multidisciplinary record that communicates the complex process of medication use. Use of the eMar requires the implementation of CPOE and CDSS. The eMar guides the nurse to use the six rights when administering medications: the right drug, the right dose, the right time, the right route, the right patient, and the right documentation. If well designed, it includes all of the pertinent documentation appropriate for the medication that is administered. Because the eMar can provide view of information in the database, the nurse can query it to display scheduled medications and medications that are pending, past due, and/or previously administered. The eMar provides a mechanism for efficient nurse time utilization as well as facilitating the delivery of safe care.

Positive Patient Identifier

The **positive patient identifier** (PPID) with bar-coded or **radio frequency identifier (RFID)**-tagged bracelets is used with the eMar for **closed-loop safe medication administration**. The term "closed loop" means that the right patient received the right medication, and it is an essential component of patient safety improvements. The Joint Commission first issued a recommendation for accurately identifying patients in 2003. The following year, the U.S. Food and Drug Administration (FDA) recommended the use of bar codes on patient identification bracelets. According to the FDA (2004), use of bar code drug administration has the potential of reducing 500,000 adverse events and saving $93 billion over a 20-year period.

The medication administration procedures when using bar coding or **passive RFID** are similar. Both procedures require the use of a bar code or RFID scanner that is either hand-held or built into a laptop or tablet computer. The nurse first scans their bar code or RFID tag on their ID badge to identify themselves in the system. Next, the nurse scans the bar code on the medication and finally scans the patient's armband prior to administering the medication. If the tag uses **active RFID**, which means that the RFID tag is battery powered and constantly transmitting signals, use of a scanning device is not necessary as the identifier will be recognized by the computer (Perrin & McAndrew, 2006). The use of active RFID would allow PPID without disturbing the patient, for example, when hanging an IV fluid when the patient was sleeping.

The outcomes of research on the use of PPID with the eMar are promising. Results of three studies conducted at a 329-bed hospital located in Pennsylvania documented 5,000 to 6,000+ potential medication errors that ranged from wrong dose, wrong frequency, not ordered, not given, and wrong patient (Ague & Schaeffer, 2007). Another study was conducted over a five-month period in a two-hospital healthcare system located in Ohio (Galvin, McBeth, Hasdorff, Tillson, & Thomas, 2007). The researchers reported that after the implementation of bar coding, 923 wrong-patient errors were prevented, resulting in an estimated $4,615,000 cost savings. Additionally, 45 allergy alerts prevented errors, which resulted in an estimated $225,000 cost savings. Bar code scanning also prevented wrong administration of additional doses of medication, resulting in a cost savings of $37,220. While the researchers noted significant patient safety improvements, they also acknowledged the need to make improvements as only 25% of the nurses reported that wristbands scanned easily.

 ## Managing Patient Flow

The patient flow is a long-standing hospital issue that must be addressed to provide safe and efficient patient care. The problems associated with patient flow are multifactorial that are based on the principle of supply (hospital beds and resources) and demand (patients). Hospitals have to operate with nearly full bed capacity for economic efficiency purposes. Staffing, supplies, and resources are budgeted according to the average occupancy. Most hospital budgets have very little flexibility.

The demand for hospital care resources is affected by the aging population, many of whom have chronic diseases such as congestive heart failure, diabetics, and chronic renal disease. This medically fragile population often has acute episodic needs as a result of their disease processes and is negatively impacted during the annual flu season. Patients expect to be treated at the time of need. If they are unable to see a physician during office hours, they use emergency services where the patient flow problems begin. Emergency beds quickly fill because of lack of available hospital beds for patients who need to be admitted causing a patient traffic jam.

On July 1, 2004, The Joint Commission issued a new recommendation requiring hospitals to discover and minimize barriers to well-organized patient flow (McBeth, 2005). Scoring on the standard went into effect on January 1, 2005. The recommendation was the result of root call analyses for sentinel events, which reported that Emergency Department (ED) over-capacity was a contributing factor in 31% of sentinel event cases (McBeth, 2005). Hospital leaders quickly recognized the difficulty in planning, tracking, and managing patient flow, and as a result many, especially the large facilities, turned to informatics bed management systems. According to the American Hospital Association Quality Center (2007), "The goal of bed management is to accurately place the patient in the right unit with the right level of staff and right level of care the first time."

TRACKING SYSTEMS SOLUTIONS

A variety of informatics solutions are available that both track the processes involved with patient flow, such as bed availability, and provide documentation of time lapses used in analysis of data and planning. As an example, Radianse Reveal™ Patient Flow by RTI™, McKesson Horizon Enterprise Visibility (2008), formerly Awarix, and the Versus® Information System (VIS™), all use RFID tags to monitor patient locations (McKesson, 2008; RTI, 2008; Versus Technology, 2008). Another example is the Hill-Rom Navicare® Care Traffic Control™, which allows for notification using the computer, a wireless device, and voice commands. Some vendors, for example, Premise Patient Flow, use a combination of phone notification and user input of computer requests to monitor patients ("One part tech, two parts process," 2007). Features common to many of the popular patient-tracking systems include the visual display of beds, which indicates the patient status (e.g., discharge, fall risk, MRSA), bed availability display, instant transport notification, and equipment (e.g., wheelchairs) locators.

Reports from a study conducted at healthcare system at a hospital located in Delaware

6. Review the Leapfrog Group Web site and then explain why the Leapfrog Group recommends the use of CPOE.

7. Review The Joint Commission Web site and at least one Web site for a company that provides informatics solutions to assist in the management of patient flow. Discuss the pertinent factors that leadership should plan to monitor to improve patient flow.

8. Does the healthcare agency where you work use a CIS? If so, do all of the nurses support the use of technology? Why or why not? Explain at least three factors that would promote the adoption of clinical systems by nurses.

REFERENCES

ADVANCE. (2007, August). Using technology to protect patients. *ADVANCE for Health Information Executives, 11*, 29–32.

Agency for Healthcare Research and Quality. (n.d.). *Computerized provider order entry.* Retrieved November 23, 2008, from http://healthit.ahrq.gov/portal/server.pt?open=514&objID=5554&mode=2&holder DisplayURL=http://prodportallb.ahrq.gov:7087/publishedcontent/publish/communities/k_o/knowledge_library/key_topics/health_briefing_02062006010308/computerized_provider_order_entry.html

Ague, T., & Schaeffer, R. (2007, December). Reaching EMR stage 6. *ADVANCE for Health Information Executives, 11*, 14–15.

American Hospital Association Quality Center. (2007). Improving patient flow patient satisfaction and patient safety. *Hospitals & Health Networks, 81*(11), 28–29.

Birkmeyer, J. D., & Dimick, J. B. (2004). *The Leapfrog Group's patient safety practices, 2003: The potential benefits of universal adoption.* Retrieved November 23, 2008, from http://www.leapfroggroup.org/media/file/Leapfrog-Birkmeyer.pdf

Breslin, S., Greskovich, W., & Turisco, F. (2004). Wireless technology improves nursing workflow and communications. *Computers, Informatics, Nursing: CIN, 22*(5), 275–281.

Centers for Medicare & Medicaid Services. (2008, November 17). *Physician quality reporting initiative.* Retrieved November 23, 2008, from http://www.cms.hhs.gov/pqri/

Certification Commission for Healthcare Information Technology. (2008). *Frequently asked questions (FAQ).* Retrieved November 23, 2008, from http://www.cchit.org/about/faq/general.asp#founding

Conn, J. (2007). Following the money. *Modern Healthcare, 37*(27), 28–30.

FierceHealthcare. (2007, April 19). *Medicare fraud cost CMS billions.* Retrieved November 23, 2008, from http://www.fiercehealthcare.com/story/medicare-fraud-costs-cms-billions/2007-04-20

FierceHealthcare. (2008). *Medicare fraud news from FierceHealthcare.* Retrieved November 23, 2008, from http://www.fiercehealthcare.com/tags/medicare-fraud

Galvin, L., McBeth, S., Hasdorff, C., Tillson, M., & Thomas, S. (2007). Medication bar coding: To scan or not to scan? *Computers, Informatics, Nursing: CIN, 25*(2), 86–92.

Hagland, M. (2006, September). *Point of care series: Part 2* [Electronic version]. *Healthcare Informatics, 23.* Retrieved November 23, 2008, from http://www.healthcare-informatics.com/ME2/dirmod.asp?sid=&nm=&type=Publishing&mod=Publications%3A%3AArticle&mid=8F3A7027421841978F18BE895F87F791&tier=4&id=18C3A5824CBB497C9F6D91FC7E4FA42A

Health and Human Services. (n.d.). *HIT certification: CCHIT.* Retrieved November 23, 2008, from http://www.hhs.gov/healthit/certification/cchit/

Kuruzovich, J., Angst, C. M., Faraj, S., & Agarwal, R. (2006, January 26). *Wireless communication role in patient response time: A study of vocera integration with a nurse call system.* Retrieved November 23, 2008, from http://www.vocera.com/downloads/UofMD_St_Agnes2.pdf

Leapfrog Group. (2008a). *The Leapfrog safety practices.* Retrieved November 23, 2008, from http://www.leapfroggroup.org/for_hospitals/leapfrog_hospital_quality_and_safety_survey_copy/leapfrog_safety_practices

Leapfrog Group. (2008b). *Our mission.* Retrieved November 23, 2008, from http://www.leapfroggroup.org/about_us/our_mission

McBeth, S. (2005). *Mitigate impediments to efficient patient flow. Nursing Management, 36*(7), 16–17.

McKesson. (2008). *Horizon enterprise visibility.* Retrieved November 23, 2008, from http://www.mckesson.com/en_us/McKesson.com/For%2BHealthcare%2BProviders/Hospitals/Interdisciplinary%2BCare%2BSolutions/Horizon%2BEnterprise%2BVisibility.html

One part tech, two parts process. (2007). *Health Management Technology, 28*(2), 34.

Perrin, R. A., & McAndrew, M. B. (2006, October). *RFID: The new strategy in healthcare IT.* Retrieved November 23, 2008, from http://www.hpnonline.com/inside/2006-10/0610-rfidcoverstory2.html

RTI. (2008). *Radianse patient flow.* Retrieved November 23, 2008, from http://www.radianse.com/patient-flow.html

U.S. Food and Drug Administration. (2004, February 25). *FDA issues bar code regulation.* Retrieved November 23, 2005, from http://www.fda.gov/oc/initiatives/barcode-sadr/fs-barcode.html

Versus Technology. (2008). *Versus.* Retrieved November 23, 2008, from http://www.versustech.com/

Electronic Healthcare System Issues

Learning Objectives

After studying this chapter you will be able to:

1. Use the EMR Adoption model to analyze the level of adoption for a healthcare agency.

2. Discuss the risks and opportunities for sharing clinical data.

3. Discuss how privacy and confidentiality of patient electronic information is currently being addressed in healthcare.

4. Discuss how the issue of interoperability affects sharing of patient health information.

5. Provide an example that demonstrates the significance of work flow redesign as it relates to a clinical documentation system.

6. Identify ways that healthcare is addressing The Joint Commission's Patient Safety Goals with the use of health information technology.

7. Provide at least two examples of strong passwords with an explanation about why the password is strong.

Key Terms

Accuracy of Data
Authentication
Biometrics
Clinical Decision Support
  System (CDSS)
Data Security
Intangibles
Interoperability
Login
Password

Return on Investment
Single Sign-On
Stark Rules
Strategic Planning
Tangibles
Unintended Consequences
Voice Recognition
Work Flow Redesign

The use of health information technology (HIT) is improving patient care outcomes. The rate of adoption of technology solutions is growing, albeit slowly. All the issues associated with its use have not been resolved. The transition from a paper record world to an automated one is a huge endeavor. Healthcare practitioners are slow to adopt new solutions that they believe could jeopardize patient care while they are "unlearning" legacy processes and "learning" new approaches. This chapter will focus on few of the issues associated with the adoption of HIT.

document that allows for flexibility. As an example, it should provide the ability to incorporate the use of new evolving technologies. The costs associated with the use of an HIT solution, such as CPOE, are often in the thousands-to-millions of dollars range, depending on the size of the institution (Conrad & Gardner, 2005). As a result, the stakeholders must be able to see that the expenditures are offset by patient outcome benefits; they must see a return on the investment. If the use of information technology is not supported by the institution's strategic plan, it will probably not be funded (Hunt, Sproat, & Kitzmiller, 2004).

Return on Investment

The **return on investment** (ROI)[1] is an important issue serving as a barrier to the adoption of electronic systems. "Chief financial officers toil to accurately present their financial counterparts with measures that capture the impact on items such as averting medication errors or reducing future cost outlays by catching illnesses in early stages" (Runy & Towne, 2005). Improving patient care outcomes and managing costs should align with the strategic plans for healthcare agencies. The process of ROI requires scrutiny regarding risks and the associated values. In other words, is risk offset by the potential value? If so, what data is available to support the value? Those persons involved in budget-making decisions must identify goals and methods for measuring achievement for both tangible and intangible values and risks.

Tangibles are those that can be clearly measured, calculated, and quantified with numerical data (Runy & Towne, 2005). Examples of tangibles include a decrease in length of stay, a decrease in anti-infective medication costs, a decrease in the number of unnecessary medications and tests, and a decrease in charges per admission. The literature reports that after implementation of CPOE for intensive care unit (ICU) patients in one set-

ting, the costs associated with anti-infective medications fell by 70%, and total hospital costs for the patients decreased by 25% (Conrad & Gardner, 2005).

Intangibles are those that are not easily calculated or in which the results cannot be directly attributed to the investment. Examples of intangibles include improved decision making, communication, and user satisfaction (Runy & Towne, 2005). Intangibles may vary between healthcare settings as a result of the differences in factors such as organizational culture, physical environments, population served, and staffing.

Fortunately, the results of a number of studies (Agency for Healthcare Research and Quality, 2001; Bates et al., 2003; Birkmeyer & Dimick, 2004; Conrad & Gardner, 2005) have spurred efforts by individual healthcare organizations and larger geographical areas to speed up the adoption of CPOE to improve patient care outcomes. The results from the research studies are being used to benchmark data and to calculate ROIs.

Reimbursement

Reimbursement is a crucial issue for healthcare agencies, physicians, and other providers. The Centers for Medicare & Medicaid services passed the Physician Self-Referral Law in an effort to prevent Medicare fraud (Centers for Medicare & Medicaid Services, 2008). The law is more commonly known as Stark Law or **Stark Rules** because Congressman Peter Stark introduced it. It has been criticized for interfering with collaborative innovations and limiting the ability of healthcare agencies and providers to design seamless solutions for sharing healthcare information using technology (Milstein, 2007). The law was relaxed in August 2006, to provide an incentive for physicians to adopt the EHR. The amended law allowed hospitals to donate "certified" interoperable systems to physicians (U.S. Department of Health and Human Services, n.d.). On the other hand, the law has been criticized for swaying physicians to use the hospital's choice of clinical information system vendor.

---

[1] Chapter 19 discusses ROI as it relates to the Systems Life Cycle.

Electronic Health Record (EHR)

The overall goal of the National Health Information Infrastructure (NHII) is to make it possible to share information and knowledge appropriately to facilitate the best possible healthcare decisions by consumers, providers, and public health personnel (National Committee Vital Health Statistics, 2001). Information embedded in the EHRs provides a strong foundation for new knowledge formation. The use of one integrated patient record for each patient in today's large healthcare enterprises is the first step in achieving this vision. Four main issues associated with the EHR are: 1) interoperability standards, 2) user design, 3) work flow redesign, and 4) quality measurement.

INTEROPERABILITY

Lack of interoperability standards interferes with the ability to share information by authorized users, including the patient. **Interoperability** is especially a significant issue as it relates to clinical information system and the EHR. Clinical information systems refer to a group of technology-enabled systems, which may or may not be originally designed to share data with one another. Purchasing from a single vendor does not assure the buyer that the system is seamlessly interoperable. Large well-known vendors commonly purchase smaller popular applications and then design interfaces with other vendor applications (Barlow, 2007). The resulting lack of interoperability requires nurses to document the same data in more than one area or application because the data does not flow over to another application. Likewise, the EHR data fields are not universally designed so that data can be shared. Many stakeholders, including government agencies, informatics professional organizations, and health-care technology companies, are working together to unravel the complexity of the healthcare delivery system to provide a foundation for authorized sharing of data, which protects the patient's confidentiality.[2] Interoperability standards may also occur at the healthcare organization level. Obtaining buy-in for use of an electronic documentation is often difficult. To obtain the support of clinicians for use of a new system, the system designers may cater to exceptions in data standards. As an example, clinicians may request the ability to chart weights and heights in the U.S. standard instead of the metric standard, or physicians may request their own specialized order sets, both of which appear to be simple requests. Many times the deviations seem minor, but in reality the deviation from system standard can become a huge issue when attempting to standardize, update, maintain (Campbell, Sittig, Ash, Guappone, & Dykstra, 2006), or to integrate applications or develop interfaces between systems. One of the many rewards of a clinical information system is the ability to share data. With that in mind, clinicians need to plan data standards accordingly, so that data can be shared.

USER DESIGN

User design of data entry screens is an issue because many healthcare providers involved in the design process have no background knowledge of or skills with database design. As a result, providers approach user design using paper chart thinking (Baron, 2007). Until all healthcare providers have some kind of education on informatics and database design basics, the issue will not be resolved. Examples of screen design issues include lack of use of uniform pain scales, pain documentation, pressure ulcer prevention programs, and falls preventions programs. These design issues impact the ability to analyze the data for evidence-based practice decisions. They also make documentation of care challenging for nurses who float to other units or who work for temporary assistance agencies. Finally, lack of uniformity introduces new opportunities

---

[2] Interoperability is addressed in Chapters 16 and 17.

for extending the time for documentation, user frustration, and documentation errors.

WORK FLOW REDESIGN

Work flow redesign is one of the many difficult issues that healthcare providers face when planning and designing the application of electronic systems. As noted several times earlier, one of the problems is lack of experience or lack of knowledge about other ways to accomplish work. Another problem relates to resistance to change. Work flow redesign also relates to the tedious processes involved in identifying how work is changed with a technology solution. It involves creating process flow diagrams that paint "before" and "after" pictures of work flow. Finally, redesign involves the nuts-and-bolts questions about the presence of computers. Common questions faced by nurses are:

▼ How many computers are needed?
▼ Where should the computers be located?
▼ Should the computers be placed on wheeled stands (computer on wheels - COWS) so that they can be moved or should they be at the bedside?
▼ What are the fire marshal regulations for storing moveable or wall-mounted computers in patient unit hallways?
▼ If laptops or tablets are used, can these be prevented from being stolen?
▼ How can the patient or their visitors be prevented from using the computer?
▼ When documenting care in public places, can unauthorized eyes be prevented from viewing the data?

QUALITY MEASUREMENT

A clinical data repository has the potential to allow us to measure quality. The goal for use of HIT is improved patient outcomes and quality of care, not the use of HIT (Milstein, 2007). A **quality measurement** issue is that the data fields have to be designed in a way that allows users to query the data for answers. According to some sources, the EHR has less than 5% of what is required for automated performance measurement (Milstein, 2007). Clinical application vendors need to work with providers to identify quality measures and design data entry windows to capture the data so that the computer can analyze it.

INTRODUCTION OF UNINTENDED CONSEQUENCES

The introduction of technology into a healthcare delivery system can result in unintended and unexpected consequences (Ash, Berg, & Coiera, 2004; Ash, Sittig, Campbell, Guappone, & Dykstra, 2007; Ash, Sittig, Poon et al., 2007). An **unintended consequence** refers to an outcome, good or bad, that was not planned or deliberate. Researchers have reported on unintended consequences for use of CPOE and CDSS. The findings from the research studies should assist nurses in avoiding these problems and recognizing the necessary compromises that must be made to ensure patient safety.

CPOE

Research investigating CPOE revealed nine types of "unintended consequences" (Ash, Sittig, Poon et al., 2007; Campbell et al., 2006). Two of the consequences related to the way work (more and new work) and work flow changed after CPOE. For example, the providers were responsible for entering orders instead of the nurses or secretaries. At least initially, work tasks took a longer time as the users learned to adjust to a new ordering system.

System demands were the third consequence. The CPOE system required unintended system design, support, and maintenance that involved personnel, software and hardware requirements. Communication and emotions were two other unintended consequences. Although patient information was readily available, some users used the computers to replace face-to-face communication, when indeed communication never occurred; there was only the appearance of communication. The information was entered into the computer, but the person who needed it didn't know. Computers should enhance, not replace other types of communication.

Emotions ranged from love to hate. Personnel who were comfortable with automated systems acclimated to CPOE, but those who were uncomfortable experienced strong negative emotions. CPOE led to power shifts, and some believed the physician was perceived as losing power, but others felt that pharmacists lost power because the physician took responsibility for ordering medications. The dependence on technology was considered an unintended consequence of problems and productivity loss associated with computer downtimes.

The research on the effects of CPOE revealed new kinds of errors, problems with confusing user screen designs, and order option presentations had the potential to result in new errors. Use of long drop-down menus had the potential for inadvertent selection of the wrong patient. Other potential errors related to medication dosing errors and orders that overlapped.

Decision Support Systems

Another research study that investigated CDSS also revealed unintended consequences (Ash, Sittig, Campbell et al., 2007). The research findings identified "patterns" of unintended consequences as: 1) those related to content and 2) those related to the way information was presented on the computer screen. Consequences related to content included the possibility of continuing unnecessary daily orders, such as chest x-rays. Content also related to the way orders had to be entered, resulting in a lack of full information from other professionals. There were problems that related to difficulties in updating the clinical decision support rules and "wrong or misleading" alerts. There were also problems related to inadequate communication between systems resulting in lack of supplies or misinformation about the costs of laboratory testing. Consequences related to clinical decision support representation on the computer screen related to order information that was required but not available and alert fatigue from too many alerts.

As in the CPOE research, CDSS research revealed unintended potential errors. Examples include the accidental selection of an auto-complete word when typing and notifications that were delivered in an untimely manner. Finally, potential errors could occur when editing and correcting a clinical decision support rule.

Rules and Regulations: The Joint Commission

The Joint Commission has challenged the healthcare organizations it surveys with annual national safety goals (The Joint Commission, 2008). Three of the top patient safety goals for years 2003 to 2008 can be augmented with the use of HIT. The first goal (2008) is to improve the accuracy of patient identification. Some agencies are using bars or armbands embedded with the radio frequency identification (RFID) chip code to meet the goal (stage 5 of the ERM Implementation Model in Figure 21.1).

The second safety goal is to improve communication. The communication goal 2B addresses notification for critical test values and standardization of abbreviations, acronyms, and symbols. Goal 2E recommends use of a *standard* approach to "hand off" communications. The goal promotes communication, which allows for questions and answers.

Healthcare agencies have begun to develop a *standardized* electronic hand-off report to supplement the verbal report. The electronic report would be used when the patient is transferred to the care of an on-call physician. For example, physicians at Columbia University reported that they developed a standardized unofficial electronic document, sign-out, to use when handing off a patient and between patient admissions. The researcher reported that the report was accessed frequently after the hand off of the patient. The researchers were able to quantify collaborative use of the document using a clinical information system logging mining technique (Stein, Wrenn, Johnson, & Stetson, 2007).

The next safety goal is to improve medication safety. Goal 3C recommends an annual review of look-alike/sound-alike drug lists. Clinical decision support could be used to alert the provider to double-check their order intent. Automatic dispensing machines should be of benefit in addressing the problem if they are stocked correctly, and if the drug vials for different concentrations are different. The nation was alerted to the problem when the infant twins of a movie star couple received 1,000 times the recommended dose of Heparin in November 2007. (Nudd & Lee, 2007). The Joint Commission clearly acknowledges the use of HIT for patient safety, but within clearly defined guidelines, still allows healthcare agencies to arrive at decisions that are the best fit for their patients and staff.

DISEASE SURVEILLANCE SYSTEMS AND DISASTER PLANNING

If and when all health records are electronic, aggregated data from the records could be trended to detect infectious disease outbreaks and bioterrorism. Currently, the National Electronic Disease Surveillance System (NEDSS) is already in place (Centers for Disease Control and Prevention, n.d.).[3] The NEDSS is a part of the Centers for Disease Control and Prevention (CDC). The goals of NEDSS are early detection of disease outbreaks and intervention using pertinent data communications with public health departments. Early detection (or potential disease) or bioterrorism health problems can be accomplished using syndromic surveillance systems.

Syndromic Surveillance

According to Mandl et al. (2004), there are four models used for syndromic surveillance. Syndromic surveillance was defined as collection of health indicators from individual and populations that present before diagnoses are made (Mandl et al., 2004, p. 141). The models vary according to the scope of population served.

One model is the Special Events Model. It was used during the 1999 World Trade Organization meeting in Seattle, the 2002 World Baseball Series in Phoenix, and the 2001 World Trade Center in New York City

terrorist attacks in which the twin towers were destroyed (Moran & Talan, 2003; "Syndromic surveillance for bioterrorism," 2002). The Special Events Model refers to events involving large numbers of people who are monitored by public health teams that collect data from regional hospitals under the legal authority of local health departments.

The second model is one that could be developed by a given region (e.g., city, county, or state) that crosses the jurisdiction of local health authorities. The proposed Public Health Information Network (PHIN) is yet a third model. The PHIN is intended to cover the entire United States with state data collected under the authority of state or local health departments. Data is exchanged through the use of interoperable information systems for both routine and emergency purposes (Centers for Disease Control and Prevention, 2008). Finally, the military model would cover a community with a large military presence or global military communities. This model is currently in place in Washington, DC, where the Department of Defense monitors military emergency department and primary care clinic patients visit diagnostic codes with the use of a centralized medical information systems database (Lewis et al., 2002).

The National Bioterrorism Syndromic Surveillance Demonstration Program (NDP) was designed to provide an alternative model to current CDC reporting methods (Lazarus, Yih, & Platt, 2006). The NDP model used no identifiable health information; instead, aggregated data counts stored on a secure server were proposed for use. Analysis would be done from the data located in a secure server. Afterwards, alerts and reports from the data analysis would be forwarded to the pertinent local public health authorities for appropriate alert distribution and care interventions.

Disaster Response and Planning

Hurricane Katrina, the disastrous storm that struck the U.S. Gulf Coast in August 2005, served to inform HIT about disaster planning. After the storm, the KatrinaHealth Web site

---

[3] NEDSS is discussed in Chapter 16.

(http://www.katrinahealth.org) was almost immediately established in conjunction with local and state governments, Dr. David Brailer, the then National Coordinator for HIT, the Markle Foundation, and pharmaceutical companies (Markle Foundation, American Medical Association, Gold Standard, RxHub, & SureScripts, 2006). The Web site served as a portal for authorized physicians and pharmacists to obtain electronic prescription medical records for victims of the storm. Reflective analysis for KatrinaHealth is available online at http://katrinahealth.org/katrinahealth.final.pdf. The report includes seven recommendations that local, state, and national policy makers and governments must consider.

- ▼ Plan for disasters now
- ▼ Use existing available resources such as the Regional Health Information Organizations (RHIOs)
- ▼ Create interoperable EHRs
- ▼ Integrate emergency response systems into nonemergent systems
- ▼ Establish systems that can be easily accessed
- ▼ Establish effective communication channels
- ▼ Overcome policy barriers

Healthcare professionals, information technology specialists, and those in leadership positions continue to learn from disasters such as Hurricane Katrina and the World Trade Center attacks. The efforts served as catalysts for improved communication channels and the development of improved informatics solutions to improve the lives of future victims.

The Regional Coordinating Center for Hurricane Response (RCC) was established in October 2005 (Mack, Brantley, & Bell, 2007). The mission for RCC was to work through the use of HIT, with the National Institute of Health's centers of Excellence in Partnerships for Community Outreach, Research on Health Disparities and Training (EXPORT), to assist with the renewing and rebuilding of the healthcare systems that were affected by hurricanes Katrina and Rita. The RCC embarked on building partnerships with local healthcare systems among the different Gulf Shore states to assist in the rebuilding process. The goals for this project

included the use of EHRs, telepsychiatry, and screening and surveillance systems. Project leaders for RCC recognized that the reconstruction process was very complicated and that it would take time to accomplish.

Protection of Healthcare Data

HEALTH INSURANCE PORTABILITY AND ACCOUNTABILITY ACT

In 1996, Congress passed a bill that continues to have a great impact on healthcare, the Health Information Portability and Accountability Act (HIPAA). The law has affected the entire healthcare entity, including HIT. The law addressed several areas pertaining to healthcare information, including simplifying healthcare claims, providing standards for healthcare data transmission, and the security of healthcare information (Centers for Medicare & Medicaid Services, 2005a). The purpose of the law was to improve the effectiveness and efficiency of healthcare. It was also designed to prevent medical fraud by standardizing the electronic exchange of financial and administrative data. The HIPAA law applies only to: 1) healthcare providers that "furnish, bill, or receive payment for healthcare in the normal business day" and who also transmit any transactions electronically; 2) healthcare clearinghouses; or 3) health plans (Centers for Medicare & Medicaid Services, 2005b).

The area that has generated the most public attention has been the privacy and security rules that address many of the privacy, confidentiality, and security issues already discussed in this chapter. There have been many areas of disagreement among the stakeholders about the rules, and legitimate concerns exist on both sides. One rule requires that in each agency, a specific person be assigned the responsibility for overseeing efforts to secure electronic data. As a result, each healthcare agency that has to abide by the rules has a person designated as the HIPAA officer. This person must be proficient in information technology, auditing, agency policies and practices, ethics, state and federal regulations, and consumer issues.

habit that can be learned as easily as locking the doors of the house or car.

Biometrics

The most secure method of authentication is **biometrics** – the use of physiological characteristics such as iris or retinal scan, fingerprint, or a voiceprint that is presumably unique to the particular person. Of these, the **iris scan** seems to hold the most promise and return the least number of false "no matches." There are more than 200 unique points on the iris that can be used for comparison (Daugman, 2007; National Center for State Courts, 2002a). For authentication purposes, users stand about 2 feet away from the scanner in a place where they can see their own eye reflection for a couple of seconds. Verification takes less than five seconds. The **retinal scan** is very accurate, but it is less beneficial in the busy healthcare environment because the users must remove their glasses, place their eye against a device, and focus on a point. The entire process takes about 10-15 seconds (National Center for State Courts, 2002b).

The rich whorls, ridges, and patterns of **fingerprints** are still useful for authentication. The users press their fingers against an optical or silicon surface reader for less than five seconds. The accuracy is improved with the use prints from more than one finger. One of the limitations of fingerprint biometrics is that the finger should be clean and not smudged with grease, dirt, or ink, such as newspaper print (Erdley, 2006). Because optical scanners require reflected light, they may fail to read fingerprints of people with dry skin, some people with dark skin, and those with fine print ridges, such as children. Improved accuracy in fingerprint authentication is achieved with ultrasound technology because it has less trouble reading a fingerprint with contaminants (Pierce, 2003). Ultrasonic print scanners are able to read fingerprints on dark skin and require no special lighting conditions. Fingerprint recognition is a common option used to authenticate access of personal digital assistants (PDAs) and laptops.

Voice recognition is another type of biometric used for security. Voice recognition creates voiceprints using a combination of two authentication factors: What is said and the way that it is said (Anderson, 2007). It can also be used at a distance with a telephone. Voice biometrics is more commonly used in the banking industry as much of banking business is done over telephone lines. Voice recognition has potential for increased use in healthcare because it is two to three times more accurate than fingerprinting and less expensive than some of the other biometric systems.

Radio Frequency Identification

RFID refers to smart labels or intelligent bar codes that can communicate with a network (Gibson & Bonsor, n.d.). RFID is designed to take the place of the Universal Product Code (UPC) that we see on almost any product we purchase, whether it is a package of CD-ROMs at the office supply store or a box of cereal at the grocery store. We may have seen or used RFID on a pass card attached to a vehicle windshield for access to toll roads. Another nonmedical use is to tag pet dogs and cats for easy identification in case they are lost. In 2006, the United States began to embed RFID chips in passports.

RFID is of two types, passive and active (VeriChip Corporation, 2006). The passive tags are lighter, less expensive ($1–3), have read-only capability, and can be read at a distance of 1–10 feet. The passive implantable[5] (inserted under the skin) tag uses a federal drug administration (FDA) chip. The active tags are more expensive ($25–50), have read-write capability, and can be read at distances from 1 to 300 feet.

Currently, RFID is used in many healthcare agencies to track patients, including newborn babies. The "Hugs" Infant Protection System by VeriChip™ Corporation is an example of how RFID is used in healthcare. Each baby receives an ankle band or a wristband with an

---

[5] The implantable VeriMed™ is discussed in more detail in Chapter 26.

embedded RFID chip. If there is an unauthorized removal of the baby, an alarm is sounded. Example of successful use was reported when a baby's abduction was thwarted from Presbyterian Hospital in Charlotte, North Carolina (Sullivan, 2005).

RFID is also used in healthcare agencies to track equipment such as wheelchairs and intravenous pumps and used to track the location of patients (Supply Insight Inc., 2006). Another use of this technology is to track hospital personnel, such as doctors and nurses (Activewave Inc., 2007). Although the use of the technology with patients and personnel has been controversial in some settings, decisions have been made in favor of improved care delivery systems and patient safety.

VeriChip also manufactures passive RFID solutions to facilitate identification and a unique identifier number of "at risk" patients who may need emergency medical treatment and to locate patients with memory impairments who may wander. The RFID tag can be implanted under the patient's skin or worn as a bracelet. The only information contained in the chip is the patient's name, address, allergies, picture, and the unique identifier, which is used to obtain health record information. The healthcare provider uses a wall or handheld scanner to obtain the information.

Data Security

The third element of healthcare data protection is **data security**. The data security issues are the responsibility of the information systems team. Data security has three aspects. The first deals with ensuring the accuracy of the data, the second with protection of the data from unauthorized eyes inside or outside the agency, and the third with internal or external damage to the data.

Informatics nurses and clinical nurses are involved in building entry screens prior to a system implementation. Nurses as well as the technical staff need to understand the principles of data security. **Accuracy of data** can be improved with methods that check the data during input.

For example, when a user chooses phrases for input from a list, the person needs to be sure that only recognized terms are entered. To check that the desired phrase was chosen before leaving the page, the user can be presented with a screen that shows the items that will be entered into the record. Another factor that must be considered is how to handle incorrect entries. Generally, provision is allowed for the entry to be corrected within a time period, but a record of all entries is kept in an **audit trail**. An audit trail provides a list of who accessed the system, the date, the time, and the activity.

Protection of the data from prying eyes involves the use of audit trails and making decisions about how much access individual users should have. Who has access to what information differs from agency to agency. For pure ease of use, all professional healthcare workers would have access to any patient record in the system. This is very helpful when patients are transferred from one department to another, and it is allowed in some institutions. Its use must be backed up by audit trails, or by a record of which individual worker accessed which record at what time and where. Additionally, those audit trails must be routinely examined to determine if breeches of security are occurring. Audit trails are closely scrutinized after the admission of persons who are well known. Making decisions about how much access users have varies from one institution to the next. Most institutions provide access only to records of those patients on the unit where the healthcare worker is stationed, and they index them by job description. Limiting access too severely will prohibit holistic care and can put patients in jeopardy.

Accuracy of the original data is also the responsibility of users. There have been situations in which clinicians have entered anything into a mandatory field just to continue in the system. Not only does this put patient care at risk, but it also compromises the integrity of the database. This cavalier attitude can be attributed to a multitude of factors: lack of awareness of what is done with the data, an unwieldy system for entering data, time pressures, and inadequate training on using the system. That being said, system designers must understand nurse work flow and require only essential mandatory fields, not ones that may be impossible to complete. Regardless of the cause, attempts to bypass mandatory data entry fields must be addressed if data are to be valid.

PROTECTION FROM SYSTEM INTRUSIONS

With the rise of the Internet and the actuality that most agencies are now connected to it, preventing outsiders from accessing institutional information has become a major responsibility of the information services department. One of the first lines of defense for protecting against unauthorized access is a firewall. A **firewall** operates in one of two ways. Either it examines all messages entering and leaving a system and blocks those that do not meet specific criteria, or it allows or denies messages on the basis of whether the destination port is acceptable. Firewalls require constant maintenance. To ensure that the system is safe from prying eyes, some agencies hire white hat hackers to try and penetrate their systems. **White hat hackers** are persons who are ethically opposed to security abuse. Their job is to attempt to penetrate systems to identify security weaknesses. Protection is then devised for any security breaches that are found.

Systems also need to be protected from outsiders who gain physical entrance to the agency and from insiders who are intent on gaining unauthorized access. Security audits completed by independent consultants are used to identify potential system security vulnerabilities. The first line of defense against this type of breach includes staff education on the importance of data security. Staff should be encouraged to expect identification from unfamiliar persons and to refuse access to anyone without recognized authorization.

PHISHING AND SPEAR PHISHING SECURITY BREACHES

The concept of phishing was discussed in Chapter 5 on email, so you may be curious about why it is being discussed again in this chapter on healthcare system issues. To steal confidential patient information, criminal hackers use phishing email tactics to lure the care provider into revealing private information. Spear phishing tactics use what appears to be legitimate business email from a person well known to the email recipient. It is a new scam that lures an employee into revealing private login information (Heuston, 2005; TechWeb, 2008). For example, in a healthcare agency, the employees might receive what appears to be a legitimate employee email from within the agency, such as from human resources, nursing services, or information services. The scam is that the email will ask the recipients to update their login and password information or to verify it. When the recipients respond, the perpetrator steals their login and password and then uses the information for criminal purposes by hacking into the hospital's information system. All phishing scams should be reported to the Antiphishing Working Group at http://www.antiphishing.org.

PROTECTION FROM DATA LOSS

Computer data need to be protected from being lost as a result of either a system problem or disaster, natural or otherwise. This latter element took on new importance after the fall of the World Trade Center on September 11, 2001, and hurricanes Katrina and Rita in 2005. To provide this protection, data must be backed up routinely and stored off-site in a secure place. These backups should be periodically examined to make sure that they are accurate and can be easily reinstalled on the system. Additionally, a disaster recovery plan needs to be devised and tested. This plan should be made in conjunction with key people in the agency to ensure adequate protection. The objective in disaster recovery is to allow work to resume using the same standards as before the disaster with the least amount of effort. One of the first tasks in planning for disaster recovery is to do a risk analysis. This analysis will determine vulnerabilities and appropriate control measures.

Identification of system weaknesses can prevent the actual occurrence of a disaster. A disaster plan should be tested at least twice a year.

 ## Conclusion

The issues associated with migration from a paper medical record to full implementation of the electronic record are extremely complex and arduous. The good news is that progress is being made one step at a time, and sometimes, one keystroke at a time. There is collaboration among the government, private and professional organizations, vendors, healthcare agencies, and healthcare professionals. The EMR adoption model developed by HIMSS Analytics serves as a roadmap for those who have undertaken or plan to undertake the electronic journey.

The healthcare organization's strategic plan serves as a foundation for successful implementation of a system. Selection decisions for health information system solutions don't come easily. In this day of financial scrutiny, stakeholders need to see a return on investment. Risks and opportunities for tangible and intangible payoffs must be explored.

The HIT steering committee should be made up of a multidisciplinary team including the top leadership, clinicians, information technology personnel, and all others whose work might be influenced by the new system. The oversight committee must address hard issues such as interoperability standards, user design of data entry screens, work flow redesign, and quality measurement desired outcomes. All users must have a clear vision of the opportunities to improve nursing outcomes, to save unnecessary avoidable hospital costs, while at the same time meet the Joint Commission's regulatory requirements. Everyone who is involved with the system design and implementation should be familiar with literature findings and research results to anticipate and avoid negative unintended consequences. No potential problem should be minimized, rather it should be addressed proactively.

As the issues of interoperability and system integration are addressed, the United States will be able to take proactive interventions to recognize communicable disease outbreaks using analysis of symptoms in a secure central database. Several initiatives addressing the creations of disease and syndromic surveillance systems can also be used for bioterrorism. As an example, the CDC NEDSS system is already in place. The EHR has the ability of expediting safe care and saving lives during a disaster if the data are stored in regional health information organization secure databases so that they are accessible wherever the victim receives care.

Issues regarding privacy, confidentiality, and data security still persist. Healthcare data privacy and security are of utmost importance to those who provide and receive care. The associated challenges are how to expedite the delivery of healthcare and communication among providers while at the same time protecting the health information system data. As new technology develops, new issues will surface. The more things change, the more they stay the same.

APPLICATIONS AND COMPETENCIES

1. Using the EMR Adoption model to analyze and describe the level of adoption for a local healthcare agency.
2. Discuss the opportunities for clinical data sharing in your city or region. Support the associated risks and opportunities with current literature.
3. Discuss the methods for assuring privacy and confidentiality of patient electronic information in a local clinical setting. Identify the penalties the agency uses for employees that breach confidentiality and security policies.
4. Interview a leadership representative from information technology at a healthcare agency to assess interoperability issues within the different health information systems. Summarize the findings in written report.
5. Conduct a literature on work flow redesign, as it relates to a clinical documentation system. Afterwards, interview a nurse on a unit that is using any method of HIT to assess any nurse work flow issues. Explain why work flow is or is not an issue for the nursing staff.
6. Analyze how a local healthcare agency is addressing The Joint Commission's Patient Safety

Goals. Is the agency using HIT to address the safety goals? Why or why not?

7. Search the Web for tools that measure the strength of a password. Use the tool to assist you to create two examples of strong passwords. Provide an explanation for how you were able to create a strong password.

REFERENCES

Activewave Inc. (2007). *Applications/solutions: Equipment tracking in hospitals*. Retrieved March 6, 2008, from http://www.activewaveinc.com/applications_hospitals.php

Agency for Healthcare Research and Quality. (2001, March). *Reducing and preventing adverse drug events to decrease hospital costs*. Retrieved March 5, 2008, from http://www.ahrq.gov/qual/aderia/aderia.htm

Anderson, N. (2007, May 13). *Voice biometrics: Coming to a security system near you*. Retrieved February 29, 2008, from http://arstechnica.com/articles/culture/voice-biometrics-come-of-age.ars/2

Ash, J. S., Berg, M., & Coiera, E. (2004). Some unintended consequences of information technology in healthcare: The nature of patient care information system-related errors. *Journal of the American Medical Informatics Association, 11*(2), 104–112.

Ash, J. S., Sittig, D. F., Campbell, E. M., Guappone, K. P., & Dykstra, R. H. (2007, November). *Some unintended consequences of clinical decision support systems*. Paper presented at the American Medical Informatics Association, Chicago, IL.

Ash, J. S., Sittig, D. F., Poon, E. G., Guappone, K., Campbell, E., & Dykstra, R. H. (2007). The extent and importance of unintended consequences related to computerized provider order entry. *Journal of the American Medical Informatics Association, 14*(4), 415–423.

Barlow, R. D. (2007). Making sense of EHR(s struggle to gain traction: Up close with McKesson provider technologies(Tom Leonard. *Healthcare Purchasing News, 31*(4), 24–25.

Baron, R. J. (2007). Improving patient care. Quality improvement with an electronic health record: Achievable, but not automatic. *Annals of Internal Medicine, 147*(8), 549–552.

Bates, D. W., Evans, R. S., Murff, H., Stetson, P. D., Pizziferri, L., & Hripcsak, G. (2003). Detecting adverse events using information technology. *Journal of the American Medical Informatics Association, 10*(2), 115–128.

Birkmeyer, J. D., & Dimick, J. B. (2004). *The Leapfrog Group(s patient safety practices, 2003: The potential benefits of universal adoption*. Retrieved March 4, 2008, from http://www.leapfroggroup.org/media/file/Leapfrog-Birkmeyer.pdf

Campbell, E. M., Sittig, D. F., Ash, J. S., Guappone, K. P., & Dykstra, R. H. (2006). Types of unintended consequences related to computerized provider order entry. *Journal of the American Medical Association, 13*(5), 547–556.

Centers for Disease Control and Prevention. (2008, February 14). *PHIN*. Retrieved March 12, 2008, from http://www.cdc.gov/phin

Centers for Disease Control and Prevention. (n.d., May 22). *National electronic disease surveillance system*. Retrieved March 12, 2008, from http://www.cdc.gov/nedss/

Centers for Medicare & Medicaid Services. (2008, January 1). *Physician self-referral*. Retrieved March 5, 2008, from http://www.cms.hhs.gov/PhysicianSelfReferral/

Centers for Medicare & Medicaid Services. (2005a). *HIPAA – General information overview*. Retrieved December 14, 2004, from http://www.cms.hhs.gov/HIPAAGenInfo/

Centers for Medicare & Medicaid Services. (2005b). *HIPAA – General information: Are you covered entity?* Retrieved December 14, 2004, from http://www.cms.hhs.gov/HIPAAGenInfo/06_AreYouaCoveredEntity.asp#TopOfPage

Conrad, D. A., & Gardner, M. (2005, May 2). *Updated economic implications of the Leapfrog Group patient safety standards: Final report to the Leapfrog Group*. Retrieved March 5, 2008, from http://www.leapfroggroup.org/media/file/Conrad_Updated_Economic_Implications_2_.pdf

Daugman, J. (2007). New methods in iris recognition. *IEEE Transactions on Systems, Man, and Cybernetics. Part B, Cybernetics, 37*(5), 1167–1175.

Erdley, W. S. (2006). Personal digital assistants, wireless computing, smart cards, and biometrics: A hardware update for clinical practice. *Journal of Obstetric, Gynecologic, and Neonatal Nursing, 35*(1), 157–163.

Gibson, C., & Bonsor, K. (n.d.). *How RFID works*. Retrieved March 6, 2008, from http://electronics.howstuffworks.com/rfid7.htm

U. S. Department of Health and Human Services. (n.d.). *HIT certification: Stark and anti-kickback in HIT*. Retrieved March 8, 2008, from http://www.hhs.gov/healthit/certification/stark/

Heuston, G. Z. (2005, November 3). *Spear phishing attacks mounting*. Retrieved February 29, 2008, from http://www.ci.hillsboro.or.us/Police/documents/SpearPhishing-11-03-05.pdf

HIMSS Analytics. (2008). *Healthcare providers: EMR adoption model*. Retrieved March 12, 2008, from http://www.himssanalytics.org/hc_providers/index.asp

Hunt, E., Sproat, S. B., & Kitzmiller, R. (2004). *The Nursing Informatics Implementation Guide*. New York: Springer-Verlag.

Lazarus, R., Yih, K., & Platt, R. (2006). Distributed data processing for public health surveillance [Electronic version]. *BMC Public Health, 6*, 235. Retrieved March 6, 2008 from http://www.biomedcentral.com/content/pdf/1471-2458-6-235.pdf

Lewis, M. D., Pavlin, J. A., Mansfield, J. L., O'Brien, S., Boomsma, L. G., Elbert, Y., et al. (2002). Disease outbreak detection system using syndromic data in the greater Washington DC area. *American Journal of Preventive Medicine, 23*(3), 180–186.

Mack, D., Brantley, K. M., & Bell, K. G. (2007). Mitigating the health effects of disasters for medically underserved populations: electronic health records, telemedicine, research, screening, and surveillance. *Journal of Health Care for the Poor and Underserved, 18*(2), 432–442.

Mandl, K., D., Overhage, J. M., Wagner, M. M., Lober, W. B., Sebastiani, P., Mostashari, F., et al. (2004). Implementing Syndromic Surveillance: A Practical Guide Informed by the Early Experience. *Journal of the American Medical Informatics Association, 11*(2), 141–150.

Markle Foundation, American Medical Association, Gold Standard, RxHub, & SureScripts. (2006, June 13). *Lessons from KatrinaHealth.* Retrieved March 6, 2008, from http://katrinahealth.org/katrinahealth.final.pdf

Milstein, A. (2007). Health information technology is a vehicle, not a destination: A conversation with David J. Brailer. Interview by Arnold Milstein. *Health Affairs, 26*(2), w236–w241.

Moran, G. J., & Talan, D. A. (2003). Update on emerging infections: News from the Centers for Disease Control and Prevention. Syndromic surveillance for bioterrorism following the attacks on the World Trade Center—New York City, 2001. *Annals of Emergency Medicine, 41*(3), 414–418.

National Center for State Courts. (2002a). *Iris scan.* Retrieved February 29, 2008, from http://ctl.ncsc.dni.us/biomet%20web/BMIris.html

National Center for State Courts. (2002b). *Retinal scan.* Retrieved February 29, 2008, from http://ctl.ncsc.dni.us/biomet%20web/BMRetinal.html

National Committee Vital Health Statistics. (2001). *A strategy for building the National Health Information Infrastructure:* U.S. Department of Health & Human Services.

Nudd, T., & Lee, K. (2007, December 4). Dennis & Kimberly Quaid sue drug company. *People.* Retrieved March 7, 2008, from http://www.people.com/people/article/0,,20164211,00.html

Pierce, F. S. (2003). Biometric identification. Ultrasonic systems can succeed where optical systems may not. *Health Management Technology, 24*(5), 38–39.

Runy, L. A., & Towne, J. (2005). Information technology + ROI: A CEO's guide to measuring and evaluating IT's financial effectiveness. *H&HN: Hospitals & Health Networks, 79*(2), 8p.

Stein, D. M., Wrenn, J. O., Johnson, S. B., & Stetson, P. D. (2007). Signout: A collaborative document with implications for the future of clinical information systems. *American Medical Informatics Association Annual Symposium Proceedings* (pp. 696–700).

Sullivan, L. (2005, July 19). RFID system prevented a possible infant abduction [Electronic version]. *Information Week.* Retrieved March 6, 2008 from http://www.informationweek.com/story/showArticle.jhtml?articleID=166400496

Supply Insight Inc. (2006, April 20). RFID applications in patient tracking. Retrieved March 6, 2008, from http://www.rfidsolutionsonline.com

Syndromic surveillance for bioterrorism following the attacks on the World Trade Center – New York City, 2001. (2002). *MMWR: Morbidity and Mortality Weekly Report, 51 Spec No,* 13–15.

TechWeb. (2008). *Phishing.* Retrieved February 29, 2008, from http://www.techweb.com/encyclopedia/defineterm.jhtml?term=phishing

The Joint Commission. (2008). *National patient safety goals.* Retrieved March 7, 2008, from http://www.jointcommission.org/PatientSafety/NationalPatientSafetyGoals/

VeriChip Corporation. (2006). RFID 101. Retrieved March 6, 2008, from http://www.verichipcorp.com/content/company/rfid101

CHAPTER 22

Carrying Healthcare to the Client

Learning Objectives

After studying this chapter you will be able to:

1. *Define the two overall classifications of technology used in telehealth.*

2. *Discuss some of the ways that telehealth can deliver healthcare.*

3. *Illustrate the opportunities for autonomous nursing practice in telehealth.*

4. *Discuss the main issues in implementing telehealth.*

5. *Analyze the ways that telehealth could impact the present healthcare system.*

Key Terms

Biometric Garment

e-Intensive Care

Portable Monitoring Devices

Real-Time

Robotics

Store and Forward (S&F)

Telehealth

Telehomecare

Telemedicine

Telemental health

Telenursing

Telepresence

Teletrauma

During the 1998 Around the World Alone sailboat race, one of the racers while in the South Atlantic developed an abscess on his elbow that could have caused him to lose his arm. Using a wireless computer and satellite technology he was put in touch with a doctor in Boston who directed his treatment and saved the arm. Not all telehealth applications are this dramatic, but the incident demonstrates the power of this emerging vehicle for delivering healthcare. Although much attention has been given to the aspect of telehealth that addresses the delivery of acute care or specialist consultations, telehealth has been shown to be far more versatile. Telehealth can be used to provide home telenursing, electronic referrals to specialists and hospitals, teleconsulting between specialists and general practitioners or nurse practitioners, minor injury consulting, and consulting through call centers (Gassert, 1996).

Terms such as "telehealth" and "telemedicine" have in the past been used interchangeably to refer to health services delivered using electronic technology to patients at a distance. According to the American Telemedicine

Association, **telemedicine** refers to the electronic exchange of patient information between two sites for the purpose of improving the patient's health status, and **telehealth**, a broader term, extends beyond the delivery of clinical services (American Telemedicine Association, 2008). The International Council of Nursing defines **telenursing** as "telecommunications technology in nursing to enhance patient care" (International Council of Nurses, 2008). This chapter will focus on emerging developments and applications using the term telehealth unless specified otherwise in the references used to support the information.

Telehealth Basics

As the sailor in the Around the World Alone sailboat race proved, the technology for delivering telemedicine does not have to be complex. Hopefully, most cases would not involve self-treatment. Generally, there are two uses of technology for delivering telehealth, either **store and forward (S&F)** or a two-way communication. The line between these two modes is becoming less and less distinct because many services use both types of communication. There is a wealth of information about telehealth on the Internet. A good place to begin is the Telemedicine Information Exchange at http://tie.telemed.org/links/specialties.asp.

STORE AND FORWARD TECHNOLOGY

In S&F technology, a still image is captured electronically by a digital camera, scanner, or technology (e.g., x-ray machine) that generates electronic images, and then that image is sent to a specialist for interpretation at a later time (American Telemedicine Association, n.d.). Radiology, dermatology, pathology, and wound care specialties lend themselves very well to this technique. S&F also includes asynchronous transmission of clinical data, such as the results of an EKG, MRI, or blood glucose levels, between two sites. This type of communication is often between healthcare providers. S&F offers the only affordable way that medicine can be practiced in remote communities, such as those in Alaska. For example, S&F is used when an x-ray is read by a radiologist located at a different site from where it was done. This method is frequently used in healthcare.

REAL-TIME TELEHEALTH

Real-time telehealth involves the patient and the provider interacting at the same time using interactive video/television. Many telecommunications devices that permit two-way communication are used to provide real-time telehealth. The oldest of these is the telephone, but current telehealth technology generally includes videoconferencing using two-way video and audio. Although videoconferencing is possible with a modem and plain old telephone service (POTS), a higher quality of service is usually preferred. The required level of service depends on the type of services offered. Some services require at least a T1 line, or line on an integrated digital network (ISDN), which must not only connect the sites but also extend to the rooms where both the patient and the distant consultant are located. Large satellite systems that have a global audience are also used in telehealth. In short, any two-way communication technology offering both audio and video has, or will find, a use in telehealth.

Real-time telehealth also makes use of special instruments that can transmit an image to a clinician at a different location. These include an ear-nose-throat scope, a camera that captures skin observations, and a special stethoscope. They can be used either in real-time or in S&F mode. In addition, using a combination of robotics and virtual reality, a surgeon with special gloves and the appropriate audio and video technology is able to actually perform surgery by manipulating surgical instruments at the remote site. This procedure uses what is known as telepresence. It is still in development and requires a 100% reliable system and a very high bandwidth. **Telepresence** is the use of technology to provide the appearance of a person's presence, although he or she is located at a remote site (Federation of American Scientists, n.d.).

Telehealth Examples

As healthcare shifts away from the hospital and into the home and community, the therapeutic uses for telehealth increase. A much broader range of healthcare professionals such as nurse practitioners, nutritionists, social workers, and home healthcare aides will have a role in the provision of telehealth. One problem that has plagued the use of telehealth in the past is that payers have focused on acute medical care; however, reimbursement for telehealth services is slowly beginning to improve. Until the reimbursement issue is completely resolved, many of our population will remain underserved. As a result, illnesses, instead of being treated in the early stages, will progress to a stage where they are very costly to treat.

TELEHOMECARE

A trend in modern healthcare is to focus on the patient instead of the provider or agency. **Telehomecare** refers to the monitoring and delivery of healthcare in the patient's home rather than the provider's work setting. The greatest use of telehomecare is that it allows the patient the comforts of his or her own home, improves quality of life, and avoids time-consuming costly visits to office appointments or hospital admissions. The ongoing monitoring allows for potential problems to be identified before they become significant problems. Because telehomecare can eliminate unnecessary emergency room visits and hospital visits, it is cost-effective.

For patients with chronic diseases, telehealth can be a powerful self-management tool. Using telehomecare devices, patients can collect and transmit vital signs, cardiac rhythm, blood glucose, and weight (see Box 22-1). The data are sent using a telephone line or broadband connection to the healthcare provider and stored in the patient's electronic health record. The healthcare provider central monitoring station can view data from all patients that they are monitoring and see any

---

Box 22-1 • Examples of Telehomecare Devices

Vendor

ViTelCare™ Health
RemoteNurse™ Patient Monitor by WebVMC
HOMMED® Health Monitoring System
Phillips Motiva remote care manager
MD.2 Medication dispensing system
VivoMetrics® Lifeshirt®
Heart Failure Management System (HFMS)

---

alerts indicating significant changes. The computer screen that the healthcare provider views looks very similar to the central monitoring station in an intensive care unit (ICU) or step-down unit. Home health monitoring services are hosted by various companies.

Portable Monitoring Devices

Portable monitoring devices, available from a number of vendors (see Box 22-1), have many similarities. For example, they include an input device and various peripheral monitoring equipments. Many of the input devices use a touch screen with text and audio to ask the patient health assessment questions. The patient can respond to questions choosing answers such as true/false, none/better/worse, yes/no, and 0–10. Some of the devices can be programmed to include branching questions. Answers to some questions may result in the display of patient education information.

There are some differences for self-monitoring equipment. While most provide access to a central monitoring station using a telephone line, others allow access using high-speed and wireless connections. The peripheral monitoring accessories can vary among vendor products. Examples of monitoring accessories include a blood pressure cuff, ECG, blood glucose meter, weight scales, fluid status monitor, pulse oximeter, monitors for PT/INR, peak flow meter, and a spirometer.

What are the future trends for home monitoring devices? We can expect vendors to design the equipment so that the monitoring data will integrate with the electronic medical record (EMR), where it can be shared with pertinent healthcare agencies and providers. For example, HOMMED® Health Monitoring System recently partnered with Procura, LLC to integrate the patient monitoring data into an EHR (Honeywell, 2007). We can also expect the devices to provide patient decision support with context-sensitive health education information, reminders to take medication and doctor's appointments, feedback regarding vital sign monitoring results, and motivational messages. One example of a home monitoring system that uses a television monitor, Phillips Motiva remote care manager, is available at http://www.medical.philips.com/goto/motiva.

Pill Dispensers/Reminders

Automatic pill dispensers/reminders are another type of telehomecare device. The pill dispensers may include auditory reminders to prompt patients to take their medications, even if the medication is not a pill. The reminders may remind the patient to take the medication with food or to take an insulin injection. If medications are not taken within a specified period of time, the caregiver is notified by telephone. If the caregiver does not answer the telephone, the device phones the support center. Compliance can be monitored remotely through a secure Web site. The systems are about the size of a coffee maker. One example of an automatic pill dispenser is the MD.2. A short video of the device can be viewed at http://www.epill.com/md2video.html.

Wearable Monitoring Garments

Our current healthcare system remains disease focused; we seek care after something has gone wrong. Emerging wearable **biometric garment** technology will allow for a proactive approach where symptoms are identified early before problems develop. Early identification of symptoms has the potential for maintaining the patient's quality of life, reducing acute exacerbations of disease processes, and avoiding unnecessary medical costs. The concept of wearable garments with built-in physiological monitoring devices is fascinating.

A lightweight, washable biometric shirt can provide telehomecare noninvasive monitoring of temperature, cardiac rhythm, and pulmonary function (see Figure 22-1). Peripheral devices for monitoring of the electroencephalogram (EEG), electrooculography (EOG), blood oxygen saturation (pO_2), blood pressure, and cough can be used with the shirt. Research from Massachusetts Institute of Technology (MIT) (Sung, Marci, & Pentland, 2005) reported that wearable garments have potential uses for symptom detection and early treatment of

- ▼ Hypothermia
- ▼ Parkinson's disease
- ▼ Epilepsy seizures
- ▼ Depression

Wearable biometric garments can also be designed for use with portable home monitoring devices (Villalba, Arredondo, Moreno, Salvi, & Guillen, 2006; Villalba, Ottaviano, Arredondo, Martinez, & Guillen, 2006). An example is available at http://www.cinc.org/Proceedings/2006/pdf/0237.pdf.

Telehomecare for Chronic Disease Management

Telehomecare used to manage the care of patients with chronic diseases such as heart failure (see Figure 22-2). Its use is associated with decrease in hospitalization rates and more efficient uses of home care services. The Centers for Medicare & Medicaid Services (CMS) have traditionally not reimbursed for telehomecare, so the studies reported in the literature are prototypes funded with grant money.

For example, home care agencies in New York began using telehomecare after receiving government grants (Telemedicine Information Exchange, 2008). Home care service reported decreases in hospitalization rates ranging from 5% to 10% after implementing the service. A home care agency in Pennsylvania successfully reported a reduction of rehospitalization rates to 1.2% and improved resource utilization by decreasing the number of skilled nursing home care visits (Schneider, 2004; Schneider & Harris, 2003).

use of telepresence of ICU intensivists in critical care is redefining the meaning of critical care remote monitoring. According to the Leapfrog Group, the mortality rates of ICU patients is 10% to 20%; however, the use of intensivists to manage or comanage patients can reduce hospital mortality by 30% and ICU mortality by 40% (Leapfrog Group, 2007). The Leapfrog Group recommends the use of ICU physician staffing (IPS) and supports the use of telemedicine intensive services to meet that need. Telepresence in critical care is currently being delivered with the use of videoconferencing tools, such as eICU® (VISICU, Baltimore, MD, U.S.), and robotics, such as RP-7 (InTouch Health, Santa Barbara, CA, U.S.).

eICU

iCare Intensive Care at North Colorado Medical Center provides telepresence using a camera, microphone, and speaker in the patient rooms (Banner Health, 2008; Trenary, 2007). The camera is activated by the bedside team during patient rounds when there is a need for the off-site intensivists and the expertise of critical care nurses located at the iCare Command Center in Banner Desert Medical Center.

The Banner Health system, which includes 20 hospitals located across 7 states, Alaska, Arizona, California, Colorado, Nebraska, Nevada, and Wyoming, and an iCare Command Center, located in Mesa, Arizona, monitored 126 critical care beds in 2007 and has plans to extend the eICU for all of the Banner system ICU beds over a two- to three-year period (Banner Health, 2007). The command center staff members have access to patient monitoring information, laboratory values, and x-rays. The cameras and microphones make it possible for the off-site experts to speak with the patients and on-site care providers using HIPAA compliant transmissions (Trenary, 2007). Patients receive information about the service upon admission to the hospital and are encouraged to ask questions or express concerns about the service. According to the Banner Health patient information, there is no additional charge for remote monitoring.

Research on the use of eICU provides promising results for the use of telehealth in critical care. Breslow et al. (2004) reported a two-year study of 2,140 ICU patients cared for using eICU. They compared economic and clinical outcomes data collected during six months of remote monitoring with data collected before the eICU was implemented. Analysis of the data showed a decrease in patient mortality from 12.9% to 9.4%. The ICU length of stay decreased from 4.35 to 3.63 days.

Nurses agree that improved patient outcomes are extremely important, but implementing **e-intensive care** had implications for the entire ICU environment. The use of these tools and robots require extensive planning and communications as well as workflow redesign. The most important factor is buy-in by all affected departments, including not only the ICU staff but also hospital leadership, information services, and respiratory therapy.

Robotics

Robotics is yet another way to provide telepresence of ICU intensivists. One example is the RP-7 robot; RP is short for remote presence (InTouch Health, n.d.). The robot is the height of a person who is 5 feet 6 inches and has a large flat screen monitor where a person's head would be; a small camera with tilt, pan, and zoom features; and a couple of antennas on top of the monitor (see Figure 22-3). The robot also has two-way audio that allows for conversations between the clinical site and the remote expert. It receives and sends data through a wireless network. It rolls about the floor on three spheres and has built-in infrared sensing devices to help guide it around obstacles.

The remote expert controls the robot using RP software and a joystick. The software can be used with either a laptop or desktop computer. Dual monitors allow the physician to view patient's electronic medical record on one monitor and to control the robot using the second monitor. The movement of the robot's camera tilt, pan, and zoom features allows the physician to examine the patient, read a chart, view x-rays mounted on a light board, or observe physiological monitor data. The robot's

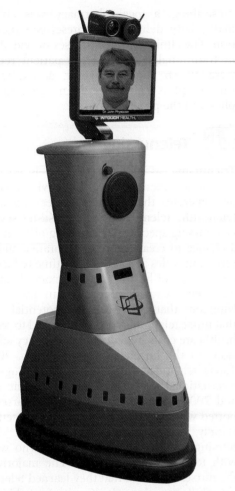

Figure 22-3 • RP-7 robot. (Reprinted with permission from InTouch Health.)

"head" (the monitor) is able to move 360°, allowing it to "face" the ICU person. The robot's audio and video features allow for real-time interaction between the physician at the remote site and the patient and care providers in the ICU.

The RP-7 robot is in use in a number of ICU settings. Childrens Hospital Los Angeles was the first hospital in the United States to use robots to support the ICU physicians and staff in the pediatric ICUs (Childrens Hospital Los Angeles, 2007). University of California Los Angeles (UCLA) reported using a robot named RONI (Robot of the Neuro ICU) in the neurological ICU (Lee, 2005). The Methodist

Hospital in Houston, Texas, reported using the RP-7 robot in the neurosurgical ICU and the stroke center (The Methodist Hospital System, 2006). The Methodist Hospital staff members affectionately named the robots MURDOC (Mobile Unit Robot Doctor) and ROHAS (Remote Operated Health Assessment System). The common goal for use in each of the ICU settings was to improve the quality of patient care by supporting the ICU physicians and staff with a real-time expert opinion.

Research on use of remote telepresence using robotics in critical care has demonstrated positive outcomes. Vespa et al. (2007) compared data for a period of time before and after using robot telepresence. They noted that the "face-to-face" response time for routine and urgent pages was reduced from 3.5 hours to less than 10 minutes. Because of the rapid response times, patient outcomes improved and the ICU length of stay was reduced. The researchers attributed a cost savings of $1.1 million to the use of robot telepresence.

TELETRAUMA CARE

Rural hospitals have been able to use telehealth to augment trauma care because they are able to obtain reimbursement for these services (American Telemedicine Association, 2007; Whitten, 2006). Known as **teletrauma**, it is used to obtain second opinions and advice from trauma care experts. Teletrauma care has also been used to deliver care in parts of the world torn by violence and war.

Rural hospitals in places like Northern California and Eastern Maine are using telehealth equipment to connect with trauma experts. The rural physicians and staff want to provide the best possible care to the patients while keeping the inconvenience of care, travel, and expense of care as low as possible. As of 2007, University of California Davis (UC Davis) pediatric intensivists had completed over 200 videoconferencing consultations with remote hospital emergency departments and ICUs (UC Davis Medicine, 2007). Thirty percent of the consultations were related to the trauma care for children. Eastern Maine

Health System (2008) has reported use of tele-conferencing to improve emergency patient outcomes. The telemedicine hub site, located at Eastern Maine Medical Center, was de-signed to provide 24/7 support for care of patients located in multiple rural care hospitals.

Research on the use of teletrauma care in rural settings has shown promising outcomes and significance for use in the rural health set-tings. Duchesne et al. (2008) reported a five-year study of 814 trauma patients comparing the outcomes before and after implementation of telemedicine in rural Mississippi settings. The trauma patients who experienced tele-trauma care had a decrease in length of stay at the local community hospital (1.5 hours vs. 47 hours) and a decrease in transfer time to trauma centers (1.7 hours vs. 13 hours). The hospital costs for the trauma patients de-creased from $7,632,624 to $1,126,683.

DISASTER HEALTHCARE

Telehealth has been used successfully in pro-viding healthcare in disasters (Garshnek & Burkle, 1999a, 1999b; Markle Foundation, American Medical Association, Gold Standard, RxHub, & SureScripts, 2006). Almost imme-diately after Hurricane Katrina hit the Gulf Shore states in the United States, the KatrinaHealth Web site was established to fa-cilitate communication and to assist victims to access their electronic prescription medication records. As a result, many nurses were able to distribute the medications in temporary living communities established across the United States where victims had been transported. One example of such a community was the Rock Eagle 4-H camp in Georgia. The home economics building was converted into a clinic and was open 24 hours to serve 240 to 500 victims. One part of the clinic was staffed by volunteer physicians and nurse practition-ers, and the other by volunteer nurses. The local health department nursing leadership co-ordinated all the care. Nurses used desktop computers with access to the Internet and se-cure logins to access information to assist the victims. With the assistance of the electronic

prescribing, a local pharmacy was able to make daily deliveries of prescribed medica-tion. The clinic volunteer nurses provided care in traditional ways, and the patient records were all on paper; however, access to the Internet played a major role in access to sup-plies and the provision of care.

Telenursing

Telenursing, as part of telehealth is not new. The project mentioned in the previous section demonstrates the use of volunteer nurses in telehealth. Telenursing in nondisaster settings is a nursing specialty. Telenursing offers nurses a chance to create more collaborative and au-tonomous roles and at the same time reduce the overall cost of healthcare. One example of this was demonstrated in a study in the United Kingdom that confirmed the potential value that nurse telephone consultation had to reduce healthcare costs by reducing emergency admis-sions to the hospital (Lattimer et al., 2000). Today, telenurses work in various settings. An international study completed between 2004 and 2005 revealed that 37% of telenurses re-ported working in hospital and college settings (Grady & Schlachta-Fairchild, 2007). Tele-nursing was described as a nurse who works with telehealth technologies. The majority of the nurses indicated that they learned telenurs-ing skills on the job (Grady & Schlachta-Fairchild, 2007; Schlachta-Fairchild, 2001). An interesting finding, given that majority of the nurses had no prior experience with telehealth before their telenursing positions, is that the majority (89.2%) of those surveyed indicated that telehealth should be included in basic nursing curriculum.

Education

Most telehealth projects have a built-in patient educational component. In some, education is delivered during the "visits," and in others through Web pages. Telehealth is also useful in the educational needs of healthcare profession-als, not only for continuing education but also for preparing practitioners. Clinical experiences for nurse practitioner and primary physician students, which often involves much driving for instructors and students, have been shown to benefit from telehealth. One such application used both S&F and real-time technology for providing clinical education. S&F methods were used to review student case presentations, while an ear-nose-throat scope, video camera, and high-quality stethoscope were incorporated into real-time use for evaluating student assessments, differential diagnoses, and management of some chronic problems (Chang & Trelease, 2001). Both faculty and student responses were generally positive with over half of the students evaluating the technology as enhancing their learning and retention a great deal. Faculty particularly expressed interest in using the technology for classroom presentations.

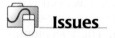 **Issues**

Telehealth in its many forms can provide many benefits such as enhanced patient care, reduced travel time, increased productivity, access to specialists, and enlarged educational opportunities for all. Many issues, however, surround this mode of healthcare delivery. Four main issues relate to 1) reimbursement, 2) medical-legal,[1] 3) technical, and 4) research.

REIMBURSEMENT

Reimbursement remains a large barrier to the widespread adoption of telehealth. Of the examples in this chapter, the majority was supported with grants. Despite successes, the telehealth projects were discontinued when the grant expired. Our healthcare system today is shaped by third party payers, both government and private. Currently, there continues to be no uniformity for reimbursement of telehealth/telemedicine services. According to the 2003 Telemedicine Reimbursement, "One of the barriers to telemedicine becoming completely integrated into the U.S. medical

system is the absence of consistent, federal and state reimbursement policies" (Center for Telemedicine Law, 2003, p. 8). For telemedicine to survive/thrive, reimbursement must be a joint effort between states, the federal government, and private payers. Reimbursement considerations must be made with the best interests of the patients' healthcare needs in mind.

A 2006 study by Whitten, which was a follow-up study on the ATA and AMD Telemedicine Study, showed progress in reimbursement for telehealth. In 2007, following a 2005 study verifying inconsistencies in Medicaid reimbursements for telehealth, the ATA published an update on CMS Medicare reimbursement policies (American Telemedicine Association, 2007) that specifies reimbursement requirements for telehealth services for 1) remote face-to-face services using videoconferencing, 2) non face-to-face services through videoconferencing and S&F technology, and 3) home healthcare services.

TECHNICAL

The safety of the patient is always a concern with developing uses of new technology. As was stated earlier in the chapter, all the projects seen thus far have been of a very high quality with no compromise in patient safety. In an endeavor to set standards in telenursing, the American Academy of Ambulatory Care Nursing (AAACN) established the Telehealth Nursing Practice Special Interest Group in 1995. The AAACN developed *Telehealth Nursing Practice Administration and Practice Standards* (American Academy of Ambulatory Care Nursing, 2007a), which address nine standards for telenursing, including staffing, competency, ethics, patient rights, and the use of the nursing process in telehealth. They followed this with publication of the *Telephone Nursing Practice Core Course Manual* (Espensen & Meeker, 2003). The organization also published the *Telehealth Nursing Practice Resource Directory* (American Academy of Ambulatory Care Nursing, 2007b). The directory includes resources and information to assist nurses to "improve the quality, efficiency, and effectiveness" of their practice. The AAACN offers certification for

---

[1] Medical-legal issues are discussed in Chapter 26.

telehealth nursing. The application can be downloaded from the AAACN Web site at http://www.aaacn.org/.

The American Telemedicine Association has adopted Core Standards for Telemedicine Operations, which addresses three types of standards: administrative, clinical, and technical. Administrative standards covers issues related to human resource management, HIPAA, research protocols, telehealth equipment use, and fiscal management. Clinical standards uphold the individual discipline standards of professional practice and standards of care as they relate to telehealth. Technical standards relate to requirements for safety and the function of telehealth equipment, the requirements for policies and procedures, and the need for redundant systems to assure network connectivity.

RESEARCH

A Cochrane Library meta-analysis of research done in the early years of this century to examine the efficacy of telemedicine versus face-to-face patient care recommendations did not demonstrate strong evidence of clinical benefits (Currell, Urquhart, Wainwright, & Lewis, 2000, 2001). A main complaint was that the number of patients in the research studies was small. The meta-analysis did note that people were satisfied with home self-monitoring and video consultations. Technology and telehealth research have matured since then, and current literature has reported studies conducted over time with larger numbers of patients (Breslow et al., 2004; Vespa et al., 2007); thus, the evidence for telehealth is now much stronger. Technology and telehealth research have matured since the meta-analysis of research was published. In addition to small case studies, current literature reports on studies conducted over time with larger numbers of patients (Breslow et al., 2004; Vespa et al., 2007).

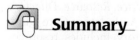

Summary

As technology improves, the possibilities for telehealth are endless. Telehealth technologies

can be classed as either S&F or real-time. S&F is an asynchronous method in which images are sent to a distant location and examined at the convenience of the specialist. Real-time telehealth, a synchronous mode, involves both the patient and the consultant interacting at the same time. Telepresence created with eICUs, two-way video teleconferencing, and robotics is being used to augment care delivered in ICUs and emergency departments. Telehomecare monitoring devices are empowering patients to live independently and to be proactive in the early detection of healthcare problems before they happen.

Telehealth offers many opportunities for nurses. Telehealth has also proved valuable in education, both professionally and for patient care and disaster care. Before telehealth becomes more widespread there are issues that need to be resolved. Medicare has been resistant to offer *uniform* payment across the United States for telehealth. The telecommunications infrastructure can also be a problem. As with many innovations, it will change the way healthcare is delivered. These changes will create opportunities for many, but if more preventive care reduces emergency room visits and hospital admissions, it has the potential to upset the financial base of the present day acute care system.

APPLICATION AND COMPETENCIES

1. Define the two overall classifications of technology used in telehealth.
2. Discuss some of the ways that telehealth can be applied to deliver healthcare.
3. Write two or three paragraphs illustrating the essential competencies for telenursing.
4. Select one of the issues in implementing telehealth and discuss the different approaches to resolving the issue.
5. Analyze two research studies done with telehealth. Compare the findings for similarities and differences.
6. Explore the ways that telehealth could have an impact on the healthcare system in your country.

REFERENCES

American Academy of Ambulatory Care Nursing. (2007a). *Telehealth nursing practice administration and practice standards* (4th ed.). Pitman, N.J.: American Academy of Ambulatory Care Nursing.

American Academy of Ambulatory Care Nursing. (2007b). *Telehealth nursing practice resource directory.* Pitman, N.J.: American Academy of Ambulatory Care Nursing.

American Telemedicine Association. (2007, January 22). *Medicare payment of telemedicine and telehealth services.* Retrieved February 15, 2008, from http://www.atmeda .org/news/Medicare%20Payment%20Of%20Services.pdf

American Telemedicine Association. (2008). *Telemedicine defined.* Retrieved November 24, 2008, from http://www .americantelemed.org/i4a/pages/index.cfm?pageid=3333

American Telemedicine Association. (n.d.). *Telemedicine/ telehealth terminology.* Retrieved November 24, 2008, from http://www.americantelemed.org/files/public/ standards/glossaryofterms.pdf

Banner Health. (2007, May 11). *Banner Health to add 50 new eICU beds in Valley.* Retrieved November 24, 2008, from http://www.bannerhealth.com/About+Us/News+Center/ Press+Releases/Press+Archive/Banner+Health+adds+ 50+eICU+beds.htm

Banner Health. (2008). *iCare intensive care, utilizing eICU technology.* Retrieved November 24, 2008, from http:// www.bannerhealth.com/Locations/Colorado/North+Col orado+Medical+Center/Programs+and+Services/iCare +Intensive+Care+Unit.htm

Bensink, M., Hailey, D., & Wootton, R. (2006). A systematic review of successes and failures in home telehealth: Preliminary results. 6th International Conference on Successes and Failures in Telehealth, SFT-6, Brisbane, Queensland, Australia, 24-24 August 2006. *Journal of Telemedicine & Telecare, 12,* S3:8–16.

Breslow, M. J., Rosenfeld, B. A., Doerfler, M., Burke, G., Yates, G., Stone, D. J., et al. (2004). Effect of a multiple-site intensive care unit telemedicine program on clinical and economic outcomes: An alternative paradigm for intensivist staffing. *Critical Care Medicine, 32*(1), 31–38.

Carmichael, M. (2005, March 1). *Combat stress teams and telemedicine: The new strategies for helping soldiers cope with war.* Retrieved November 24, 2008, from http://www .pbs.org/wgbh/pages/frontline/shows/heart/readings/ telemedicine.html

Center for Telemedicine Law. (2003). *Telemedicine reimbursement report.* Retrieved November 24, 2008, from http://www.hrsa.gov/telehealth/pubs/reimbursement.htm

Chang, B. L., & Trelease, R. (2001). Nursing informatics. Can telehealth technology be used for the education of health professionals? *Western Journal of Nursing Research, 23*(1), 107–114.

Childrens Hospital Los Angeles. (2007). *Virtual robotic doctor working with intensive care staff at Childrens Hospital Los Angeles.* Retrieved November 24, 2008, from http://www .childrenshospitalla.org/site/apps/nlnet/content2.aspx?c=ip INKTOAJsG&rb=3793521&ct=4909875

Currell, R., Urquhart, C., Wainwright, P., & Lewis, R. (2000). Telemedicine versus face to face patient care: Effects on professional practice and health care outcomes. *Cochrane Database Systematic Reviews* (2), CD002098.

Currell, R., Urquhart, C., Wainwright, P., & Lewis, R. (2001). Telemedicine versus face to face patient care: Effects on professional practice and health care outcomes. *Nursing Times, 97*(35), 35.

Daley, S. (2007). Riding the technological wave. *Health Management Technology, 28*(11), 18, 20.

Duchesne, J. C., Kyle, A., Simmons, J., Islam, S., Schmieg, R. E., Jr., Olivier, J., et al. (2008). Impact of telemedicine upon rural trauma care. *The Journal of Trauma, 64*(1), 92–97; discussion 97–98.

eHealthNews.eu. (2007, November 2). *St. Lucas Andreas Hospital to start home monitoring of cardiac patients.* Retrieved November 24, 2008, from http://www .ehealthnews.eu/content/view/805/26/

EMHS. (2008). *EMHS telehealth: Improving access to healthcare in Maine's rural communities.* Retrieved November 24, 2008, from http://www.emh.org/dynamic .aspx?id=14710

Espensen, M., & Meeker, P. (2003). *Telehealth nursing practice core course* (2nd ed.). Pitman, N.J.: American Academy of Ambulatory Care Nursing.

Federation of American Scientists. (n.d.). *Glossary.* Retrieved November 24, 2008, from http://www.fas.org/ spp/military/docops/usaf/2020/app-v.htm

Garshnek, V., & Burkle, F. M., Jr. (1999a). Applications of telemedicine and telecommunications to disaster medicine: Historical and future perspectives. *Journal of the American Medical Informatics Association, 6*(1), 26–37.

Garshnek, V., & Burkle, F. M., Jr. (1999b). Telecommunications systems in support of disaster medicine: Applications of basic information pathways. *Annals of Emergency Medicine, 34*(2), 213–218.

Gassert, C. A. (1996). Defining information requirements using holistic models: Introduction to a case study. *Holistic Nursing Practice, 11*(1), 64–74.

Grady, J. L., & Schlachta-Fairchild, L. (2007). Report of the 2004-2005 international telenursing survey. *Computers, Informatics, Nursing: CIN, 25*(5), 266–272.

Honeywell. (2007, December 11). *Integration of systems improved healthcare providers' telehealth connectivity.* Retrieved November 24, 2008, from http://www.hommed .com/News/ProcuraAnnc.asp

International Council of Nurses. (2008). *Nursing matters: Telenursing.* Retrieved November 24, 2008 from http:// www.icn.ch/

InTouch Health. (n.d.). *RP-7 Robot.* Retrieved November 24, 2008, from http://www.intouchhealth.com/products_ rp7robot.html

Lattimer, V., Sassi, F., George, S., Moore, M., Turnbull, J., Mullee, M., et al. (2000). Cost analysis of nurse telephone consultation in out of hours primary care: Evidence from a randomised controlled trial. *British Medical Journal, 320*(7241), 1053–1057.

Leapfrog Group. (2007, February 21). *Factsheet: ICU physician staffing (IPS).* Retrieved November 24, 2008, from http://www.leapfroggroup.org/media/file/Leapfrog-ICU_Physician_Staffing_Fact_Sheet.pdf

Lee, C. (2005). Meet RONI the robot [Electronic version]. *UCLA Today, 25.* Retrieved November 24, 2008, from http://www.today.ucla.edu/2005/050322campus_ meetroni.html

Markle Foundation, American Medical Association, Gold Standard, RxHub, & SureScripts. (2006, June 13). *Lessons from KatrinaHealth.* Retrieved November 24, 2008, from http://katrinahealth.org/katrinahealth.final.pdf

Mattia, J. (2007, May 21). *How Piedmont Hospital cut heart failure patient readmissions by 75 percent.* Retrieved November 24, 2008, from http://www.healthleadersmedia.com/content/89750/topic/WS_HLM2_TEC/How-Piedmont-Hospital-Cut-Heart-Failure-Patient-Readmissions-by-75-Percent.html

NCSBN. (2007, March). *Participating states in the NLC.* Retrieved November 24, 2008, from https://www.ncsbn.org/158.htm

NCSBN. (2008). *Background information about the RN and LPN/VN nurse licensure (NLC).* Retrieved November 24, 2008, from https://www.ncsbn.org/156.htm

Puskin, D. S. (2001). Telemedicine: Follow the money. *Online Journal of Issues in Nursing, 6*(3), 13p.

Schlachta-Fairchild, L. (2001). Telehealth: A new venue for health care delivery. *Seminars in Oncology Nursing, 17*(1), 34–40.

Schneider, N. M. (2004). Clinicians' forum. Managing congestive heart failure using home telehealth. *Home Healthcare Nurse, 22*(10), 719–722.

Schneider, N. M., & Harris, D. K. (2003). Telemedicine success story. *Telemedicine Journal and e-Health, 9*(1), 115–116.

Sung, M., Marci, C., & Pentland, A. (2005). Wearable feedback systems for rehabilitation. *Journal of Neuroengineering and Rehabilitation, 2*, 17.

TeleHealth Connections for Children and Youth. (2005, July). *Telemedicine for CSHCN: A state-by-state comparison of Medicaid reimbursement policies and Title V activities.* Retrieved November 24, 2008, from http://www.ichp.ufl.edu/documents/Telemedicine%20in%20Medicaid%20and%20Title%20V%20Report.pdf

Telemedicine Information Exchange. (2008, January 9). *Telemedicine and telehealth news.* Retrieved November 24, 2008, from http://tie.telemed.org/news/#item1608

The Methodist Hospital System. (2006). *Mobile robots offer 24/7 care to neurosurgical ICU, stroke patients.* Retrieved November 24, 2008, from http://www.methodisthealth.com/tmhs/newsItem.do?channelId=1073829253&contentId=1073946287&contentType=NEWS_CONTENT_TYPE

Todder, D., Matar, M., & Kaplan, Z. (2007). Acute-phase trauma intervention using a videoconference link circumvents compromised access to expert trauma care. *Telemedicine Journal and e-Health, 13*(1), 65–67.

Trenary, K. (2007). Advances in technology affects nursing: iCare Intensive Care, Banner Health: Remote telepresence in the critical care setting. *Arizona Nurse, 60*(2), 6–6.

Tschirch, P., Walker, G., & Calvacca, L. T. (2006). Nursing in tele-mental health. *Journal of Psychosocial Nursing and Mental Health Services, 44*(5), 20–27.

UC Davis Medicine. (2007, Spring). *Telemedicine extends trauma care to rural areas.* Retrieved November 24, 2008, from http://www.ucdmc.ucdavis.edu/ucdavismedicine/issues/spring2007/features/3.html

Vespa, P. M., Miller, C., Hu, X., Nenov, V., Buxey, F., & Martin, N. A. (2007). Intensive care unit robotic telepresence facilitates rapid physician response to unstable patients and decreased cost in neurointensive care. *Surgical Neurology, 67*(4), 331–337.

Villalba, E., Arredondo, M. T., Moreno, A., Salvi, D., & Guillen, S. (2006). User interaction design and development of a heart failure management system based on wearable and information technologies. *Conference Proceedings of IEEE Engineering in Medicine and Biology Society, 1,* 400–403.

Villalba, E., Ottaviano, M., Arredondo, M. T., Martinez, A., & Guillen, S. (2006). Wearable monitoring system for heart failure assessment in a mobile environment [Electronic version at http://www.cinc.org/Proceedings/2006/pdf/0237.pdf]. *Computers in Cardiology, 33,* 237–240.

Wachter, G. (2002, July). *Malpractice and telemedicine – Telemedicine liability: The uncharted waters of medical risk.* Retrieved November 24, 2008, from http://tie.telemed.org/legal/other/malpractice0702.pdf

Whitten, P. (2006, July). *Private payer reimbursement for telemedicine services in the United States.* Retrieved November 24, 2008, from http://www.liebertonline.com/doi/abs/10.1089/tmj.2006.0028

Young, T. L., & Ireson, C. (2003). Effectiveness of school-based telehealth care in urban and rural elementary schools. *Pediatrics, 112*(5), 1088–1094.

UNIT VI

Computer Uses in Healthcare Beyond Clinical Informatics

CHAPTER 23   Educational Informatics: e-Learning
CHAPTER 24   Administration Tools for Efficiency
CHAPTER 25   Informatics and Research
CHAPTER 26   Legal and Ethical Issues

The information that we gain from healthcare informatics allows us to become knowledge workers so that we can improve the welfare of others. The process of transforming data into knowledge is the crux of informatics, but it does not end there. The combination of knowledge and critical thinking skills is empowering and provides rich opportunities to improve nursing decision making and practice settings. The theme for this unit is computer uses in healthcare beyond clinical informatics.

Chapter 23 explores the use of computers for online learning, whether in the pursuit of nursing education or to meet the ongoing clinical education requirements for employment. Chapter 24 looks at the nurse administrator's role in the use of computers and information systems to analyze data and make business decisions and the nurse's role as it relates to clinical information systems. Chapter 25 addresses basic competencies in data analysis and research that provide a foundation for decision making in nursing and healthcare. Finally, Chapter 26 addresses the legal and ethical responsibilities of the nurse as they relate to informatics. Topics that are discussed include the professional codes of ethics, Health Insurance Portability and Accountability Act of 1996 (HIPAA), Web 2.0, telehealth, the implantable patient identifier, and copyright issues.

Educational Informatics: e-Learning

Learning Objectives

After studying this chapter you will be able to:

1. Describe how different online teaching methodologies contribute to learning using Bloom's taxonomy of learning.

2. Compare computerized quizzing and survey features with that of a print version.

3. Describe how online databases of teaching/learning resources such as the MERLOT project benefit learners.

4. Identify the strengths and weaknesses of e-Learning.

5. Interpret the factors affecting distance education outcomes.

6. Discuss the role of the learner in distance education.

7. Discuss three essential characteristics that contribute to success of learners who take courses online.

Key Terms

Animation
Avatar
Bloom's Taxonomy of Learning
Computer-Aided Instruction (CAI)
Computer-Based Learning (CBL)
Drill and Practice
e-Learning
Hybrid Courses
Instructional Games
Learning Assessment
Learning Content Management System
Learning Management System
Learning Style
Multimedia
Simulation
Sharable Content Object Reference Model (SCORM)
Simulation-Based Learning (SBL)
Streaming Video
Tutorial
Virtual Reality (VR)

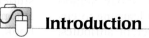

Introduction

You may have heard or read e-Learning (electronic learning) advertisements – "go to school in your pajamas" or "earn a college degree without ever leaving your home." You may be taking courses that are offered completely online or with parts of the course online (hybrid courses). You may be earning an online degree. But then again, you may be taking classes at a traditional brick and mortar school where you have schoolwork that requires use of a computer for learning activities and quizzing functions. If your learning falls into any of these situations, you have critical thinking. The best use of the drill and practice method is as an aid for memorization. Pure memorization provides learning at Bloom's Taxonomy *knowledge* level, which is essential in many areas to provide a foundation for higher-level learning. For example, it is essential to memorize information such as medical terminology along with rules for combining the terms to create other words to understand the nursing information in texts and articles. Alternative Medicine at http://nursing.iweb.bsu .edu/bbcourses/201/flashcards is an example of a Web site designed to assist with learning facts at the knowledge level.

Tutorials

Tutorials are step-by-step programs designed to guide learners to understand information. Well-designed tutorials are interactive when the learner is presented with learning content and then provided with self-assessment multiple choice questions to assess the learning. Most are patterned on a programmed learning model. The quality of a tutorial is evident with the use of branching techniques. At the low end of the continuum are programs that just inform the learner whether the answer is correct. Those at the high end offer more than one explanation for the same phenomenon and provide feedback on incorrect answers.

Tutorials do not have to "tell" the learners what they need to know. Learners can instead be presented with a situation, given the tools necessary to discover the answer, and then allowed to proceed at their own pace. An example of a tutorial is Congestive Heart Failure at http://www.nlm.nih.gov/medlineplus/tutorials/congestiveheartfailure/htm/index.htm. The interactive tutorial provides an opportunity for the learners to review the different modules and test their learning.

Simulations

Simulations imitate actual experiences. Simulations have many uses, such as part of an orientation or in-service, a face-to-face classroom or clinical laboratory setting, or as a part of a homework assignment. Effective simulations match the learner's knowledge background, or at least are only slightly above it, and the point of view addresses the learning needs. Simulations are available on CD-ROM and the Internet.

The Internet provides simultaneous use by a large number of learners. An online flash simulation, Painless (http://www2.cdl.edu/painless/), allows the learner to manage postoperative pain for a cancer patient, using morphine and patient-controlled analgesia (PCA). The simulation includes a history and physical, doctor's orders, and a blank nurse's notes page. Management of pain is a complex skill. Assessing blood pressure is also a complex skill for the novice healthcare provider student. The simulation, Assessing Blood Pressure at http://132.241.10.14/bp/bp.html, provides essential knowledge about how to take blood pressure and interpret the sounds. The student uses a mouse to "pump" the virtual blood pressure bulb, and then releases the valve to hear the sounds. An interactive quiz provides feedback on the learning.

Animations

Animations provide visual representations of difficult concepts, processes, and models. Animations can be created in a number of file formats. One common format used is called Flash. A Flash player, a free download from http://www.macromedia.com/software/flash/about/, may be used to view the files. Animations are best used as a supplement to written information. The kidneypatientguide (http://www.kidneypatientguide.org.uk/site/treatment.php) uses several animations to demonstrate concepts related to dialysis, transplants, and diet. The animation is designed for patients but can also be used with nursing students.

Instructional Games

Online **instructional games** can add a competitive contest aspect to learning. The purpose for use of games is to provide motivation to students to learn the needed information. Learners must be clear about the purpose when using games. They should also be sure that they have the technology hardware and software necessary to play the game. Games that are successful must meet instructional requirements and be enjoyable for players.

Many different types of games and software are used to create them. Hot Potatoes™ software provides a variety of game formats; it is free for educators and available for a fee for noneducators. Some examples of games include those that select letters to identify words or phrases, similar to a popular television show, crossword puzzles, and fill-in-the-blank (Half-Baked Software Inc., 2008a). Quandary allows faculty to create action mazes, which are interactive online case studies (Half-Baked Software Inc., 2008b). StudyMate Author® allows faculty to create games such as crossword puzzles, fill-in-the-blank, and pick-a-letter that can be uploaded into LMSs (Respondus®, 2007).

Games are also available on the Web. The online game, Outbreak at Water's Edge: A Public Health Discovery Game at http://www.mclph.umn.edu/watersedge/ uses a Java applet, a program written in Java programming language, to play a game to discover the source of contamination making residents in the local community sick. The game is available in both English and Spanish. The Nobelprize.org Web site (http://nobelprize.org/educational_games/medicine/) offers fun interactive games on topics difficult for learners to understand, such as blood typing, malaria, and the immune system.

Computerized Quizzes and Surveys

Computers allow for many testing functions. Quizzes and surveys provide a means for assessing learning; therefore, termed **learning assessment**. LMSs and numerous companies include tools to create quizzes and anonymous surveys. Quizzes can be generated using the forms function of word processing software or more sophisticated proprietary software. Quizzes found on the Web are often self-tests associated with tutorials. Self-tests are categorized as *formative* tests because they provide information about ongoing learning. Quizzes associated with course grades are *summative* tests because they sum up learning. Summative tests are given in a secure testing environment.

Quiz Software.   Quiz software is specially designed database software with a variety of uses. It allows faculty to create online quizzes either administered on the Web or integrated for use as a testing function within an LMS. Quiz software can also be useful in creating paper tests. Sophisticated testing software allows for the feedback for right and wrong answers, the ability to categorize questions, test item analysis, and student performance. Quiz software may allow the teacher to create a test bank of questions for reuse in various classes. Most test scoring software is capable of providing a file for the instruction that can be imported into a spreadsheet or database as a part of an electronic grading book.

Question Writer from http://www.questionwriter.com/free-quiz-software.html is a free (for noncommercial use) program that allows the creation of multiple choice quizzes that can be posted to the Internet. Users are able to print out a results report and to view question feedback for correct/incorrect responses.

Surveys.   Surveys provide a way to aggregate information anonymously from learners. They are often used in LMSs for learning assessment, such as "the muddiest point" technique and course evaluations. The "muddiest point" assessment is one where the student describes a topic that is least clearly understood. Surveys are a tool that provides evaluation information. Several survey services are available on the Web. For example, SurveyMonkey at http://www.surveymonkey.com/ provides free and for-purchase survey tools.

SCORM Tools.   **Sharable content object reference model (SCORM®)** refers to a learning module that can be imported into any SCORM-compliant LMS; think of it as one design fits all (Advanced Distributed Learning, 2007). Typically the SCORM module is designed to include a self-test associated with one or more learning tools such as flash cards, games, and tutorials. The learner has an opportunity to interact with the learning tools and then take the associated self-test. The self-test resides within the SCORM module, as

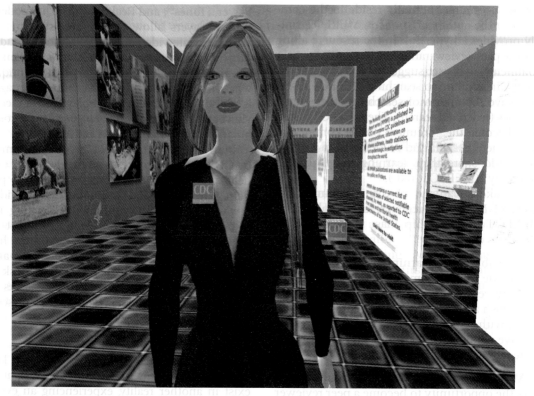

Figure 23-5 • CDC in second life.

endoscope simulation use: "You need to realize that looking to the right translates into steering to the left. Don't be surprised if it takes a while to get the hang of "driving" [the endoscope] – or that the OR is a high-stress place to learn this skill."

Students can use VR to enhance learning using online sites such as Croquet™ or Second Life. Both Croquet and Second Life are online 3D VR environments. Croquet (http://www .opencroquet.org) is open source software. Second Life participants must first register on the site (http://www.secondlife.com/) to obtain a login id and password, and then download Second Life software. Participants interact using avatars. An **avatar** is a fictionalized computer representation of self. Avatars can be custom designed with different looks. Because avatars can fly, they can "teleport" to different locations.

The CDC has a presence on Second Life at http://slurl.com/secondlife/Juwangsan/216.253/ 205.835. Figure 23-5 shows Hygeia Philo, the CDC's lead avatar in the virtual CDC site. The CDC avatar's name is based on the Greek meaning – "lover of health." Hygeia Philo serves as the lead spokesperson and health educator for the CDC virtual world.

HealthInfo Island at http://infoisland.org/ health_info/ is a virtual library complete with access to Medline Plus and nursing instructional videos. Some disease symptoms, such as hallucinations associated with schizophrenia, are difficult to imagine. Virtual Hallucinations at http:// www.ucdmc.ucdavis.edu/ais/ virtualhallucinations/ is an educational Second Life environment that allows users to experience hallucinations.

There are strengths and limitations for using virtual worlds as a part of instruction.

Because avatars fictionalize representations of the users, any user disabilities are invisible. Everyone can walk and fly. The sites provide many opportunities for experimentation and research (Skiba, 2007). A potential limitation is that virtual world learning has technical requirements and computer skills that all learners may not have. Navigating in a virtual world is a learned skill; fortunately tutorials and videos are available for use. Learners should have specific learning goals prior to engaging with the learning content. Learners must also be very self-directed; otherwise they could become lost in VR and end up very frustrated.

VR may soon become a standard alternative for learning in higher education. The Kentucky Community and College System is blazing trails in the use of **simulation-based learning (SBL)** (News Blaze, 2008). The global Interactive Digital Center (IDC) Consortium began showcasing SBL technology for use in higher education and workforce development. SBL used interactive realistic visualizations. The learner can view or "enter" the visualization, for example, the cardiovascular system. According to the IDC Consortium, SBL interactions engage the learner and result in "40% greater retention of the subject content with the learner" (Eon Reality, 2008).

A number of resources are available on the use of VR. Ambient Intelligence.org at http://www.ambientintelligence.org/ provides a good starting point. The site links to other Web sites, journal articles, and books about the use of VR in healthcare. Although the use of VR in healthcare and nursing education is still in its infancy, we can anticipate that it will become commonplace in the future.

PATIENT SIMULATORS

Patient simulators allow the learner to practice a patient encounter by providing care to a computerized mannequin. This problem-based learning approach provides opportunities for the learner to develop higher-order thinking skills. The primary objective for use of patient simulators is to allow the learner to be an actual participant in a patient care situation that would be either too difficult, dangerous, or time consuming to provide in a real clinical setting (Childs & Sepples, 2006). Patient simulators, such as Human Patient Simulator™ made by Medical Education Technologies, Inc. and SimMan® made by Laerdal, are used in many nursing programs.

Bearnson and Wiker (2005) reported the use of patient simulators with nursing students using three different postoperative pain scenarios in three simulated patients. One patient was a healthy adult, and the other two patients had significant comorbidities, such as obesity, coronary artery disease, and hypertension. The students were expected to assess and provide postoperative care based on the different patient responses. As a result of the learning simulation experience, students reported increased knowledge about side effects of medications and different patient responses. They also reported that their self-confidence in medication administration skills had improved.

Research reports on the use of patient simulators indicate that students consistently value the learning experiences. There are, however, downfalls to the use of more complex simulators. Purchase costs, mannequin, hardware, software, and training costs can be prohibitive. Moreover, time is an issue; time is required for faculty training and learning content development (Nehring & Lashley, 2004).

Activating Learning Using Clicker Technology

Clicker technology refers to the personal response systems used in the traditional classroom to provide assessment-centered instruction. Clickers look similar to remote control devices used to control television sets and other media devices (see Figure 23-6). Clickers are useful in both small and large classrooms. The two basic requirements for clicker technology are that faculty must have response software loaded on the computer used in the classroom and the students must each have a clicker (Educause, 2005; Skiba, 2006). Examples of companies that produce clicker software and hardware are iRespond™ (http://www.irespond.com) and Senteo™ (http://www2.smarttech.com).

Box 23-1 • Advantages and Disadvantages of Distance Learning

Advantages of Distance Learning

1. Depending on the structure, students can participate in their schedule.
2. Students without easy access to a college can participate.
3. Some agencies have found that offering distance learning as a perk increases retention.
4. Classes in a limited specialty can be offered because of an expanded audience.
5. Access to class is available 24 hours a day, 7 days a week.
6. Learners must think before they express their ideas, thus they cannot speak impulsively. Organizing one's ideas increases learning.
7. All learners must participate.

Disadvantages of Distance Learning

1. Additional resources are needed to assist instructors and students.
2. Lack of face-to-face contact.
3. May not be suitable to all contents.
4. The technology may contribute to frustration.

Box 23-2 • Successful Online Learners

Successful Online Learners

LEARNING TECHNOLOGY AND ENVIRONMENT. THE LEARNER:

- Must be very committed and focused on learning. Work and home obligations can be very distracting and can interrupt the learning environment.
- Must give online learning a priority in daily activities.
- Must have access to a working computer with antivirus and antispam protection, an Internet connection, required e-Learning software, and a printer. The computer becomes an essential tool for online learning. A computer is as important to an online learner as a motorized vehicle is to a nurse commuting to work in a healthcare agency. To maintain a functioning computer, the learner should:
  - Restrict the use of the personal computer from any other user who may inadvertently download a virus or corrupt the operating system.
- Have a "backup strategy" in case of computer problems. For example, using the college, community library, college, or hospital computer laboratory, or renting a laptop.

LEARNER QUALITIES. THE LEARNER SHOULD:

- Be self-motivated and exercise self-discipline; own responsibility for learning.
- Be able to communicate effectively in writing.
- Be open-minded about sharing experiences and willing to learn from others.
- Be willing to ask for help.
- Be respectful of others in the learning environment.
- Participate in the virtual classroom 4–7 days/week.
- Be willing to apply learning to everyday life.
- Have the ability to commit the required number of hours/week for completing assignments and class participation.

---

access course content anywhere in the world from a computer with an Internet access. Online learning accommodates shift work, family obligations, and military duty deployment. Before signing up for a course that uses e-Learning, students should make sure that they have the qualities leading to success (see Box 23-2).

Students can access the learning resources when they are best able to learn. Online learning allows learners to participate in learning experiences that otherwise are not available outside of real life. It also permits the learners to set their own pace. Another advantage is that, unlike a traditional lecture, learners never have to miss a class; the learning content and class discussion are online. ADA-compliant courses make learning accessible to students who are physically unable to attend class. Courses can be designed to accommodate vision- and hearing-impaired students.

Online learning also has disadvantages. Learners need the required software and hardware. They also need to have a backup plan in case of a computer problem. They need to have sufficient technology skills to allow them to access online courses and to troubleshoot technology glitches. Online learning is a disadvantage to the learner who is not motivated to learn and who does not exercise self-discipline.

Distance Learning and Hybrid Courses

Distance learning is a phenomenon that has been with us since Roman times whenever and wherever a reliable postal service was available. In the United States, correspondence courses have been available since the 18th century. Although correspondence courses are used in many parts of the world, online courses continue to grow in popularity. Face-to-face courses that have a virtual presence in LMSs are known as **hybrid courses**.

Distance learning means education in which the learners and students are in different locations. Distance education formats differ in the time frames that they use; some are asynchronous, and others synchronous (see Table 23-1). In the asynchronous format, learners use the learning resources at a time and place that is convenient for them. The asynchronous format is the most common use of LMSs. In synchronous learning, class is held at set times and all participants are "present," either online or in the classroom. Web conferencing and webinars, often used to provide an educational session, are examples of synchronous learning.

There are many uses for distance learning in healthcare. One of the most widespread uses is for CE. This type of learning is available in different formats; some CE modules are free, and others are available for a small fee. The American Nursing Association provides a comprehensive listing of online CE learning resources at http://nursingworld.org/ce/cehome.cfm. Some of the CE resources are free for members. Most nursing journals that have an online presence provide access to journal articles and an associated quiz for CE credit. Staff educators may find that many of these offerings could be made a part of a staff education program for career ladder programs or other necessary learning.

Full degree programs are also offered online. Accreditation of distance learning is offered by the major college-accrediting bodies just as if the programs were all in a regular classroom. Several certificate programs are also offered online. The various programs vary in their requirements for a presence on campus during the program; some require none, others may require a weekend presence during each course, or a given on-campus presence sometime during the program.

Future Trends

Ward once said, "If you can imagine it, you can achieve it; if you can dream it, you can become it" (ThinkExist.com Quotations, 2006). In

TABLE 23-1 • Time Criteria Continuum in Distance Learning

Functions	Synchronous	Asynchronous
Meeting times	Set meeting times	No set meeting times
Assignments (includes quizzes and tests)	Set due dates	Students complete assignments when they have time; there is no due date beyond that of the end of the course
Time period of course	Starts and ends on a given date	Starts and ends at convenience of students (most have a given time length from beginning to end of the course)
Type of learning	Instructor-led/class discussions	Independent, only feedback is on assignments

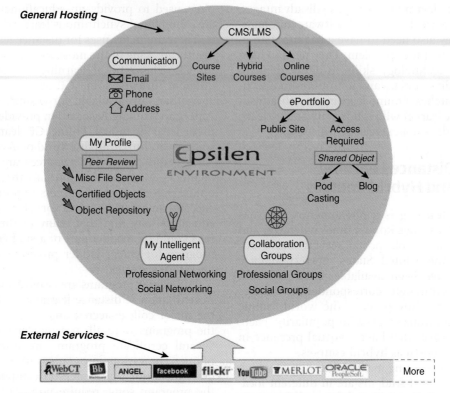

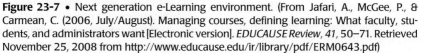

Figure 23-7 • Next generation e-Learning environment. (From Jafari, A., McGee, P., & Carmean, C. (2006, July/August). Managing courses, defining learning: What faculty, students, and administrators want [Electronic version]. *EDUCAUSE Review, 41*, 50–71. Retrieved November 25, 2008 from http://www.educause.edu/ir/library/pdf/ERM0643.pdf)

1993, futurist Marc Smith described cyberspace and virtual communities (Smith, 1993). In 1996, Chris Dede portrayed the social aspect of e-Learning based on Smith's work: "Social network capital (an instant Web of contacts with useful skills), knowledge capital (a personal, distributed "brain trust" with just-in-time answers to immediate questions), and communion (psychological/spiritual support from people who share common joys and trials) are three types of "collective goods" that bind together virtual communities enabled by computer-mediated communication" (Dede, 1996). The imaginations of Smith and Dede helped to set the stage for the Web 2.0 e-Learning environment.

Technological advances will continue to impact e-Learning and the design of the learning environment. Futurists are now depicting the future of learning/course management systems for "next generation" learners (Jafari, McGee, & Carmean, 2006, July/August). Some predictions are:

▼ The free Web 2.0 tools will continue to direct future trends in e-Learning. LMSs will integrate with other systems.
▼ The learning environment will have educational equivalents of free Web 2.0 tools such as Facebook, wikis, RSS feeds, blogs, and more.[1]
▼ Educational Web 2.0 tools will allow learners to collaborate with others across the world, not simply within a given course.
▼ The design of instruction and technology used to deliver the instruction will center on the learner's needs (see Figure 23-7).

[1] Web 2.0 social networking tools are described in Chapter 6.

▼ LMSs will take on some of the smart features of Amazon.com.

▼ LMSs will "remember" the students' profile, what they like, and how they learn.

▼ LMSs will incorporate decision support tools to "remember" where a student was when he or she last exited the course and make recommendations for pertinent learning resources.

The New Media Consortium and EDUCAUSE Learning Initiative qualitative research study described six technologies likely to impact teaching and learning. The technologies were 1) shared grassroots (taken by anyone) videos; 2) collaboration Webs where users can share documents, data, work with others using free applications on the Web; 3) mobile broadband using handheld computers; 4) data mashups with Web sites that include combinations of different Web resources such as photos, videos, and blogs; 5) collective intelligence using tools like wikis, community tagging, and data mashups; and 6) social operating and networking systems (The New Media Consortium & EDUCAUSE Learning Initiative, 2008). Technological advances and free Web-enabled creative resources are empowering the learners to custom design their personal learning environment.

Summary

In the Information Age it is imperative that higher education prepare learners to be active, independent learners and problem solvers. e-Learning, when used appropriately, facilitates this process and provides a venue for lifelong learning. e-Learning can be classified by the learning method or the technology. There are numerous learning methods including drill and practice, tutorials, simulations, gaming, and testing. Effective learning methods, whether used online or face-to-face, must provide interactivity and prompt feedback to learners. The technology includes multimedia, VR, patient simulators, and clicker technology; each meets different needs.

Using e-Learning successfully depends on how it is integrated into the total learning program. The level of interactivity also needs to be considered and matched with program goals. Like all teaching methods, e-Learning has advantages and disadvantages. Advantages include interactivity and the flexibility of the medium. Disadvantages can include lack of familiarity with the technology, technology glitches, lack of access, and cost.

With the advent of the Internet, distance learning has become a much more popular method for educational offerings. Programs offered via distance learning vary from correspondence courses and magazine articles to full degree programs. Distance learning requires the development of skills that are not always needed in traditional education including the ability to discipline oneself to set aside time for the program and the ability to communicate effectively in writing.

APPLICATIONS AND COMPETENCIES

1. Discuss uses for multimedia and VR in nursing education.
2. Differentiate between the characteristics of the learning methods, drill and practice, tutorial, and game, providing an example that is related to nursing for each one.
3. Identify and analyze an online nursing simulation.
4. Compare the different modes of computerized testing and give examples for appropriate use.
5. Search for an online learning resource of value to nursing and then add it to MERLOT collection.
6. Discuss the current status of distance education for nursing. Make a list of essential competencies and qualities for successful learners and then compare your list with those listed in this chapter.
7. Evaluate one of your learning experiences using the seven principles for good practice in undergraduate education. If you are a graduate student, discuss if and how the principles apply to graduate education.
8. One of your functions in a 100-bed hospital is to provide staff education. You wish to integrate e-Learning into your organization. Write a proposal that:
   a. Interprets the various choices for e-Learning.

b. Discusses the advantages and disadvantages of each.

c. Provides reasons for using two of these methods.

REFERENCES

Advanced Distributed Learning. (2007). *SCORM® 2004*, 3rd ed. Retrieved November 25, 2008, from http://www .adlnet.gov/scorm/index.aspx

Bearnson, C. S., & Wiker, K. M. (2005). Human patient simulators: A new face in baccalaureate nursing education at Brigham Young University. *Journal of Nursing Education, 44*(9), 421–425.

Bloom, B. S. (1956). *Taxonomy of educational objectives, handbook 1: Cognitive domain.* New York: Addison Wesley Publishing Company.

Bluetooth Laser Keyboard. (2008). Retrieved November 25, 2008, from http://www.thinkgeek.com/computing/ input/8193/

Chickering, A. W., & Ehrmann, S. C. (1996). *Implementing the seven principles: Technology as lever.* Retrieved November 25, 2008, from http://www.tltgroup.org/ programs/seven.html

Childs, J. C., & Sepples, S. (2006). Clinical teaching by simulation: Lessons learned from a complex patient care scenario. *Nursing Education Perspectives, 27*(3), 154–158.

Clark, R. C., & Mayer, R. E. (2003). *e-Learning and the Science of Instruction.* Hoboken, NJ: John Wiley & Sons.

Dede, C. (1996). The evolution of distance education: Emerging technologies and distributed learning. *American Journal of Distance Education, 10*(2), 4–36.

Educause. (2005). *7 things you should know about clickers.* Retrieved November 25, 2008, from http://www .educause.edu/ir/library/pdf/ELI7002.pdf

Eon Reality. (2008). *i3D symposium.* Retrieved January 30, 2008, from http://www.eonreality.com/i3DSymposium/ SiMT/FlorenceSC/

Greenberg, L. (2002, December 9). *LMS and LCMS: What's the difference?* Retrieved November 25, 2007, from http://www.steptwo.com.au/columntwo/lms- and-lcms-whats-the-difference/

Half-Baked Software Inc. (2008a). *Hot Potatoes™.* Retrieved November 25, 2008, from http://hotpot.uvic.ca/

Half-Baked Software Inc. (2008b). *Quandary.* Retrieved November 25, 2008, from http://www.halfbakedsoftware .com/quandary.php/

Jafari, A., McGee, P., & Carmean, C. (2006, July/August). Managing courses, defining learning: What faculty, students, and administrators want [Electronic version]. *EDUCAUSE Review, 41*, 50–71. Retrieved November 25, 2008 from http://www.educause.edu/ir/library/ pdf/ERM0643.pdf

Lord, T., & Baviskar, S. (2007). Moving students from information recitation to information understanding: Exploiting Bloom's taxonomy in creating science questions. *Journal of College Science Teaching, 36*(5), 40–44.

Medical Education Institute. (2006). Kidney school™: Unique CKD education tool [Electronic version]. *In Control, 3,* 4. Retrieved November 25, 2008 from http://www.lifeoptions.org/catalog/pdfs/news/icv3n2.pdf

MERLOT. (n.d.). *About us.* Retrieved November 25, 2008, from http://taste.merlot.org/

NCSBN. (n.d.). *Computerized adaptive testing (CAT) overview.* Retrieved November 25, 2007, from https://www.ncsbn .org/CAT_Overview.pdf

Nehring, W. M., & Lashley, F. R. (2004). Current use and opinions regarding human patient simulators in nursing education: An international survey. *Nursing Education Perspectives, 25*(5), 244–248.

News Blaze. (2008). *EON Reality and Kentucky Community and Technical College System create first statewide simulation-based learning collaboration.* Retrieved November 25, 2008, from http://newsblaze.com/story/ 2008010909561100001.mwir/newsblaze/EDUCATIO/ Education.html

Nyswaner, A. (2007). "Driver's ed" for the OR nurse. *RN, 70*(3), 45–48.

Pastore, R. S. (2003). *Principles of teaching.* Retrieved November 25, 2008, from http://teacherworld.com/ potdale.html

Respondus®. (2007). *Studymate Author 2.0.* Retrieved November 25, 2008, from http://www.respondus.com/ products/studymate.shtml

Schatell, D., Klicko, K., & Becker, B. N. (2006). In-center hemodialysis patients' use of the internet in the United States: A national survey. *American Journal of Kidney Diseases, 48*(2), 285–291.

Shegog, R., Bartholomew, L. K., Parcel, G. S., Sockrider, M. M., Masse, L., & Abramson, S. L. (2001). Impact of a computer-assisted education program on factors related to asthma self-management behavior. *Journal of the American Medical Informatics Association, 8*(1), 49–61.

Skiba, D. J. (2006). Emerging technologies center. Got large lecture hall classes? Use clickers. *Nursing Education Perspectives, 27*(5), 278–280.

Skiba, D. J. (2007). Nursing education 2.0: Second life. *Nursing Education Perspectives, 28*(3), 156–157.

Smith, M. (1993). *Voices from the WELL: The logic of the virtual commons.* Los Angeles: University of California.

Thalheimer, W. (2006, May 1). *People remember 10%, 20%. Oh really?* Retrieved November 25, from http://www .willatworklearning.com/2006/05/people_remember.html

The New Media Consortium & Educause Learning Initiative. (2008). *The horizon report: 2008 edition.* Retrieved November 25, 2008, from http://www.nmc.org/ publications/2008-horizon-report

Thede, L. (1995). *Comparison of a constructivist and objectivist framework for designing computer-aided instruction.* Unpublished manuscript, Ann Arbor, MI.

ThinkExist.com Quotations. (2006). *William Authur Ward quotes.* Retrieved November 25, 2008, from http://thinkexist.com/quotes/william_arthur_ward/

United States Access Board. (n.d.). *E-Learning: Conforming to section 508.* Retrieved November 25, 2008, from http://www.access-board.gov/sec508/e-learning.htm

Administration Tools for Efficiency

Learning Objectives
After studying this chapter you will be able to:

1. *Identify the tools necessary to manage business processes in nursing services.*

2. *Demonstrate basic competencies in spreadsheets and flowcharting in nursing administration.*

3. *Discuss data management to improve outcomes using quality improvement, benchmarking, and patient care.*

4. *Explore the use of specialized applications in nursing administration, including scheduling systems and patient classification systems.*

Key Terms

Benchmarking

Business Intelligence

Clinical Information Systems

Consumer Assessment of Health Providers and Systems

Core Measures

Dashboards

Employee Scheduling Systems

Financial Management

Flowcharting

Forecasting

Gantt Chart

Human Resource Management Systems

National Database of Nursing Quality Indicators®

Patient Classification Systems

Patient Throughput

Process Improvement

Quality Improvement

There is little doubt that nurse administrators and managers must have competency in a wide range of technology skills to be effective in their roles. According to the American Organization of Nurse Executives (AONE, 2005), one of the five leadership domains is **business skills**, which includes information management and technology. The use of email, word processing, spreadsheets, and the Internet are basic skills. Beyond these, nurse administrators use management information systems for the purposes of **financial management, process improvement, human resource management, quality improvement, benchmarking,** and **business intelligence.** Because of the nurse administrator's unique role as leader of nursing services, knowledge of **clinical information systems** is important as well. Box 24-1 specifies the competencies needed by nurse managers and nurse executives (AONE).

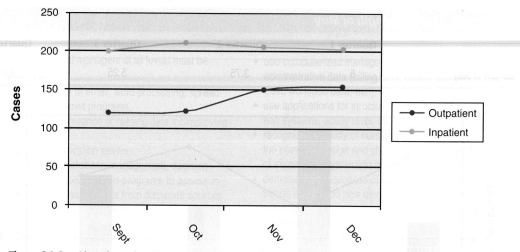

Figure 24-2 • Line chart showing number of surgical cases in four months. (Reprinted with permission from Microsoft Corporation.)

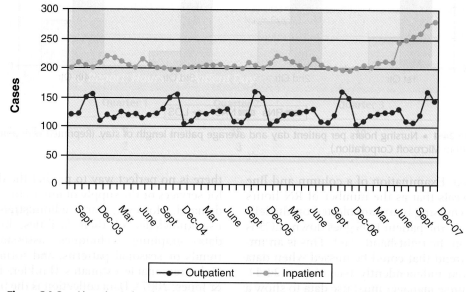

Figure 24-3 • Line chart showing number of surgical cases in five years. (Reprinted with permission from Microsoft Corporation.)

When viewed within the five-year period, the administrator can clearly see a seasonal pattern: outpatient surgeries increase during the months of November and December and return to a level of approximately 120 per month during the rest of the year (Figure 24-3). However, inpatient surgeries begin to increase around July 2007. The administrator knows that a new orthopedic surgeon and a new urologist were recruited to the hospital during that time, which accounts for the increase in inpatient surgeries. This increase can be expected to persist in future years.

PROCESS IMPROVEMENT

Process improvement is the application of actions taken to identify, analyze, and improve existing processes within an organization to meet requirements for quality, customer satisfaction, and financial goals. Administrators can use a particular strategy such as total quality management, six sigma, or a general process improvement framework called plan-do-check-act (PDCA) (Yoder-Wise, 2006). Whatever the strategy used for improvement, an organized approach is necessary to understand the current state of the process and plan for changes to improve outcomes. Process improvement should be an analytical process where tools such as flowcharts, cause-and-effect charts, and other control methods are used to make changes to targeted processes.

Analysis of Processes with Flowcharting

Flowcharting software applications can be useful because nurse administrators can map processes in nursing services. There are many instances in healthcare where care processes need to be examined to make them more efficient or to reduce unwanted variation in care. For example, the movement of patients from the emergency department into a hospital inpatient room for admission is a complicated process. Delays in starting care are unnecessary and costly; analysis through flowcharting may reveal opportunities for improvement in the admission process. In Figure 24-4, unnecessary delays can be avoided if the path from

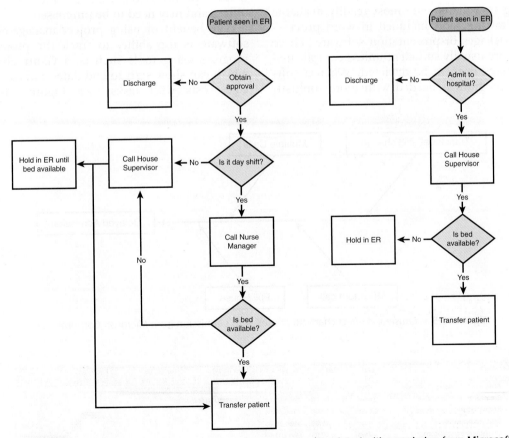

Figure 24-4 • Flowchart of admission from emergency room. (Reprinted with permission from Microsoft Corporation.)

decision to admit and the transfer of the patient is a straight line. When multiple decisions need to be made or multiple people are involved, the process becomes more complicated, and delays occur. The use of flowcharting is a powerful way to identify steps in a process that can be reorganized for better flow.

A **cause-and-effect chart** is another useful diagram for nurse administrators to make so that relationships among complex processes are examined. The cause-and-effect chart places the effect at one end of the chart with the many suspected causes branching out from it. The resulting chart resembles a fishbone, thus it is commonly referred to as a fishbone chart. Figure 24-5 depicts a simple cause-and-effect chart; more complex charts show multiple related causes under each branch.

There are many software options for developing flowcharts. The most readily available are drawing tools included in word processing packages or presentation software. These tools are usually sufficient unless complicated processes need to be depicted. When a software program is needed with more sophisticated flowcharting abilities, the nurse administrator should analyze the products on cost and capabilities. The Microsoft® product is called Visio®, and other similar products are WizFlow (from Pacestar software©), SmartDraw®, EDrawSoft©, and ConceptDraw (from Computer Systems Odessa Corp©), to name a few. Most of the products are $50 to $200 for a single-user license.

Project Management

Nurse administrators often oversee planning and implementation of complex projects with numerous stakeholders, resources, and financial implications. In many cases, the use of project management software can provide needed organization to keep projects on time and in budget. This type of software is not one that is typically used in nursing administration offices and may need to be purchased.

The benefit of using project management software is the ability to track the project's progress using tools such as a **Gantt chart**, which can show start to end dates and associated costs with tasks (see Figure 24-6).

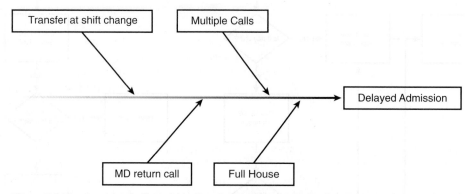

Figure 24-5 • Cause-and-effect chart. (Reprinted with permission from Microsoft Corporation.)

Task Name	Duration	Start	Finish
Analysis of ER admission process	8 days	Wed 1/23/08	Fri 2/1/08
Setup ER process committee	2 days	Mon 1/21/08	Tue 1/22/08
Review results of first analysis	2 days	Mon 2/4/08	Tue 2/5/08
Draft recommendations	1 day	Wed 2/6/08	Wed 2/6/08
Circulate recommendations	3 days	Thu 2/7/08	Mon 2/11/08

Figure 24-6 • Gantt chart. (Reprinted with permission from Microsoft Corporation.)

Milestones can be marked on the chart so that important parts of a task are highlighted. Links can be made between tasks to depict when tasks need to be completed before others start. Linking tasks is a good practice to use because when a date changes in one task, all other dates are updated to linked tasks. Some project management software can be set to send email reminders to individuals responsible for milestones or tasks within the project. This automation frees the administrator to focus on the big picture and leaves the details to the software.

Reports of tasks and costs can be generated. These reports provide a snapshot of the progress, resources, and finances for the project. Depending on the level of integration, these reports can be exported to a spreadsheet application for sharing with others in the organization.

There are many vendors who make project management software for personal computers including Microsoft Project®, Standard Register that produces SmartWorks®, Inuit® that produces QuickBase®, and Experience In Software, Inc. that develops Project Kickstart™. Other options include purchasing a Web-based service if the nurse administrator needs to collaborate with others in a multi-hospital network. Several factors should be considered when making a decision about purchasing project management software. The first is the degree of integration with other administrative tools such as spreadsheets, email, and calendars. The second is the number of users who would access the information contained in the project management software. The third is the security of Web-based systems compared with other deployment methods. Finally, cost of the software should be considered: single-user licenses are relatively inexpensive but do not encourage collaboration. If a nurse administrator needs collaboration and has a secure Web solution, the cost of a multi-user license may be well worth the investment.

HUMAN RESOURCE MANAGEMENT

Personnel management is one of the most important parts of the job of a nurse manager. Using a **human resources management system (HRMS)** is essential to planning and staffing nursing services appropriately. Nursing personnel, staffing, and employment data can be managed with HRMS, which generally includes four categories: personnel profiles including demographic data, daily work schedule and time-off requests, payroll data, and educational and skill qualifications as well as licensure information.

Not only can an HRMS serve as a scheduling system and repository of personnel data, but a productivity module can also be purchased, which can pull nursing data (hours of care-and-skill mix) together with patient data (patient days, average LOS, and patient acuity). This productivity information is critical for nurse managers and nurse administrators to track, trend, and analyze productivity for meaning within their organizations and benchmark against similar organizations across the United States. This is likely the most powerful information that is produced for managers and administrators in healthcare today.

Because regulators and accreditation agencies require information about employees such as competencies, certifications, and evaluations, HRMS may provide a solution to managing these data too. Many HRMSs will contain employee appraisals, orientation checklists, employee competency checklists, development plans, compensation adjustments based on achievement of personal, unit or organization goals, and possibly succession plans. The HRMS may also generate reports for the Joint Commission.

Nurse administrators who might be involved in the decision to purchase an HRMS should be certain to see demonstrations from vendors whose products are specialized to healthcare. Because the work of nursing services is so different from manufacturing or other service-related industries, it is important to have systems that meet many specifications. The human resource management system needs to meet the following minimal requirements: 1) handle scheduling for 24 hours per day, 7 days per week; 2) accommodate different scheduling rules for units across an entire organization or network; 3) allow for staff self-scheduling; 4) determine the right number and mix of nursing staff for patient needs; 5) provide analysis of nursing staff usage to manage productivity and support quality patient outcomes; 6) track time and attendance; 7) connect to the payroll system; 8) retain certification and licensure information; and 9) serve as repository for competency assessments and annual employee appraisals.

Using Data to Improve Outcomes

QUALITY IMPROVEMENT AND BENCHMARKING

Patient safety has risen on the national agenda owing to mortality statistics that have shown that between 44,000 and 98,000 deaths occur in U.S. hospitals each year as a result of errors in care (Institutes of Medicine [IOM], 2000). In a report to Congress, Michael Leavitt, Secretary of Health and Human Services, declared that Medicare would begin "pay[ing] in a way that expresses our commitment to supporting providers and practitioners for doing the right thing – improving quality and avoiding unnecessary costs, and promoting competition to improve quality and lower costs – rather than directing more resources to less effective care" (Centers for Medicare and Medicaid Services [CMS], 2006). This initiative has become known as pay for performance. Because hospitals want to do the right thing and to be paid for services rendered, the pay-for-performance initiative proposed by the CMS has begun to exert significant pressure on hospitals to examine how patient care can be improved so that the right care can be provided to every patient, every time.

In the past, nurses have been viewed as overhead to hospital organizations because revenue was generated by admissions to the hospital, not by the quality of patient care that was provided. This view is changing with pay-for-performance initiative. Nurses are in pivotal positions to improve quality, prevent errors, and improve patient satisfaction in hospitals. According to a recent research report on healthcare staffing shortages (PricewaterhouseCoopers, 2007), nurses will become the "rainmakers" for revenue generation when pay-for-performance initiative is implemented. For example, if nurses prevent nosocomial infections in postoperative patients, the hospital will receive full reimbursement allowed under CMS regulations for those patients. However, if a patient develops a nosocomial infection, the hospital's reimbursement is reduced for that patient. In order for excellence in patient care to be the norm for hospitals, nurse administrators must follow the progress of improvements in care and keep nursing staff informed about how their performance affects the hospital's reimbursement.

Not only do nurse administrators engage in quality improvement projects specific to their hospitals, but they also must provide leadership for the hospital's required participation in improvement initiatives mandated by the CMS. These mandated programs include **Core Measures** and **Consumer Assessment of Health Providers and Systems**, Hospital Survey (HCAHPS) (CMS, 2008). In addition, nurse administrators may choose to join the **National Database of Nursing Quality Indicators**® (NDNQI®). These quality improvement initiatives require the nurse administrator to designate staff and resources to the collection of data, aggregation of data for submission to databases, and response to reports.

Core Measures

In 1998, the Joint Commission in cooperation with the CMS and the Hospital Quality Alliance (HQA) established standardized core measurements required for all accredited healthcare organizations. A few standardized core measurements were required in the first year. In subsequent years, more core measures were added in areas including myocardial infarction, congestive heart failure, pneumonia, pregnancy, treatment of asthma in children, and surgical care improvement project. In

2008, the prevention and care venous thromboembolism and inpatient psychiatric care services were added (Joint Commission, 2007). Each of these core measures requires extensive data collection, aggregation, and reporting to stay in compliance. Once reported, the core measures are available for the public at http://www.hospitalcompare.hhs.gov.

Consumer Assessment of Health Providers and Systems: Hospital Survey

Beginning in 2007, the CMS in collaboration with the HQA required hospitals to survey patients and families to gather information about their experiences with healthcare (CMS, 2008). The tool, known as HCAHPS, was developed by the Agency for Healthcare Research and Quality (AHRQ) and is a standardized survey tool designed to be administered to a sample of discharged patients. Hospitals are required to submit data to the CMS Web site so that patients' experiences can be trended over time within one hospital and benchmarked to other hospitals. These data will be available to the public to provide accountability in healthcare at http://www.hospitalcompare.hhs.gov.

Hospitals may use a vendor to survey patients or elect to conduct surveys with its employees. Regardless of this choice, surveyors must use a standardized method of collecting data, use a core set of questions (hospitals can add other questions to customize the survey), and submit data within specified time frames so that comparisons can be made. Of the 18 core questions, 10 were first publicly reported in March 2008. These include six composite topics, one topic on cleanliness, one topic on quietness, and two overall ratings (CMS, 2008).

National Database of Nursing Quality Indicators®

The quality of nursing care has an influence on a hospital's performance in some of the areas of core measures and patients' experiences in healthcare as measured by HCAHPS. A more direct measurement of the quality of nursing care is possible when nurse administrators choose to participate in the NDNQI®. The American Nurses Association (ANA) in partnership with the University of Kansas, School of Nursing began development of its safety and quality initiative, which resulted in NDNQI®. After a development period of approximately four years, the NDNQI® began accepting data for comparison from hospitals in 1998. The service was free until 2001 when a fee was established for joining the database. In 2008, over 1,200 hospitals participated in the service (ANA, 2008).

The NDNQI® is a national database to which hospitals submit nursing-sensitive data about structure, process, and outcomes of nursing care. The NDNQI® aggregate the data quarterly and returns reports to participating hospitals. Nurse administrators and managers receive unit-level information that is compared across time periods and benchmarked to similar units from other hospitals. The NDNQI® data include nursing hours per patient day, staff mix, falls, nursing turnover, pressure ulcers, infections, restraint use, intravenous infiltration, and nosocomial infection, to name a few (ANA, 2008). More information can be found at http://www.nursingquality.org.

BUSINESS INTELLIGENCE

Nursing services collect thousands of data elements every day in the delivery of patient care and in management processes such as utilization review, case management, and infection control. More measurements are not needed. In fact, nurse administrators need to focus on a few measurements that are the key drivers of effective, quality care (Fitzpatrick, 2006). Decisions about quality measurements need to be aligned throughout the hospital organization so that they provide information about the outcomes of patient care, patient satisfaction, costs, and revenue. This alignment and linking of data to transform them into information for the purpose of decision making is called **business intelligence** (Elliot, 2004).

hospitals in the United States have clinical documentation systems (HIMSS Analytics, 2008). Nurse administrators, in hospitals both large and small, will be faced with the purchase of some type of module for the current information system, bar coding for medication administration, scheduling system, or any number of business applications. Although the nurse administrator may not have knowledge of technical aspects, the administrator must be the voice of nursing when purchases are considered. Products need to be selected that enhance the work of nursing, not impede it. The nurse administrator is in the best position to advocate for all of nursing services and place nurses on purchase committees to make product selections that streamline work processes and put information in the hands of nurses.

The AONE released the guiding principles for the role of the nurse administrator in the selection and implementation of information systems (AONE, 2006). This document clearly states that although nurse administrator may delegate operational aspects of the acquisition and implementation of an information system, the administrator retains accountability for the process. Some key points include: 1) describe the strategic nursing plan so that the chief information officer and members of the task force understand the information needs of nurses now and in the future; 2) know about the planned technology purchases that will occur during the information system acquisition, and consider the implications on nursing services; 3) develop an understanding of contracts and legal issues surrounding data ownership; 4) make site visits to hospitals where proposed information systems have been implemented and talk to the chief nurse executives at those facilities; 5) get a clear understanding of the responsibility for training (when, where, how long, who provides, and who pays); 6) develop metrics for implementation and monitor the implementation process using them; 7) include deans from schools of nursing, pharmacy, and others to lessen the impact on their programs; and 8) be prepared for system downtimes.

Summary

Nurse administrators, like all other healthcare professionals, use computer applications in their daily work to communicate by email, find resources on the Internet, and develop documents with word processors and spreadsheets. Use of these tools, in addition to applications that can assist in the analysis of processes and in the planning for change, is an essential competency for today's nurse administrator. Moreover, nurse administrators are routinely involved in monitoring data from quality improvement studies (core measures, HCAHPS, NDNQI®, and other measures) to implement change in nursing practice and patient care.

The nurse administrator's need for tools and information to support decisions on financial matters, to develop strategies for improvement in patient care, and to meet regulatory requirements has never been greater. Systems that support administrative work include human resource management systems, scheduling systems, patient management systems, and acuity systems. Information from these systems assists the nurse administrator to use nursing services wisely and assess the effectiveness of decisions over time.

The nurse administrator should always have a strong voice in the decision to purchase an information system, whether it is a management system or clinical system. This involvement begins well before an information system is selected and continues after implementation to evaluate the performance metrics, costs, and vendor responsibility. The nurse administrator must ensure that decisions regarding clinical information systems, expert systems to support clinical decision making, medical technology, databases, and data warehousing systems, which affect nursing services, remain within the authority of the nurse administrator because it is this role that retains responsibility and accountability for providing the resources to accomplish patient care in a safe, efficient manner.

APPLICATIONS AND COMPETENCIES

1. Copy the data from the table below into a spreadsheet. Develop a chart (custom type) with line column on two axes. Place the patient outcomes (falls and pressure ulcers) in the columns and the percentage of RNs in the line.

	Quarter 1	Quarter 2	Quarter 3	Quarter 4
Number of falls	5	8	9	4
Number of pressure ulcers	4	6	7	5
Percentage of registered nurses	0.80	0.75	0.76	0.81

2. Using drawing tools in a word processing software or presentation software, diagram the process for hiring an RN in your organization.
   a. Analyze the process.
      i. Are there ways that the hiring process can stagnate?
      ii. Are there steps that can be streamlined?
   b. Draw the ideal process.
   c. Consider ways to implement change in your organization.
3. Search the Internet and find five software vendors for project management.
   a. List the strengths and weaknesses of each.
   b. Download a trial version of at least two project management software packages.
   c. Develop a Gantt chart for a simple project in your organization to learn to use the software.
4. Go to http://www.hospitalcompare.hhs.gov and compare your hospital's outcome on core measures to three others in your area and two from different areas that have services similar to your own.
   a. Review the following outcomes:
      i. Surgical care improvement/surgical infection prevention
      ii. HCAHPS
      iii. Pneumonia

   b. Develop a plan for improvement in areas where the hospital is below the state and national average.
5. Investigate the use of dashboards in your organization. If dashboards are in use, clarify your understanding of the metrics included on dashboard. If dashboards are not currently used, develop necessary knowledge of dashboards.
   a. Read more about dashboards from publications in nursing and business.
   b. Look for vendors offering healthcare dashboard services on the Internet.
   c. Discuss options with the chief information officer.

REFERENCES

American Nurses Association. (2008). *NDNQI® history.* Retrieved February 1, 2008, from http://www.nursingworld.org/MainMenuCategories/ThePractice ofProfessionalNursing/PatientSafetyQuality/NDNQI/NDNQI_1.aspx

American Organization of Nurse Executives. (2005). AONE nurse executive competencies. *Nurse Leader, 3*(1), 15–22. Retrieved January 9, 2008, from http://www.aone.org/aone/pdf/February%20Nurse%20Leader—final%20draft—for%20web.pdf

American Organization of Nurse Executives. (2006). *Role of the nurse executive in the acquisition, implementation, and evaluation of information technology.* Retrieved, January 14, 2008, from http://www.aone.org/aone/resource/home.html

Association of Perioperative Registered Nurses. (2007). Hospitals adopting technology allowing bidding for open shifts. *AORN Management Connections, 3*(11), 1–3.

Centers for Medicare and Medicaid Services. (2006). *Report to Congress: Improving the medicare quality improvement organization program – Response to the Institute of Medicine study.* Retrieved, October 7, 2007, from http://www.cms.hhs.gov/QualityImprovementOrgs/downloads/QIO_Improvement_RTC_fnl.pdf

Centers for Medicare and Medicaid Services (CMS). (2008). *HCAHPS and IPPS payment provisions.* Retrieved February 1, 2008, from http://www.hcahpsonline.org/default.aspx#currentnews

Elliot, T. (2004). *Choosing a business intelligence standard.* Retrieved, January 21, 2008, from http://www.businessobjects.com/pdf/solutions/evaluate/evaluating_bi.pdf

Finkler, S., Kovner, C., & Jones, C. (2007). *Financial management for nurse managers and executives* (3rd ed.). St. Louis, MO: Saunders Elsevier.

Fitzpatrick, M. (2006). Using data to drive performance improvement in hospitals. *Health management technology, 27*(12), 10–16. Retrieved, January 10, 2008, from www.healthmgttech.com

HIMSS Analytics (2008). *Electronic medical record (EMR) adoption model.* Retrieved, January 28, 2008, from http://www.himssanalytics.org/

Institutes of Medicine. (2000). *To err is human: Building a safer health system*. Washington, DC: National Academy Press.

Joint Commission (2007). *Performance measurements initiatives*. Retrieved, June 18, 2007, from http://www.jointcommission.org/PerformanceMeasurement/PerformanceMeasurement/default.htm

Malik, S. (2005). *Enterprise dashboards, design and best practices for IT*. New York: John Wiley & Sons.

Mazzella-Ebstein, A. S. R. (2004). Web-based nurse executive dashboard. *Journal of Nursing Care Quality, 19*(4), 307–315. Retrieved January 9, 2008, from www.cinahl.com/cgi-bin/refsvc?jid=454&accno=2005028750http://search.ebscohost.com/login.aspx?direct=true&db=rzh&AN=2005028750&site=ehost-live

PricewaterhouseCoopers. (2007). *What works: Healing the healthcare staffing shortage*. Retrieved January 14, 2007, from http://www.pwc.com/extweb/pwcpublications.nsf/docid/674D1E79A678A0428525730D006B74A9

Thomas, R. (2006). Information-based transformation: The need for integrated, enterprisewide informatics. *Healthcare Financial Management, 60*(9), 140–142. Retrieved February 1, 2008, from http://search.ebscohost.com/login.aspx?direct=true&db=buh&AN=22510816&site=ehost-live

Yoder-Wise, P., & Kowalski, K. (2006). *Beyond leading and managing: Nursing administration for the future*. St. Louis, MO: Mosby.

Informatics and Research

Learning Objectives

After studying this chapter you will be able to:

1. *Demonstrate basic competencies in statistical analysis software.*

2. *Identify sources of data for research.*

3. *Discuss the use of data to conduct research in nursing service, education, and administration.*

4. *Synthesize research findings in healthcare informatics as evidence for decision making in nursing.*

Key Terms

Agency for Healthcare
Research and Quality
Argument
Business Intelligence
Centers for Medicare and
Medicaid Services
Codebook
Computerized Decision
Support Systems
DataFerrett
Descriptive Data Analysis
Electronic Medical Records
Evidence-Based Practice

Formula
Healthcare Analytics
Integrative Review
Meta-analysis
Microdata
National Institute of
Nursing Research
Output
Personal Digital
Assistants
Research Utilization
Statistical Analysis

I n this data-rich healthcare environment, the need to turn data into useable information is imperative. There is a movement to develop **business intelligence** (also known as **healthcare analytics**), which can integrate financial data, patient data, and quality data to produce predictive analytics for decision makers in healthcare (Fitzpatrick, 2006). Nurse informatics specialists need to understand this next wave of innovation. Moreover, nurses in all roles need skills and tools to summarize sets of numbers into understandable pieces of information and to interpret the meaning of evidence produced through research. The purpose of this chapter is to develop basic competencies in data analysis and research to form a foundation for decision making in nursing and healthcare.

The History of Data Analysis and Research in Medicine and Nursing

The use of data analysis and research in medicine has an interesting history, which began in France and England (Chen, 2003). One of the first instances wherein statistical procedures were used to influence medical decision making was in the early 19th century to demonstrate the harm of performing bloodletting to treat infection. Physicians debated the appropriateness of using mathematics to understand the individual responses of humans to treatments. They argued that medicine was an art that could not be subjected to methods used in science such as astronomy. Even in 1870 when Joseph Lister published his findings on the effect of antiseptic methods in surgery on mortality rate of patients, physicians rejected the use of statistical methods in medicine. As a professor at the University College in London, Dr. Karl Pearson developed the first inferential statistical methods in the 1880s. The first statistics department was established as the Lister Institute for Preventive Medicine at the turn of the century where Major Greenwood furthered the work of Lister and Pearson (Chen, 2003).

Unfortunately the use of statistical analysis in medicine was not accepted until the 1920s, nearly 100 years after the first use of statistics in medicine (Chen, 2003). By that time, others joined Pearson and Greenwood in their call for the use as a useful tool that should be taught to premedical students. Later in the 1940s, the first clinical trial was conducted by the British Medical Research Council to test the effectiveness of streptomycin compared with the usual treatment of bed rest for tuberculosis. Patients' clinical condition and radiological findings improved when treated with an antibiotic. Following this study, the acceptance of statistics in medicine was secured (Chen, 2003).

The use of statistics and research in nursing has a similar history. The pioneer of statistical thinking was Florence Nightingale, whose work in the 1850–1860s showed that clean condition in field hospitals in the Crimean War reduced the mortality rate for soldiers (Brown, 1993). Despite Miss Nightingale's groundbreaking work, the use of statistical analysis and research did not develop until the 1920s when case studies were used to describe the effectiveness of nursing interventions (Gortner, 2000). Afterward, between 1930 and 1960, nursing research in the United States was generally concentrated on nurses, nursing education, and the practice of professional nursing. In 1952, *Nursing Research* was first published; however, the emergences of nursing as a clinical science did not develop until nearly a quarter century later. **The National Institute of Nursing Research**, which provided federal funding to nursing studies aimed at prevention of illness, promotion of healthy lifestyles, and support of quality of life, was established in the mid-1980s (Gortner, 2000). Since that time, nurse scientists have been providing research evidence to change traditional ways of caring for patients. This emphasis on **evidence-based practice** is an important step in the development of nursing science and the improvement in patient care.

Use of Technology

Today, **statistical analysis** and research in nursing are increasing in complexity in large part as a result of the availability of personal computers and statistical analysis programs. Nurse researchers can collect data, manage them in databases, and analyze them with specialized programs. With attention to the principles of data analysis, other nurses (e.g., nurse informatics specialists, managers, educators, clinical nurses, and advanced practice nurses) can benefit from the use of statistical analysis to improve decision making and outcomes.

Personal computers are capable of performing any complex statistical analyses. Commercial statistical analysis programs can be purchased, spreadsheet programs can be used, or free programs can be downloaded from the Internet. Most commercial programs are comparable. Cost and user preference are likely to be the deciding factors. The most popular commercial programs are Statistical Package for Social

Sciences (SPSS® provided by SPSS Inc.), Statistical Analysis Software (SAS® provided by SAS Institute Inc.), and Minitab® Statistical Software (provided by Minitab Inc.). Microsoft Excel® (included with Microsoft Office) and Quattro Pro® (included in Corel® WordPerfect® Office product) are useful because many nurses have this software readily available. Free statistical analysis programs are available on the Internet. A comparison of analysis capabilities of free programs is available at http://freestatistics .altervista.org/en/comp.php. Most of these programs are not as user friendly as commercial software because they do not have a graphical user interface. Instead, they require the use of command lines to input data and run analyses. BrightStat© overcomes this problems, does not require the download of a program because it is an Internet-based program, and provides commonly used statistical procedures.

Statistics Basics

Because data is readily available in healthcare settings today, nurses have an obligation to use it responsibly. Data must be collected, aggregated, analyzed, and interpreted correctly. Nurses who wish to analyze data should refresh their knowledge of statistics either through an academic course or by using reliable sources such as printed textbooks or online textbooks. Several online sources (listed below) are excellent sources of information about the basics of statistics and correct application of statistical procedures to data. Readers are encouraged to review one of the following online sources to understand statistical concepts before undertaking an analysis.

▼ Statsoft at http://www.statsoft.com/ textbook/stathome.html?esc.html&1
▼ Online Statistics: An Interactive Multimedia Course of Study at http:// onlinestatbook.com/
▼ Rice Virtual Lab in Statistics at http:// onlinestatbook.com/rvls.html
▼ Research Methods Knowledgebase at http://www.socialresarchmethods.net/kb/ index.php

▼ National Library of Medicine: National Information Center on Health Services Research and Health Care Technology at http://www.nlm.nih.gov/nichsr/outreach .html

USING STATISTICAL SOFTWARE

Simple **descriptive data analysis** can be completed using a spreadsheet. The first step in any data analysis is to put data in the correct format. Enter data on the row with variable labels in the columns. Data that are categorical should be coded with numbers. For example, gender is male or female, but statistical programs only understand numbers. Change the word "female" into the number "0" and "male" into "1." Make a **codebook** to remember what the numbers mean. The next step is to create or insert **formulas** into the spreadsheet. Fortunately, spreadsheets have built-in formulas for many statistical procedures such as mean, median, standard deviation, variance, and correlation. Users can select a cell on the spreadsheet and insert a formula using the "Insert" menu and clicking "Function." A formula is added by typing the name of the statistical procedure or selecting a category of formula using the drop-down menu. If the category "Statistical" is chosen, a list of statistical formulas is displayed. Users can scroll down until the desired formula is shown. Finally, the numbers that are to be used in the statistical formula are defined by adding them to the "**argument.**" This is accomplished by clicking the icon inside the number field. The window minimizes, and the user can select the numbers that are needed. Once the formula is inserted and the arguments are defined, the result of the statistical procedure is displayed.

Spreadsheets also provide graphical presentation of data. As described in Chapter 9, charts can be easily created using the chart wizard. Besides pie, bar, and line charts, scatter charts are used to show relationships between two pieces of data.

Even though spreadsheets can be used to calculate many descriptive statistics, data analysis can be more efficient if a program

(http://dataferrett.census.gov/). A video and tutorial are provided on the Web site to guide users. DataFerrett is an application that must be downloaded and installed in a local computer. Once installed, users can access public **microdata** (individual responses – not aggregated) from various federal agencies.

Another useful site for health information on the Internet is the **Agency for Healthcare Research and Quality** (AHRQ) at http://www.ahrq.gov/data. The AHRQ also provides tools (software downloads), evaluation toolkits, and databases for conducting research. Nurses can use tools to mine for data in several national initiatives (see list below). In addition, nurses can find research on quality, access, cost, and information technology at the AHRQ site. Research findings are synthesized or provided in fact sheets for easy reading.

▼ Medical Expenditure Panel Survey (MEPS)
▼ Healthcare Cost and Utilization Project (HCUP)

▼ HIV and AIDS Costs and Use
▼ Safety Net Monitoring Initiative

The **Centers for Medicare and Medicaid Services** (CMS) provide access to research, statistics, data, and systems at its site http://www.cms.hhs.gov/home/rsds.asp. Nurses can locate information on patient satisfaction, outcomes of care, and cost. Findings from the newly required Hospitals Consumer Assessment of Health Providers and Systems (H-CAHPS) are available for review and comparison.

No discussion of research on the Internet would be complete without looking at the National Institute of Nursing Research (NINR) located at http://www.ninr.nih.gov/. Publications from the NINR provide the latest scientific evidence on clinical topics. Monthly summaries of research are made available at http://www.medscape.com/index/section_1221_0. Other Internet sites where useful health statistics can be found are provided in Table 25-1.

TABLE 25-1 ● *Helpful Internet Sites to Find Health Statistics*	
Name of Internet Source	**URL**
Agency for Healthcare Research and Quality	http://www.ahrq.gov/data/
Behavioral Risk Factor Surveillance System (CDC)	http://apps.nccd.cdc.gov/brfss/
Bureau of Labor Statistics	http://www.bls.gov/bls/safety.htm
Centers for Medicare and Medicaid Services	http://www.cms.hhs.gov/home/rsds.asp
Department of Health and Human Services Gateway to Data and Statistics	http://www.hhs-stat.net/
FedStats	http://www.fedstats.gov/
FirstGov	http://www.usa.gov/
Health Insurance Information from the Census Bureau	http://www.census.gov/hhes/www/hlthins/hlthins.html and http://www.census.gov/hhes/www/hlthins/cps.html
Health Resources and Services Administration Geospatial Data Warehouse	http://datawarehouse.hrsa.gov/
Healthy People 2010	http://www.healthypeople.gov/Data/
Morbidity and Mortality Weekly Report	http://www.cdc.gov/mmwr/weekcvol.html
National Cancer Institute	http://www.cancer.gov/statistics/finding
National Center for Health Statistics	http://www.cdc.gov/nchs/express.htm
National Program of Cancer Registries	http://www.cdc.gov/cancer/npcr/
Substance Abuse and Mental Health Services Administration: National Outcome Measures	http://www.nationaloutcomemeasures.samhsa.gov/outcome/sa_pre.asp
National Vital Statistics Survey	http://www.cdc.gov/nchs/nvss.htm
Web-Based Injury Statistics Query and Reporting System (WISQARS)	http://www.cdc.gov/ncipc/wisqars/

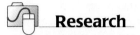 **Research**

RESEARCH UTILIZATION IN NURSING

Research utilization is critical to the advancement of nursing care and patient outcomes. The consequences of failing to apply research in clinical practice can be harmful to patients. For example, when deaths from Sudden Infant Death Syndrome (SIDS) were noticed in the 1970s, it took over 20 years to change the practice of positioning babies during sleep to prevent SIDS (Fredriksen, 2006). Even after the American Academy of Pediatrics made the recommendation in 1992 for babies to sleep supine, half of maternal-child nurses did not change the practice of positioning babies (Moos, 2006). It is the responsibility of every nurse to keep current in practice by using research evidence. There are several ways to stay current: read research literature in the specialty area, subscribe to clinical practice journals, attend professional meetings, and read source documents for new guidelines.

There are other reasons for the failure of clinicians to use research findings to change clinical practice. The first is that research is published in journals to which clinicians might not subscribe. Second, studies with important findings may not be replicated. Single studies are not usually the basis for changing practice. Third, when multiple studies are conducted on a topic, the methods may be so disparate that combining findings into an **integrative review** or **meta-analysis** may not be possible. Stronger evidence is built through replication and synthesis of findings to change practice. A good example of the strength of a meta-analysis to change practice is the study of low-dose warfarin as prophylaxis for central venous catheter in patients with cancer (Rawson & Newburn-Cook, 2007). The researchers located randomized control trials by searching Medline, Embase, Cancerlit, CINAHL, and the Cochran Library. After conducting a meta-analysis procedure, the researchers reported that low-dose warfarin failed to prevent thrombus formation in central venous catheters and was associated with adverse patient outcomes. This study provides clear evidence used to change clinical practice.

The skills needed to find research reports, read, and critique them for use in practice begin in a nurse's basic educational program. Faculty in nursing education programs face challenges when introducing evidence-based practice to nursing students. Morgan, Fogel, Hicks, Wright, and Tyler (2007) reported their experiences of teaching students how to search databases for quantitative research associated with health disparity. They reported that undergraduate students need practice and positive reinforcement to improve their health information literacy skills to prepare for the workplace. Students who practice should be able to overcome the challenges of finding and using research in clinical practice. Table 25-2 provides some learning strategies.

Even though research utilization is clearly important to keep clinical practice safe, there is evidence that nurses in all practice specialties fail to use research. In a recent study, McCloskey (2008) found that nurses report having little access to research findings in their work settings, state that little research is conducted in their clinical areas, and believe that colleagues do not discuss research findings. McCloskey analyzed responses by education (Associates, Bachelors, Masters), years of experience, and roles in the healthcare setting (management, advanced practice, and staff nurse). Nurses with a higher educational preparation and those in management or advanced practice roles reported using research findings more than that by staff nurses and those with an associate degree in nursing. Years of clinical experience were not related to utilization of research findings in changing clinical practice. This research report shows the need for leaders in the healthcare to support, recognize, and reward nurses who use research in clinical practice. Moreover, leaders must develop processes whereby patient outcomes are always viewed through the lens of research literature to ensure that opportunities to implement best practices are not missed. Not only does this benefit patient safety, but it

TABLE 25-3 • Research Studies on CDSS

Authors	Function of CDSS	Outcome	Improvement
Lee & Bakken (2007)	Diagnosis and management of adult obesity	Adherence to clinical practice guideline	No
Farion et al. (2008)	Diagnosis of acute abdomen	Comparison of accuracy of CDSS and physician to recommend correct triage plan	No
Sintchenko, Iredell, Gilbert, & Coiera (2005)	Antibiotic prescribing in critical care	Patient length of stay	Yes
		Defined daily doses	Yes
		Mortality	Same
Ruland (2002)	Preference-based care planning	Nursing care plans consistent with patient preference	Yes
Kroth et al. (2006)	Documentation of erroneous patient temperature	Improvement in accurate patient temperature	Yes
Cimino (2007)	Information management at the point of care	Provider satisfaction with context-specific information.	Yes
		Provider perception of improvement in patient care	Yes
Garg et al. (2005), review of 100 studies from 1977–2003	• Systems for diagnosis • Clinical reminders for preventative care • Disease management • Drug prescribing	Improvement in provider performance	40% of studies 76% of studies 18% of studies 62% of studies
Smith, DePue, and Rini (2007), review of nine studies from 1986–2006	Diagnosis of pain Management of pain	Information for provider use	Feasibility studies— no comparisons made

most commonly used criteria for information system selection. Among the 22 research reports used in the review, 5 broad evaluation categories were found: system quality (ease of use and time savings), information quality (accuracy and completeness), user satisfaction, individual impact (work practices, shifts in responsibilities, and use of informa-

tion in work), and organizational impact (communications, collaboration, patient care, and costs). As expected, studies of information system evaluation were mostly descriptive or correlational and varied in measurements that were made, and comparisons among research studies were difficult to make.

Adoption of EMRs does not automatically improve outcomes. User support and education are necessary to successful implementation and maintenance. Nelson, Evans, Samore, and Gardner (2005) reported that education, monitoring, and performance feedback yielded a significant increase in bedside and real-time charting of medications compared with a unit where no educational intervention was implemented. Even when support and education are present, some implementations can be uneven. Ammenwerth, Mansmann, Iller, and Eichstadter (2003) reported that acceptance of an EMR was influenced by previous acceptance of the nursing process and confidence with using computers. Nurses on one implementation unit had declining acceptance scores as a result of lower confidence and impediments to work flow that were created with the EMR, whereas, nurses on other units were accepting of the new system.

Researchers who plan to study the impact of using an EMR need to build upon the research base already in place. Assessments of user satisfaction, clinical outcomes, and financial impact are the most widely studied aspects, but there is little consistency in methods or measures. This severely limits the ability to synthesize findings to determine the best practices in EMR planning, implementation, and evaluation. Nahm, Vaydia, Ho, Scharf, and Seagull (2007) suggested tools and methods to study outcomes following EMR rollout. Otieno, Toyama, Asonuma, Kanai-Pak, and Naitoh published results of a new instrument to measure nurses' perceptions on use, quality, and satisfaction with EMRs in 2007. Nurse informatics specialists should use published instruments (if validity and reliability are acceptable) and employ standardized evaluation techniques whenever possible to address the identified shortcomings in the informatics literature.

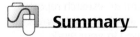 ## Summary

Research in medicine and nursing has a short history. Most scholars point to the beginning

of clinical trials in the 1940s as a significant marker. Since that time, healthcare professionals have engaged in research to find the best way to produce good patient outcomes. Personal computers are now capable of performing complex statistical analyses that were not possible before the 1990s. Data is available in healthcare settings through EMRs, administrative databases, and the Internet. These advances in technology make the need to produce evidence more urgent. Decision makers at the bedside, in board rooms, and in educational settings need to understand what effects current practice has upon outcomes to assess the need for change. The ability to provide meaningful information from discrete data is here and must be used.

Evidence to guide the practice of nursing informatics is beginning to emerge, and informatics specialists need to keep their knowledge current. Research on PDAs, computerized decision support systems, and EMRs are predominant at this point. Yet, the research methodology used in existing studies is mostly descriptive. More rigorous designs are needed to test the effectiveness of technology to improve patient care and outcomes. Nurse informatics researchers are in a good position to lead change through the use of evidence produced in research.

APPLICATIONS AND COMPETENCIES

1. Copy the data from the table below into a spreadsheet. Perform a statistical analysis to obtain descriptive statistics that summarize the data (complete using spreadsheet or BrightStat©). Remember to split the data by hospital first.
   a. Obtain the mean, median, minimum, maximum, and standard deviation for length of stay (LOS) and age.
   b. Find the frequency count of male and female patients and for type of hospital.
   c. Write a paragraph to summarize the length of stay of patients at the rural and city hospitals.
   d. Write a paragraph to describe the age of the patients at both hospitals

LOS	Age	Gender	Hospital	LOS	Age	Gender	Hospital
3	50	Male	City	4	65	Male	Rural
7	72	Female	City	5	72	Male	Rural
2	45	Male	City	2	68	Male	Rural
8	82	Female	City	7	70	Male	Rural
5	72	Female	City	4	50	Male	Rural
7	85	Male	City	6	62	Male	Rural
3	67	Male	City	5	65	Male	Rural
7	66	Male	City	8	80	Female	Rural
5	62	Female	City	8	71	Female	Rural
10	78	Female	City	5	55	Male	Rural
7	77	Male	City	5	47	Male	Rural
8	81	Male	City	10	77	Female	Rural
6	70	Male	City	10	82	Female	Rural
4	63	Female	City	9	85	Female	Rural
8	90	Male	City	8	76	Female	Rural
8	77	Male	City	7	77	Female	Rural
6	79	Female	City	10	81	Female	Rural
7	82	Female	City	8	67	Female	Rural
3	55	Male	City	7	73	Male	Rural
9	57	Male	City	6	66	Male	Rural
4	60	Male	City	10	63	Female	Rural
5	62	Male	City	9	74	Female	Rural
6	78	Male	City	10	80	Female	Rural
6	73	Female	City	6	72	Female	Rural
7	69	Male	City	6	72	Female	Rural
7	70	Female	City	7	67	Female	Rural
9	77	Female	City	3	73	Male	Rural
2	57	Male	City	4	76	Male	Rural
6	59	Male	City	7	72	Male	Rural
7	52	Male	City	10	88	Female	Rural
6	83	Female	City	3	67	Male	Rural

2. Using the same data set, determine the relationship of age and LOS in each hospital.
   a. Make a scatter chart for both hospitals
   b. Calculate the correlation of age and length at both hospitals.
   c. Write a paragraph to describe the findings.
3. Compare the LOS for males and females at both hospitals.
   a. Run a t-test to determine if there is a significant difference in mean LOS.
   b. Write a paragraph to describe the findings.
4. Search for research findings at the AHRQ located at http://www.ahrq.gov/research/

   a. Find a fact sheet regarding the health of minority women in the United States and summarize the findings.
   b. Look for research synthesis on hospital nurse staffing and quality of care. Summarize the main findings.
5. Search for current nursing informatics research in databases at your local hospital, college, or university. Find at least three research reports in your area of interest. Think about how the research could be used in your work setting.

REFERENCES

Ammenwerth, E., Mansmann, U., Iller, C., Eichstadter, R. (2003). Factors affecting and affected by user acceptance of computer-based documentation: Results of a two-year study. *Journal of the American Medical Informatics Association, 10*(1), 69–84.

Brown, P. (1993). *Florence Nightingale: The tough British campaigner who was the founder of modern nursing.* Watford, England: Exley Publications, Ltd.

Chen, T. (2003). The history of statistical thinking in medicine. In Ying Lu & Ji-Qian Fang (Eds.), *Advanced medical statistics*. World Scientific Publishing Company. Retrieved March 13, 2007 from http://www.worldscibooks.com/lifesci/etextbook/4854/4854_chap1.pdf

Cimino, J. (2007). An integrated approach to computer-based decision support at the oint of care. *Transactions of the American Clinical and Climatological Association, 188*, 273–288.

Farion, K., Michalowski, W., Rubin, S., Wilk, S., Correll, R., & Gaboury, I. (2008). Prospective evaluation of the MET-AP system providing triage plans for actue pediatric abdominal pain. *International Journal of Medical Informatics, 77,* 208–218.

Fitzpatrick, M. (2006). Using data to drive performance improvement in hospitals. *Health Management Technology, 27*(12), 10–16. Retrieved, January 10, 2008 from www.healthmgttech.com

Fredriksen, S. (2006). Tragedy, utopia and medical progress. *Journal of Medical Ethics, 32*, 450–453.

Garg, A., Adhikari, N., McDonald, H., Rosas-Arellano, M., Devereaux, P., Beyene, J., Sam, J., & Haynes, R. (2005). Effects of computerized clinical decision support systems on practicitioner performance and patient outcomes. A systematic review. *Journal of the American Medical Association, 293*(10), 1223–1238.

Gortner, S. (2000). Knowledge development in nursing: Our historical roots and future opportunities. *Nursing Outlook, 48*(2), 60–67.

Harris Interactive, Inc. (2002). European Physician Especially in Sweden. Netherlands and Denmark lead U.S. in use of electronic medical records. *Health Care News, 2*(16). Retrieved March 13, 2008 from http://www.harrisinteractive.com/news/newsletters/healthnews/HI_HealthCareNews2002Vol2_Iss16.pdf

HIMSS Analytics™ EMR adoption model. Retrieved January 17, 2008 from http://www.himssanalytics.org

Kroth, P., Dexter, P., Overhage, M., Knipe, C., Hui, S., Belsito, A., McDonald, C. (2006). A computertized decision support system improves the accuracy of temperature capture from nursing personnel at the bedside. *AMIA Annual Symposium proceedings, 444–448.*

Lee, N., & Bakken, S. (2007). Development of a prototype personal digital assistant-decision support system for the management of adult obesity. *International Journal of Medical Informatics, 765*, 281–292.

McCloskey, D. (2008). Nurses' perceptions of research utilization in a corporate health care system. *Journal of Nursing Scholarship, 40*(1), 39–45.

McCormick, K., Delaney, C., Brennan, P., Effken, J., Kendrick, K., Murphy, J., Skiba, D., Warren, J., Weaver, C., Winer, B., & Westra, B. (2007). Guideposts to the future – an agenda for nursing informatics. *Journal of the American Medical Informatics Association, 14*(1), 19–24.

Menachemi, N., Perkins, RM., van Durme D. J., & Brooks, R.J. (2006). Examining the adoption of electronic health records and personal digital assistants by family physicians in Florida. *Informatics in Primary Care, 14,* 1–9.

Moos, M. (2006). Responding to the newest evidence about SIDS. *AWHONN Lifelines, 10*(2), 163–166.

Morgan, P., Fogel, J., Hicks, P., Wright, L., & Tyler, I. (2007). Strategic enhancement of nursing students information literacy skills: Interdisciplinary perspectives. *The ABNF Journal, 18*(2), 40–45.

Nahm, E., Vaydia, V., Ho, D., Scharf, B., & Seagull, J. (2007). Outcomes assessment of clinical information system implentation: A practical guide. *Nursing Outlook, 55*(6), 282–288.

Nelson, N., Evans, R., Samore, M., & Gardner, R. (2005). Detection and prevention of medication errors using real-time bedside nurse charting. *Journal of the American Informatics Association, 12*(4), 390–397.

Otieno, O. G., Toyama, H., Asonuma, M., Kanai-Pak, M., & Naitoh, K. (2007). Nurses' views on the use, quality, and user satisfaction with electronic medical records: Questionnaire development. *Journal of Advanced Nursing, 60*(2), 209–219.

Pew Research Center. (2006). *Maturing internet news audience – Broader than deep.* Retrieved March 13, 2008 from http://people-press.org/reports/pdf/282.pdf

Rawson, K., & Newburn-Cook, C. (2007). The use of low-dose warfarin as prophylaxis for central venous catheter thrombosis in patients with cancer: A meta-analysis. *Oncology Nursing Forum, 34*(5), 1037–1043. Retrieved January 18, 2008, from CINAHL database.

Ruland, C. (2002). Handheld technology to improve patient care: Evaluating a support system for preference-based care planning at the bedside. *Journal of the American Medical Informatics Association, 92,* 192–201.

Sintchenko, V., Iredell, J., Gilbert, G. & Coiera, E. Handheld computer-based decision support r patient length of stay and antibiotic prescrib critical care. *Journal of the American Inform Association, 12*(4), 398–402.

Smith, M., DePue, J., & Rini, C., (2007). C decision-support systems for chronic in primary care. *Pain Medicine, 8*(53)

Stroud, S., Erkel, E., & Smith, C. (2007) bene personal digital assistants by nurs on size and faculty. *Journal of the Ameri* 5(5), 1–19. *Practitioners, 12*(2), 67–75.

Thakkar, M., & Davis, D. (2006) (2003). fits of EHR systems: A com ical information of hospital. *Perspectives in of the American* (3), 235–243.

Van der Miijden, A., Tange, Determinants of succe systems: A literature *Medical Informatics*

Google Book Search at http://books .google.com/ provides a way to search, browse, purchase, or borrow a book from a library on-line (Google, 2008a). Google has partnered with a number of large libraries internation-ally, including Columbia University Library, Harvard University, and Oxford University, for the liberty to scan their book collections and make that information available online. Proponents of Google Book Search state that Google is actually helping publishers and authors by making the books available to the public and that the project is assisting in the sale of books. It allows access to rare books that are otherwise unavailable and too fragile to be viewed by the public. The Google book project moves the access to books residing in a ital library to the user.

Those opposed to the project state that the Book Project is a copyright infringe- and violates fair use practice. The prob- that Google has not asked for permis- authors of copyrighted books. As a several lawsuits, including those by hors Guild, were filed against Google Journal, 2006). Google now allows owners to "opt out" of the Google by notifying them of their wishes included in the database (Bracha,

EXCEPTIO

According to are four *excep*

Book Search Help Center notes

▼ Work that it does respect the copyright law not well defie books are displayed. If Google recorded mue permission from authors or without prepaticipants, the only book infor- recorded or wrd is that similar to a card cata-

▼ Composites of oogle suggests that use of author(s). Exananalogous to visiting a book- height and weiging through the books. The and information ct has challenged copyright

▼ "Titles, names, shme time changed to cohab- familiar symbols otion of copyright law. of typographic orna coloring; mere listin Copyright Office, 20

▼ "In the case of sound ed with multiple legal perform the work pub chapter has focused on digital transmission" (t addressed in previous Office, 2006a).

chapters. Informatics ethical issues have been addressed by the professional organizations codes of ethics. As technology matures and evolves, professional codes of ethics must be updated to ensure that patient information issues are clearly addressed. Professionals are constantly being asked to balance the risks as-sociated with patient autonomy and the greater good. Use of RFID technology using the im-plantable MediChip with patient and medical record number identification is an example that was explored. Telehomecare monitoring is another example that was provided. Does tele-homecare monitoring invade the patient's privacy and/or does it provide unnecessary opportunities for security breaches?

There are strengths and weaknesses of the HIPAA law. The law was crafted with the elec-tronic transmission of patient record informa-tion for CMS billing. Because nurses and the general public have heard so much about the law, we have begun to develop misconceptions that HIPAA protects all patient information. There are concerns about the lack of adequate protection for electronic health records and personal health records. We can expect to see changes in the law to address the evolving technologies.

Because boards for professional nursing prac-tice rules vary from state to state, there is no uni-form way to license practice that crosses state lines. The NCSBN did develop the compact li-censure agreement, but the decision to have a licensure agreement is still at the state level. The implication for nursing is that the telehealth nurse may have to obtain a license to practice in each state practice area, if those states do not have an agreement. Nurses who practice across state lines must also be aware of the differen-ces in state board rules and regulations for all states in which they are licensed.

Finally, there are legal and ethical issues associated with copyright. Copyright law has evolved so that it now covers all fixed tangible media whether or not the owner has paid a fee and registered their copyright with the gov-ernment office. Copyright registration pro-vides a mechanism for the owner to sue for infringements on unauthorized use. There is still no agreement on what constitutes fair use; the answers lie in "it depends" when, where, why, and how the information is used. We are cautioned to notify the copyright owner to clarify any question about fair use. Even if the medium is not copyrighted, as is the case with government documents, we must always provide credit to the source to avoid plagiarism. Plagiarism is ethically wrong because it entails stealing the creation of others.

The legal and ethical aspects associated with informatics are very complex and constantly changing. Ignorance of the law has never provided any protection. What it means is that in addition to changes in practice, nurses must also stay abreast of the associated legal and ethical issues. It also means that to protect patient information, we must advocate for the necessary technology and policy changes.

APPLICATIONS AND COMPETENCIES

1. After reviewing the different codes of ethics discussed, select one for nursing and one other. Discuss the similarities and differences. Is nursing management of patient health information explicit enough? If not, make at least one recommendation for a change in the code.

2. Explore the Privacy Rights Clearinghouse Web site at http://www.privacyrights.org/ on the subject of data breaches. Discuss at least three recent health information breaches and identify strategies to prevent those breaches.

3. Discuss the strengths and weaknesses of HIPAA.

4. Identify one strategy that could be used to protect the privacy of the electronic health record and the personal health record. Explain how the strategy could be applied.

5. Discuss the pros and cons of the implantable patient identifier that uses RFID microchip technology.

6. Conduct a search for nurse-authored features that use Web 2.0 applications. Were you able to identify any legal or ethical issues for the content that was displayed? Discuss your findings.

7. Compare and contrast use of copyright law when writing a journal article versus the design of a personal blog space.

REFERENCES

ATA. (2007, March). *Licensure portability*. Retrieved November 24, 2008, from http://www.americantelemed .org/files/public/policy/Licensure_Portability.pdf

Beard v. City of Chicago, 299 F. Supp. 2d 872 C.F.R. (N.D. Ill., 2004).

Blanchard, J. (2004). Ethical considerations of home monitoring technology [Electronic version]. *Home Health Care Technology Report, 1*, 53, 63–64. Retrieved November 24, 2008, from http://tie.telemed.org/ articles/article.asp?path=homehealth&article= ethicsAndHomeTech_jb_hhct04.xml

Bracha, O. (2007). Standing copyright law on its head? The googlization of everything and the many faces of property. *Texas Law Review, 85*(7), 1799–1869.

Curtin, L. L. (2005). Ethics in informatics: The intersection of nursing, ethics, and information technology. *Nursing Administration Quarterly, 29*(4), 349–352.

Dobbins, W. N., Souder, E., & Smith, R. M. (2005). Living with fair use and TEACH: A quest for compliance. *Computers, Informatics, Nursing: CIN, 23*(3), 120–124.

Dunlop, L. (2006). Electronic health records: Interoperability challenges patient's right to privacy [Electronic version]. *Shidler Journal of Law, Commerce & Technology, 3*. Retrieved November 24, 2008, from http://www .lctjournal.washington.edu/Vol3/a016Dunlop.html

Gibson, C., & Bonsor, K. (n.d.). *How RFID works*. Retrieved March 6, 2008, from http://electronics.howstuffworks .com/rfid7.htm

Google. (2008a). *About Google Book Search*. Retrieved November 24, 2008, from http://books.google.com/ googlebooks/about.html

Google. (2008b). *Google Book Search: News & views*. Retrieved November 24, 2008, from http://books.google .com/googlebooks/newsviews/history.html

iHealthBeat. (2007, September 4). *VeriChip to offer free microchips to Florida Alzheimer's patients*. Retrieved November 24, 2008, from http://www.ihealthbeat.org/ articles/2007/9/4/VeriChip-To-Offer-Free-Microchips- to-Florida-Alzheimers-Patients.aspx?topicID=59

Jones, J. M. (2007, December 10). *Lobbyists debut at bottom of honesty and ethics list*. Retrieved November 24, 2008, from http://www.gallup.com/poll/103123/Lobbyists- Debut-Bottom-Honesty-Ethics-List.aspx

Morrissey, S. (2007, October 18). *Are microchips safe?* Retrieved November 24, 2008, from http://www .verichipcorp.com/news/1192716360

NCSBN. (2007, March). *Participating states in the NLC*. Retrieved November 24, 2008, from https://www.ncsbn .org/158.htm

NCSBN. (2008). *Background information about the RN and LPN/VN nurse licensure (NLC)*. Retrieved November 24, 2008, from https://www.ncsbn.org/156.htm

Privacy Rights Clearinghouse. (2008, November 20). *A chronology of data breaches*. Retrieved November 24, 2008, from http://www.privacyrights.org/ar/ ChronDataBreaches.htm#2007

Spychips.com. (2006, May 31). *Wisconsin bans forced human RFID chipping*. Retrieved November 24, 2008, from http://www.spychips.com/press-releases/verichip- wisconsin-ban.html

Swedberg, C. (2008, February 15). *Washington State House gives nod to privacy bill.* Retrieved November 24, 2008, from http://www.rfidjournal.com/article/articleview/3928/

Tech Law Journal. (2006). *District court rules in Perfect 10 v. Google.* Retrieved November 24, 2008, from http://www.techlawjournal.com/topstories/2006/20060217b.asp

Terry, N., & Francis, L. P. (2007). Ensuring the privacy and confidentiality of electronic health records [Electronic version]. *University of Illinois Law Review, 2.* Retrieved November 24, 2008, from http://lawreview.law.uiuc.edu/publications/2000s/2007/2007_2/index.html

The dark world of blogs. (2005). *Nursing Standard, 19*(50), 12–12.

The Library of Congress. (n.d.). *Timeline of copyright milestones.* Retrieved November 24, 2008, from http://www.loc.gov/teachers/copyrightmystery/text/files/

The University of Melbourne. (2008, February 14). *Academic honesty and plagiarism.* Retrieved November 24, 2008, from http://academichonesty.unimelb.edu.au/advice.html

U.S. Copyright Office. (2006a, July). *Copyright basics.* Retrieved November 24, 2008, from http://www.copyright.gov/circs/circ1.html#wci

U.S. Copyright Office. (2006b, July). *Copyright fair use.* Retrieved November 24, 2008, from http://www.copyright.gov/fls/fl102.html

USG Online Library Learning Center. (n.d.). *Plagiarism.* Retrieved November 24, 2008, from http://www.usg.edu/galileo/skills/unit08/credit08_03.phtml

VeriChip Corporation. (2006). *Physician demo.* Retrieved November 24, 2008, from http://www.verimedinfo.com/demo3/index.html

VeriChip Corporation. (n.d.). *VeriChip physician office demo.* Retrieved November 24, 2008, from http://www.verimedinfo.com/demo3/index.html

Wachter, G. (2002, July). *Malpractice and telemedicine – Telemedicine liability: The uncharted waters of medical risk.* Retrieved November 24, 2008, from http://tie.telemed.org/legal/other/malpractice0702.pdf

Zinn, J. (2007). The benefits and problems of using health care blogs [Electronic version]. *Nurse Author and Editor Newsletter, 17.* Retrieved September 29, 2007, from http://www.nurseauthoreditor.com/article.asp?id=87

Index

AACN. *See* American Association of Colleges of Nursing (AACN)

AAFP. *See* American Academy of Family Physicians (AAFP)

ABC. *See* Alternative Billing Codes (ABC)

Absolute formula, spreadsheets, 148

Accessibility factors, Web page design, 261
  color blindness, 262
  screen readers, 261–262

Active cell, spreadsheets, 146

Active RFID, 354

Active Server Page (ASP), 89

Active X, 89

Admission, discharge, and transfer (ADT) system, 349–350

Adobe Acrobat Reader®, 90

Adobe Captivate®, 398

ADSL. *See* Asymmetric digital subscriber lines (ADSL)

Adult CPR Anytime™ Personal Learning Program, 402

Advanced Research Projects Agency Network (ARPANET), 81

Advanced search, 207–208

Adware, online security and, 93

Agency for Healthcare Research and Quality (AHRQ), 417, 428

Aggregated data, 8, 161, 351

AHIC. *See* American Health Information Community (AHIC)

AHIMA. *See* American Health Information Management Association (AHIMA)

Alkaline (AAA) batteries, 218

Alliance for Nursing Informatics (ANI), 325–326

Alternative Billing Codes (ABC), 274, 275

Alt tags, 262

ALU. *See* Arithmetic logic unit (ALU)

American Academy of Family Physicians (AAFP), 331

American Association of Colleges of Nursing (AACN), 9, 186

Americans With Disabilities Act (ADA), 402

American Health Information Community (AHIC), 275–276

American Health Information Management Association (AHIMA), 322, 324–325, 349

American Medical Informatics Association (AMIA), 322, 324, 325, 341

American National Standards Institute (ANSI), 180, 272

American Nurses Association (ANA), 6, 193, 312
  CNPII, 293–294
  NIDSEC, 294
  role in standardization, 293–294
  terminologies recognized by, 294–301
    developed by nursing, 296–299
    minimum data set, 294–296
    multidiscipline standardization, 299–301

American Nursing Informatics Association (ANIA), 322

American Society for Testing and Materials (ASTM) international, 270, 271, 331

American Standard Code for Information Interchange (ASCII), 30

AMIA. *See* American Medical Informatics Association (AMIA)

ANA. *See* American Nurses Association (ANA)

ANA Web site, 195

ANGEL® Learning, 392

ANI. *See* Alliance for Nursing Informatics (ANI)

ANIA. *See* American Nursing Informatics Association (ANIA)

Animations, 396
  in professional presentation, 140

ANSI. *See* American National Standards Institute (ANSI)

Antivirus software
  against computer malware, 94–95

Anxiety, computer, 23–24

AONE Information Management and Technology Competencies, 410, 420

Apple, 216

Application tools, for efficiency
  clinical information systems, 419–420
  employee scheduling system, 419
  financial management, 410–412
  hospital survey, 417
  human resource management, 415–416
  NDNQI®, 417–418
  patient classification systems, 419
  process improvement, 412–415
  quality improvement and benchmarking, 416
  standardization of core measurements, 416–417

Area charts, 155–156

Arithmetic division, in spreadsheets, 149

Arithmetic logic unit (ALU), 29

ARPANET. *See* Advanced Research Projects Agency Network (ARPANET)

Articulate®, 398

ASCII. *See* American Standard Code for Information Interchange (ASCII)

ASP. *See* Active Server Page (ASP)

Asterisk (*), spreadsheet formula, 149

ASTM. *See* American Society for Testing and Materials

Asymmetric digital subscriber lines (ADSL), 84

Atomic level data, 178

Attachments, email, 113

Attributes, texts, 122, 137

ATutor, 392

Authentication, 368

Automatic backups, of object/document, 68

Automatic log-out, 369

Automatic numbering, in word processors, 128–130

AutoNumber, 163, 164

Avatar, defined, 400

Background layers, of professional presentation, 136

Backups, of object/document, 68–69
  automatic, 68
  purposeful, 69

Backward compatibility, 41, 113
  files, 70

Banner Health patient information, 382

Bar
  scroll, 60
  status, 60–61
  task, 62
  vertical, 60

Bar charts, 154, 155

Basic input–output system (BIOS), 28

Batteries
  handheld computers
    alkaline, 218
    rechargeable, 218
  lithium ion, 28
  nickel-based, 27–28
  self-discharging, 28

Bcc. *See* Blind carbon copies (Bcc)

Beaming, 219–220

Best-of-breed approach, to vendor selection, 348

Big-bang conversion, 344–345

Billing standardization
  ABC, 275
  DRG, 274
  HCPCS, 274–275
Biometrics, 370
Bits, 29, 30
Black hat hacker, 41
Blind carbon copies (Bcc), 110
Blog, 105
Bloom's Taxonomy of learning,
  394–395
Bluetooth, 220–221, 399
Body mass index (BMI), calculation, 149
Boolean logic, 168–169
Booting, 41
Braille reader, 262
BrightStat©, 426
British Computer Society Nursing Specialist
  Group, 325
Broadband, 83–84, 260
Bug, 41
Bullets, in word processors, 128–130
Bus, 29
Business intelligence, 423
Bytes, 30

Cache memory, 31
Capital Area Roundtable Informatics Nursing
  Group (CARING), 322
Carbon copy (Cc), 110
Cards, 29
Caret (^), spreadsheet formula, 149
CARING. *See* Capital Area Roundtable
  Informatics Nursing Group (CARING)
Case sensitivity, 22
Cause-and-effect chart, 414
Cc. *See* Carbon copy (Cc)
CCC. *See* Clinical Care Classification (CCC)
CCD. *See* Continuity of care document
CCHIT. *See* Certification Commission
  for Healthcare Information
  Technology (CCHIT)
CD. *See* Compact disk (CD)
CDA. *See* Clinical Document Architecture
CDC. *See* Centers for Disease Prevention
  and Control
Cell phones, 216
Cells, spreadsheets, 145
  address, 146
  formatting with content type, 150
  linking from other source, 151
  range for, 146
CEN. *See* Comité Européen de
  Normalisation (CEN)
Center for Nursing Advocacy
  Web site, 437
Centering, vertical, in word processing, 124
Centers for Disease Control and Prevention
  (CDC), 10
  Web site, 192
Centers for Medicare and Medicaid Services
  (CMS), 348, 428
Central processing unit (CPU), 28, 29
Certification Commission for Healthcare
  Information Technology (CCHIT),
  280, 348
Certified Professional in Healthcare
  Information and Management
  Systems (CPHIMS), 324
Change theories, informatics, 314–316
  Lewin's field theory, 315–316
  Roger's diffusion of innovation theory,
  314–315

Chaos theory, informatics, 316–317
Charts
  area, 155–156
  bar, 154, 155
  basics, 152–156
  column, 154
  creation of, 156–157
  cumulative, 154, 155
  defined, 152
  line, 155–156
  pie, 153–154
  in professional presentation, 139
  stacked, 154
CHESS. *See* Comprehensive Health
  Enhancement Support
  System (CHESS)
CHI. *See* Consolidated Health
  Informatics (CHI)
Child tables, 176, 177
Chip, 29
CINAHL. *See* Cumulative Index to Nursing
  and Allied Health Literature (CINAHL)
CiteULike, 201
Classification systems, terminologies, 293
Clicker technology, 401–402
Client/server architecture, 79
Clinical Care Classification (CCC), 297
Clinical decision support system (CDSS),
  354, 360
Clinical Document Architecture (CDA), 330
Clinical documentation, 351
Clinical information systems (CIS). *See also*
  Healthcare information systems
  ancillary systems, 350–351
  clinical documentation, 351
  computerized provider order entry
    (CPOE), 351–354
  use in medication administration, 354–355
Clinical monitors, 38
Clinical practice, handheld computers in,
  224–226
Clipboard, 66–67
Clock speed, 29
Closed-loop safe medication
  administration, 354
CNPII. *See* Committee for Nursing Practice
  Information Infrastructure (CNPII)
Cochrane, Archie, 206
Cochrane Library, 206
Code of ethics
  for informatics specialists, 437–438
  for nurses, 437
Cognitive science, informatics, 317–318
Cold boot, 41
Collective intelligence tools, 103–105
  applications, 105
  folksonomy, 105
  sharing media, 104
  Web 2.0 office suites, 104
  Wikis, 104
Color
  blindness, 262
  in professional presentation, 139–140
Column
  charts, 154
  spreadsheets, 146
    freeze, 150
  in word processors, 127
Combo box, spreadsheets, 151
Comité Européen de Normalisation
  (CEN), 273
Committee for Nursing Practice Information
  Infrastructure (CNPII), 9, 293–294

Common Currency Project, 399
Compact disk (CD), 36
Compatibility
  backward, 41
  forward, 41
Comprehensive Health Enhancement
  Support System (CHESS), 259
CompuServe, 108
Computer-aided instruction (CAI), 392
Computerized provider order entry (CPOE),
  10, 330, 348, 351–354, 364–365
Computerized quizzes and surveys, 397–398
ComputerLink project, 258
Computer-projected visuals
  lecture replacement model, 135
  lecture support model, 134–135
Computers
  anxiety, 23–24
  characteristics, 23
  connecting peripherals, 38–39
  and consumers, 256–257
  fluency, 16–17
  hard disk, 32
  in healthcare, 12–14
  malware. *See* Malware
  memory in, 30–36
  misconceptions, 22
  peripherals, 37–38
  point-of-care (POC) data entry, 27
  processing components, 27–28
  related terms, 40–41
  types of, 24–27
  viruses, online security and, 92–93
  works with data, 29–30
Conferences, themes and locations of, 325
Confidentiality, 368
  of data, 240
  of private information, 369–370
Connecting peripherals
  firewire, 38–39
  USB port, 38
Connections, 79–80
  connection to Internet, 83
  types of, 83–85
Consolidated Health Informatics (CHI),
  280–281
Consumer Assessment of Health Providers
  and Systems, 416
Consumer-Driven Healthcare, 248
Consumer informatics, 249
Consumers
  computers and, 256–257
  empowerment, 249–250
  PHR, 238
Content layers, of professional
  presentation, 136
Context-sensitive help, 65, 343
Contingency plan, 344
Continuity of care document (CCD), 331
Continuum, nursing informatics, 213
Coordinated Licensure Information System,
  439–440
Copy
  files, 73
  object, 66–67
  texts, 122
Copyright law, 441–444
Corel Office®, 46
Cost benefit, 339
Costs, healthcare informatics, 10–11
CPOE. *See* Computerized provider
  order entry
CPU. *See* Central processing unit (CPU)

Cracker, 41
Critical thinking, and information literacy, 187–88
Cross-referencing, in word processors, 130
Ctrl key, 59
Cumulative chart, 154, 155
Cumulative Index to Nursing and Allied Health Literature (CINAHL), 201, 204
Cutting, texts, 122
Cyberchondriacs, 254

Dale's Cone of Experience, 393–394
Data. *See also* Databases
  analysis and research, 424
    application of statistical procedures, 425–426
    in informatics, 430–433
    in nursing, 429–430
    use of technology, 424–425
    using web, 426–428
  atomic level data, 178
  dump, 36
  entry. *See* Data entry
  mining, 179–180
  nursing informatics, 212
  presentation, PHR, 238
  protection, spreadsheets, 151
  queries, 167–168, 173–175
    Boolean logic, 168–169
    mathematical operators, 173
    SQL, 180
  requirements, 169–171
    structured format, 170–171
  secondary use, 179
  security. *See* Data security
  sorting, 171–172
    primary, 172
    secondary, 172
    tertiary, 172
  standards, PHR, 237–238
  warehouse, 179–180
Database management system (DBMS), 178
Databases
  data entry forms, 165–166
  data in, 162
    saving, 167
  date arithmetic, 162
  DBMS, 178
  defined, 161–162
  digital. *See* Online library databases
  flat, 175
  hierarchical, 175
  KDD, 179
  network model, 175–176
  object-oriented, 178
  object/relational, 178
  paper, 162
  queries, 167–168, 173–175
    Boolean logic, 168–169
    mathematical operators, 173
    SQL for, 180
  record requirements, 169–171
  relational, 162, 176–178
  reports, 166–167
  scope creep, 176
  tables in, 162–164
    antibiotics, 163, 164
    AutoNumber, 163, 164
    lookup, 164
    master, 163, 164
    relationship, 164

Data entry
  forms, 165–166
  handheld computers, 219
  spreadsheets, 150–151
Data security
  handheld computers, 226
  PHR, 237
  spreadsheets, 151
DBMS. *See* Database management system (DBMS)
Debugging, 342
Decision support, 251
Default, 59
De-identified data, 234
Department of Health and Human Services (DHHS), 287
Designing spreadsheets, 151–152
Desire2Learn, 392
Desktop model, 27
DHHS. *See* Department of Health and Human Services (DHHS)
Diagnosis-related groups (DRG), 274
Dialog box, 62
  tabs on, 63
Dial-up connections, 260
DICOM. *See* Digital Imaging and Communications in Medicine (DICOM)
Digital divide, 251–252
Digital camera, 37
Digital Imaging and Communications in Medicine (DICOM), 272–273
Digital library. *See* Online library databases
Digital Subscriber Lines (DSL), 84
  versus cable, 84–85
Digital versatile disk (DVD), 36
Diskettes, 32–33
Disk Operating System (DOS), 45
Disk organization, files, 70–72
Disk wiping, 36
Display, handheld computers, 217–218
Docking stations, 27
Document, word processing, 121
Documentation, 288
  classification, 288–289
  labeling, 290
  standardization. *See* Terminologies, standardization
  traditional *vs.* data-driven, 289
DOS. *See* Disk Operating System (DOS)
DRG. *See* Diagnosis-related groups (DRG)
Drill and practice software, 395–396
Driver, 41
Drop-down menus, 62
DSL. *See* Digital Subscriber Lines (DSL)
DVD. *See* Digital versatile disk (DVD)

E-books, 221
ED. *See* Emergency department
Editing, text, 62–64
  erasing text, 63
  moving insertion point, 63
  word wrap, 63–64
Education (nursing), handheld computers, 222–223
E-encounters, 241
  email. *See* Email communication implementation, 243–244
EFMI. *See* European Federation for Medical Informatics (EFMI)
EHR. *See* Electronic health record; Electronic health records

EICU®, 382
E-intensive Care Units, 381–382
E-Learning
  basics, 392
  distance learning and hybrid courses, 405
  and educational programs, 402–403
  evaluation process, 403
  learner's perspective, 393–398
  pros and cons, 403–405
  resources, 398–399
  role of instructor, 403
  successful online learners, 404
  technology
    disability-compliant, 402
    multimedia, 399
    patient simulators, 401–402
    virtual reality (VR), 399–401
  time criteria continuum in, 405
  trends, 405–407
Electronic health record (EHR), 5, 233–234, 330–331. *See also* Personal health record (PHR)
Electronic health technology, issues with, 348
  adoption model, 360–361
  concept of phishing, 372
  confidentiality, 368–370
  CPOE, 364–365
  data loss, 372–373
  data security, 371–372
  decision support systems, 365
  disaster response and planning, 366–367
  interoperability standards, 363
  patient privacy, 368
  protection of healthcare data, 367–370
  quality measurement issues, 364
  radio frequency identification (RFID), 370–371
  reimbursement, 362
  return on investment (ROI), 362
  rules and regulations, 365–366
  strategic planning for, 361–362
  syndromic surveillance, 366
  system intrusions, 372
  unintended consequences, 364
  user design, 363–364
  workflow redesign, 364
Electronic mailing list, 258
Electronic medical record (EMR), 233, 330
  real-time information, 333
Electronic medication administration record (eMAR), 336, 350, 354, 361
Electronic numerical integrator and computer (ENIAC), 12
Electronic personal health record (ePHR), 330, 349. *See also* Personal health record (PHR)
Electronic records
  benefits of, 332–334
  need for, 335
Email, 107–108
  accounts, 109
    planning, 109–110
  acronyms, 112–113
  addresses, 109
  attachments, 113
  barriers to
    liability, 242
    privacy, 242
    workload, 242–243
  benefits, 241–242
  configuration, 109
  contracts, 244

Email (*continued*)
creating, 110
do's and don'ts of contents, 111
emoticons, 112–113
etiquette, 111–112
file format, 111
listserv, 115–116
managing, 113
out-of-office replies, 113–114
overview, 241
privacy issues, 111
retrieving email, remote email account, 115
sending, 110
signature, 110
software, 108–109
spam, 114–115
triage messages, 244
user name, 109
virus, online security and, 93
EMAR. *See* Electronic medication administration record
Embedding, 74–75
Emergency department (ED), 332
Emoticons, 112–113
Employee scheduling system, 419
Empowerment, consumers, 249–250
EMR. *See* Electronic medical record
Endnotes, in word processors, 127
ENIAC. *See* Electronic numerical integrator and computer
Enter key
word wrap, 64
Erasing text, 63
Ergonomics, 39–40
European Federation for Medical Informatics (EFMI), 324
Evidence-based care, 5, 211
Evidence-based nursing, 195
Evidence-based practice (EBP), 195
challenges to adoption of, 211–212
Internet resources, 195–196
Excellence in Partnerships for Community Outreach, Research on Health Disparities and Training (EXPORT), 367
Extensible Markup Language (XML), 86–87, 331
Extensible markup language (XML), 331
External reference, spreadsheets, 151
Extranet, 91, 260
Ezines, 194

Factual databases, 200
FASM. *See* Fast Analysis of Shared Multidimensional Information (FASM)
Fast Analysis of Shared Multidimensional Information (FASM), 180
FAT. *See* File allocation table (FAT)
Favorites (Bookmarks), 89–90
FDA. *See* Food drug administration
Federal efforts, healthcare informatics, 8–9
Federal Health Architecture (FHA), 281
FHA. *See* Federal Health Architecture (FHA)
Fiber optic cable, 83–84
File allocation table (FAT), 32
Filename extension, 70
Files, 69–73
backward compatibility, 70
copying/moving, 73
different files open in one program, 74
in different formats, 70
disk organization, 70–72

embedding and linking, 74–75
file extensions, 70
format
HTML, 111
RTF, 111
TXT, 111
list, viewing, 72
saving
in different formats, 70
at specific location, 73
tags, 72–73
viewing list of, 72
File Transfer Protocol (FTP), 80
Financial systems, 350
desktop computer application tools, 410–412
Find and replace tool, in word processors, 127
Fingerprint recognition, 370
Firewalls, 372
against computer malware, 94
Firewire, 38–39
Flame, 117
Flash® animation, 260
Flashcard Friends, 395
Flash drive, 34–35, 231
Flash memory, 34–35
handheld computers, 219
Flat database, 175
Flesch-Kincaid Grade Level tests, 190
Flesch Reading Ease, 190
Flickr™, 106
Flowcharting software applications, 413–414
Flow chart symbols, 338, 341
Folksonomy, 105
Fonts, 122
sans-serif, 137
serif, 137
sizes, 122
Food and Drug Administration (FDA), 10
Footers, word processing, 125
Footnotes, in word processors, 127
Forecasting, 411
Formulas, spreadsheets
absolute formula, 148
arguments, 149
calculation, 149
expression, 149
functions, 149
order of mathematical operation, 149–150
relative formula, 148
symbols, 148
Forward compatibility, 41
Forward slash (/), spreadsheet formula, 149
Freebase, 105
Freeware, 56
Freeze, spreadsheets
columns, 150
defined, 150
rows, 150
FTP. *See* File Transfer Protocol (FTP)
Function keys, 59

Gantt chart, 414
Garbage in, garbage out (GIGO) principle, 23
General systems theory, informatics, 316–317
GHz. *See* Gigahertz (GHz)
Gigahertz (GHz), 29
GIGO. *See* Garbage in, garbage out (GIGO) principle
Google Android OS, 217
Google Docs™, 104

Google Docs Spreadsheets, 147
Google Groups™, 106
Google Image Labeler, 105
Google Maps, 106
Google Print Library Project, 444
Government sponsored organizations, 192–193
Gradient background, in professional presentation, 139
Grammar checkers, in word processors, 126
Granularity, 292
Graphical user interface (GUI), 45–46, 145
Graphics, in word processors, 127
Grass Roots Media, 106–107
Groupware, 52
GUI. *See* Graphical user interface (GUI)

Hacker
black hat, 41
white hat, 41
Handheld computers, 216
battery, 218
in clinical practice, 224–226
connectivity features, 219–221
beaming, 219–220
Bluetooth, 220–221
WiFi networking, 221
data entry, 219
data security, 226
display, 217–218
in education, 222–223
future trends, 227
in library searches, 223–224
memory, 218–219
operating systems (OS), 217
in research, 226–227
synchronization, 219
uses, 221–222
vs. PCs, 217
Handout creation, 141
Hanging paragraphs, 124
Hard disk, 32
Hard drive, 33
Hard wired, 79
transmission *vs.* wireless transmission, 80
HCAHPS, 416–417
Headers, word processing, 125
Health
literacy, 255, 256
defined, 186
readability and, 190–191
skills development, 186–187
numeracy, 255, 256
portals, 251
Healthcare
agency strategic planning, 361–362
analytics. *See* Business intelligence
informatics. *See also* Informatics
costs, 10–11
description of, 6
early systems, 12–13
federal efforts, 8–9
nursing, 9–10
patient safety, 10
standardization. *See* Healthcare standardization
Healthcare Common Procedure Coding System (HCPCS), 274–275
Healthcare Effectiveness Data and Information Set (HEDIS), 250
Health Care Financing Administration (HCFA). *See* Centers for Medicare and Medicaid Services (CMS)

Healthcare Information and Management
    Systems Society (HIMSS), 322,
    324, 349
Healthcare information systems (HIS),
    334–336. *See also* Electronic health
    technology, issues with
  admission, discharge, and transfer (ADT)
      system, 349–350
  benefits of electronic record, 332–334
  clinical information system, 350–355
  EHR, 330–331
  EMR, 330
    real-time information, 333
  ePHR, 330
  financial system, 350
  in management of patient flow, 355–356
  meaning, 347
  multidisciplinary documentation, 356
  need for electronic record, 335
  point-of-care systems, 356–357
  project management, 336–337
  project requirements of, 340
  quality measures, 348, 349
  selection of vendor system, 348
  strengths of paper records, 334
  systems life cycle, 337–340
  technological competencies, 336
  weaknesses of paper records, 334–335
  workflow redesign, 335–336
Healthcare standardization
  for billing
    ABC, 275
    DRG, 274
    HCPCS, 274–275
    ICD-CM, 274
  CEN, 273
  DICOM, 272–273
  HL7, 272
  ICD, 271–272
  ICF, 272
  IHTSDO, 273
  SNOMED CT, 273
  US efforts for. *See* United States
      standardization, for healthcare
Health information and management systems
    society (HIMSS), 331
Health Information Exchange (HIE),
    277–278
Health Information Portability and
    Accountability Act (HIPAA), 36,
    367–368, 438–439
Health information technology (HIT), 5,
    348–349, 359
  need for interoperability in, 332
Health Information Technology Standards
    Panel (HITSP), 279, 280
Health Insurance Portability and
    Accountability Act (HIPAA),
    235, 271
Health Level Seven (HL7), 272, 330
HEDIS. *See* Healthcare Effectiveness Data
    and Information Set (HEDIS)
HELP. *See* Help evaluation logical processing
Help, 64–66
  context-sensitive, 65
  read the screen, 65–66
  Wizards, 65
Help evaluation logical processing (HELP), 13
Hertz, 29
Hibernation, 75
HIE. *See* Health Information Exchange (HIE)
Hierarchical database, 175

Hill-Rom Navicare® Care Traffic
    Control™, 355
HIMSS. *See* Healthcare Information and
    Management Systems Society (HIMSS)
HIMSS Analytics, 349, 360
HIPAA. *See* Health Information Portability
    and Accountability Act (HIPAA);
    Health Insurance Portability and
    Accountability Act (HIPAA)
HIS. *See* Healthcare information systems (HIS)
HIT. *See* Health information
    technology (HIT)
HL7. *See* Health Level Seven (HL7)
Hoaxes, 95–96
  damaging, 95–96
  urban legends, 95
  viruses, 95
Home monitoring, 244–245
Home page, 89
Hospital Quality Alliance (HQA), 416
Hot Potatoes™ software, 397
Hotspot, 221
HTML. *See* HyperText Markup
    Language (HTML)
HTTP. *See* Hypertext Transfer
    Protocol (HTTP)
Hugs Infant Protection System, 369
Human Patient Simulator™, 401
Human resource management, 415–416
HyperText Markup Language (HTML),
    86, 111
Hypertext Transfer Protocol (HTTP), 87

ICAHN. *See* International Corporation for
    Assigning Names and Numbers (ICAHN)
ICD. *See* International Classification of
    Disease (ICD)
ICF. *See* International Classification of
    Functioning, Disability and
    Health (ICF)
ICNP. *See* International Classification of
    Nursing Practice (ICNP)
Icons, 64
IEC. *See* International Electrical
    Commission (IEC)
IFIP. *See* International Federation for
    Information Processing (IFIP)
IHTSDO. *See* International Health
    Terminology Standards Development
    Organisation (IHTSDO)
Images
  map, 262
  in professional presentation, 138–139
IMAP. *See* Internet Mail Access
    Protocol (IMAP)
IMIA. *See* International Medical Informatics
    Association (IMIA)
Impermanence, of storage media, 36
Indenting, margins, 124
Index, 200
  subject headings, 201
  MeSH, 201, 203
Index of Learning Styles Questionnaire,
    The, 394
Individual changes, Roger's theory, 215
Infection control, computer, 40
Informatics. *See also* Nursing informatics
  benefits of
    for healthcare, 14–15
    to nursing profession, 15
  contributions of theories to, 319
  definition of, 4

educational preparation, 321–323
healthcare, 6
nursing. *See* Nursing informatics
organizations, 324–326
  multidisciplinary groups, 324–325
  nursing informatics groups, 325–326
social, 313–314
specialist
  programs for, 323–324
  role for, 318–321
tasks, categories of, 311
theories supporting, 312–318
  change theories, 314–316
  chaos theory, 317
  cognitive science, 317–318
  general systems theory, 316–317
  learning theories, 318
  nursing informatics theory, 312–313
  sociotechnical theory, 313–314
usability, 318
Information
  literacy, 17–18
    critical thinking and, 187–188
    defined, 186
    healthcare consumer, 188–189
    information technology skills, 191
    skills development, 186–187
  management tool, 11–12
  nursing informatics, 212
  systems progression, 13–14
Information services (IS), 24
Information technology skills
  current, 191
  foundational, 191
  intellectual capabilities, 191
Infrared (IR) port, 39
Insert, in word processing, 121
Insertion point
  Status bar, 60–61
  text editing, 63
Instant messaging (IM), text based, 102
Institute of Medicine (IOM), 8, 206, 332
Instructional games, 396–397
Intangibles, 362
Integrated enterprise system, 348
Integrated vendor selection
    approach, 348
Interface, 347
  terminology, 282, 292
International Classification of
    Disease (ICD)
  codes, 271–272
  ICD-1, 271
  ICD-6, 271
International Classification of Functioning,
    Disability and Health (ICF), 272
International Classification of Nursing
    Practice (ICNP), 299
International Corporation for Assigning
    Names and Numbers (ICAHN), 82
International Electrical Commission
    (IEC), 270
International Federation for Information
    Processing (IFIP), 324
International Health Terminology Standards
    Development Organisation
    (IHTSDO), 273
International Medical Informatics
    Association (IMIA), 324
International Organization for
    Standardization (ISO), 269–270
  naming conventions in, 270

Internet, 81–85, 252–253. *See also* Web sites; World Wide Web (WWW)
applications and competencies of, 97
beginning of, 81–82
broadband, 260
connections to, 83
types of, 83–85
dial-up connections, 260
evidence-based care resources on, 195–196
extranet, 260
in healthcare, 233
health information on, 191
Internet domains, 82–83
IP address, 82
ISP, 82
journals on. *See* Online journals
network neutrality, 85
nursing knowledge on, 191–192
online security, 91–97
computer malware, 92–95
hoaxes, 95–96
security pitfalls, 96–97
pharmacies, 254–255
RIA and, 85
support groups, 257–258
teleconferencing, 103
Internet Freedom Preservation Act (2008), 85
Internet Mail Access Protocol (IMAP), 109
Internet Protocol (IP), 80
address, 82
Internet service provider (ISP), 82, 108
Interoperability
in HIT, 332
standards, 363
Interoperable digital file, 235. *See also* Smart cards
Intranet, 91
Inuit®, 415
IOM. *See* Institute of medicine; Institute of Medicine (IOM)
Iomega Corporation, 33
IP. *See* Internet Protocol (IP)
iPhone™, 216
iPod®, 216
IR. *See* Infrared (IR) port
iRespond™, 401
Iris scan, 370
IS. *See* Information services (IS)
ISO. *See* International Organization for Standardization (ISO)
ISP. *See* Internet service provider (ISP)
iTunes®, 399

Java, 89
JavaScript, 89
Jaz disks, 33
Journal of Online Learning and Teaching (JOLT), 193
Journal of the American Medical Association, 288
Journals, on Internet. *See* Online journals
Justification, paragraphs, 123

KatrinaHealth Web site, 366–367
KDD. *See* Knowledge discovery in databases (KDD)
Keys, 59
ctrl, 59
function, 59
redo (Ctrl + Y), 64
tab, 64
undo (Ctrl + Z), 64
Keywords, 200

KLAS, 349
Knowledge, 213
generation, 188
quest, online library databases
advanced search, 207–208
for appropriate evidence, 207–209
critical analysis of findings, 209–211
evaluating results and effectiveness of implementation, 211
implementing findings into practice, 211
recognizing information need, 206–207
sharing, 188
Knowledge-based digital databases, 200
Knowledge discovery in databases (KDD), 179

Laboratory systems, 350–351
LAN. *See* Local Area Network (LAN)
Language translation, in word processing, 131
Learning management systems (LMS), 102
Laws, rules, and regulations
associated with telehealth, 439
copyright law, 441–444
data security breach, 438
doctrine of fair use, 441–442
HIPAA, 438–439
issues of privacy, 440–441
Web 2.0 applications, 441
Layout layers, of professional presentation, 136
Leapfrog Group, 382
Learning management system (LMS), 392, 394
Learning style, 393–394
Learning theories, informatics, 318
Lecture replacement model, 135
Lecture support model, 134–135
Lewin's field theory, informatics, 315–316
moving, 316
refreezing, 316
unfreezing, 315
Line charts, 155–156
Line spacing, in word processors, 127
Linking, 74–75
Listserv, 115–116
etiquette, 117
nursing, 116
topography, 116
Lithium ion batteries, 28
LMS. *See* Learning management systems (LMS)
Local Area Network (LAN), 78
Logical, 41
Logical Observations: Identifiers, Names, Codes (LOINC), 300–301
Login names, 109, 368–369
LOINC. *See* Logical Observations: Identifiers, Names, Codes (LOINC)
Lookup tables, in databases, 164
Lotus SmartSuite®, 46

Mac OS X, 217
Macro, in word processors, 130
Magnetic disks, 32
Magnetic resonance imaging (MRI), 333
Magnetic storage, 32
Mail merge, in word processors, 128
Mainframes, 26
Malware, 92–94
adware, 93
computer viruses, 92–93
phishing and pharming, 92
protection against, 94–95
antivirus software, 94–95
firewalls, 94
spyware, 93–94

Mapping, 292–293
MAR. *See* Medication administration record
Margins, in word processing, 124
Markup language, 86–87
Mashup, 106
Massachusetts medical society (MMS), 331
Medical subject headings (MeSH), 201, 203
tree structure, 203
Medicare fee-for-service (FFS) providers, 368
Medication administration record (MAR), 336
Medication error reporting and prevention (MERP), 334
MEDLINE, 205–206
Memory
cache, 31
handheld computers, 218–219
flash memory, 219
RAM, 218
ROM, 218
measurement of, 31–32
random access memory, 30–31
read-only memory, 30
temporary, 30
Menu tabs, 62
MERP. *See* Medication error reporting and prevention
MeSH. *See* Medical subject headings (MeSH)
Message content analysis, 258
Meta-analysis, 206
Mice, 60
Microprocessor
process, 29
technology, PC, 26
Microsoft Excel®, 425
Microsoft 2007 Excel worksheet, 147
Microsoft Office®, 46
Microsoft Office Suite™, 55
Microsoft Project®, 415
Microsoft Vista®, 46, 50
Microsoft Windows®, 46–51
accessories and utilities in, 49
easy access, 49–50
exiting, 50
handling problems, 50–51
maximizing and minimizing, 48–49
multiple windows, 46–48
opening program in PC, 46
working with program in PC, 46
Microsoft Word 2007®, 46
Military healthcare, 381
Minicomputers, 26
Minimum data set, 294–296
NMDS, 295–296
NMMDS, 296
Minitab® Statistical Software, 425
Mission critical systems. *See* Financial systems
MMS. *See* Massachusetts Medical Society (MMS); Multimedia messaging (MMS)
Mobile devices. *See* Handheld computers
Modem, 83
Moodle, 392
Motherboard, PC systems, 28
MRI. *See* Magnetic resonance imaging
Multidisciplinary groups, informatics, 324–325
Multimedia Education Resource for Online Learning and Teaching (MERLOT), 398–399
Multimedia messaging (MMS), 102
Multitasking, 73–75
different files open in one program, 74
embedding and linking, 74–75
sleep (stand by)/hibernate, 75

NANDA. *See* North American Nursing Diagnosis Association (NANDA)

National Alliance for Health Information Technology (NAHIT), 349

National Bioterrorism Syndromic Surveillance Demonstration Program (NDP), 366

National Committee for Quality Assurance (NCQA), 250, 348

National Committee on Vital and Health Statistics (NCVHS), 271, 281

National Council of State Boards of Nursing (NCSBN), 192

National Database of Nursing Quality Indicators®, 416–418

National Database of Nursing Quality Indicators™ (NDNQI), 250

National Electronic Disease Surveillance System (NEDSS), 281, 366

National Health Information Infrastructure (NHII), 276

National Health Information Network (NHIN), 233, 332

National Information and Data Set Evaluation Center (NIDSEC), 9

National Library of Medicine (NLM), 205, 282, 300

National Work Group on Literacy and Health, 189

Nationwide Health Information Network (NHIN), 276–277
  basic elements of, 276
  benefits of, 277

Navigation bars, 262

NCVHS. *See* National Committee on Vital and Health Statistics (NCVHS)

NDNQI. *See* National Database of Nursing Quality Indicators™ (NDNQI)

NEDSS. *See* National Electronic Disease Surveillance System (NEDSS)

Needs assessment, 339–340

Networks, 78–80
  architecture, 78–79
  connections, 79–80
  databases, 175–176
  neutrality, 85
  protocols, 80

New Media Consortium and EDUCAUSE Learning Initiative qualitative research study, 407

NHII. *See* National Health Information Infrastructure (NHII)

NHIN. *See* National health information network; Nationwide Health Information Network (NHIN)

NIC. *See* Nursing Intervention Classification (NIC)

Nickel-based batteries, 27–28

NIDSEC. *See* National information and data set evaluation center; Nursing Information and Data Set Evaluation Center (NIDSEC)

NIWG. *See* Nursing Informatics Working Group (NIWG)

NLM. *See* National Library of Medicine (NLM)

NMMDS. *See* Nursing Management Minimum Data Set (NMMDS)

NOC. *See* Nursing Outcomes Classification (NOC)

Noncompliance with treatment, 188

Nonlinear presentation, of professional presentation, 140–141

North American Nursing Diagnosis Association (NANDA), 297–298

Nosology, 291

Notepad, 121

Not-for-profit organizations, 192–193

Nurse Licensure Compact (NLC), 439

Nursing informatics, 310–312
  ANA definition, 312
  cognitive science in, 7–8
  computer fluency, 16–17
  continuum, 313
  data, 312
  definitions of, 7–8
  description of, 6–7
  focus of, 7
  groups, 325–326
  information, 312–313
  information literacy, 17–18
  information technologies in, 7
  knowledge, 313
  skill set in, 17
  wisdom, 313

Nursing Informatics Working Group (NIWG), 325

Nursing Information and Data Set Evaluation Center (NIDSEC), 294

Nursing Intervention Classification (NIC), 296, 298

Nursing Management Minimum Data Set (NMMDS), 296

Nursing Outcomes Classification (NOC), 296, 298

OASIS. *See* Outcome and Assessment Information Set (OASIS)

Object-oriented databases, 178

Objects, 41
  copy, 66–67
  moving, 66–67
  selection, 66–67
  working with created, 67–69
    automatic backups, 68
    purposeful backups, 69
    saving, 67–68

Office of the National Coordinator for Health Information Technology (ONC), 275

OLAP. *See* Online Analytical Processing (OLAP)

Omaha System, 292, 296–297
  using, 302

ONC. *See* Office of the National Coordinator for Health Information Technology (ONC)

Online Analytical Processing (OLAP), 180

Online Journal for Issues in Nursing (OJIN), 193

Online journals, 193
  difficulties, 193–194
  factors affecting, 193–194
  print journal articles, 194
  scholarly articles, 194–195

Online library databases
  CINAHL, 204
  Cochrane Library, 206
  factual, 200
  guides and tutorials, 201
  knowledge-based, 200
  knowledge quest
    advanced search, 207–208
    for appropriate evidence, 207–209
    critical analysis of findings, 209–211
    evaluating results and effectiveness of implementation, 211

implementing findings into practice, 211
  recognizing information need, 206–207

MEDLINE, 205–206

personal reference managers, 200–201

PsycINFO, 206

search interface (engines) use, 203–204
  online help resources, 203
  stop words, 203, 204
  subject headings, 201

Online medical opinions, 260

Online personal videos, 106–107

Online photos, 106

Operating systems (OS), 45–46
  DOS, 45
  graphical user interfaces (GUI), 45–46
  handheld computers, 217
  Microsoft Windows®, 46–51
  Palm operating system, 45

OPSN. *See* Outcomes potentially sensitive to nursing (OPSN)

Optical disks, 36
  caring for, 37

Outcome and Assessment Information Set (OASIS), 281

Outcomes potentially sensitive to nursing (OPSN), 287

Outlook® 2007, 109

Out-of-office replies, email, 113–114

Overtype, in word processing, 121

Overtype mode, status bar, 61

Page, word processing
  breaks, 124–125
  numbers, 125
  orientation, 124
  properties, 123–124

Palm Garnet OS, 217

Paper records
  strengths of, 334
  weaknesses of, 334–335

Paragraphs, in word processing
  formatting, 123
  justification, 123

Parallel conversion, 344

Parallel port, 38

Passwords, 368–369

Pasting, texts, 122

Patient
  classification systems, 419
  portals, 251
  safety, healthcare informatics, 10

PC. *See* Personal computer (PC)

PDA. *See* Personal digital assistants (PDA)

PDF. *See* Portable Document Format (PDF)

Peer-reviewed articles, 194, 204

Peer-to-peer network, 78

Perioperative Nursing Data Set (PNDS), 299

Peripherals, computers
  clinical monitors, 38
  digital camera, 37
  scanners, 37–38

Personal computer (PC)
  formats, 27
  systems, 28

Personal digital assistant (PDA), 215.
  See also Handheld computers
  in advance practice, 226
  basics, 216
  in clinical practice, 224–226
  in education, 222–223
  history, 216
  uses, 221–222

Personal digital assistants (PDA), 27
Personal health record (PHR), 233, 234–241
  barriers to implementation, 236–238
    consumers, 238
    costs, 238
    data presentation, 238
    data security, 237
    data standards, 237–238
    unique patient identifier, 237
  benefits, 236
  computerized, 235
  practitioner instituted, 241
  self-created, 238–239
  smart cards, 239–240
Personal identification number (PIN), 238
Personal information managers (PIM), 216
Personal reference manager, 200–201
  CiteULike, 201
  for formatting search findings, 209
  Zotero, 201, 202
Pharmacy system, 351
Pharming, 114
  and phishing, 92
Phased conversion, 344
PHIN. *See* Public Health Information
  Network (PHIN)
Phishing, 114
  and pharming, 92
PHR. *See* Personal health record (PHR)
Physician Consortium for Performance
  Improvement®, 348
Physician Quality Report Initiative (PQRI), 348
Physician Self-Referral Law, 362
Piconet, 220
Picture archive and communication system
  (PACS), 351, 360
Pie charts, 153–154
Pilot conversion, 344
PIM. *See* Personal information
  managers (PIM)
PITAC. *See* President's information
  technology advisory committee
Plagiarism, 443
Plain old telephone service (POTS), 83
Plain text (TXT), 111
Plan-do-check-act (PDCA), 413
Plug-ins, 90, 261
PMBK. *See* Project Management Body of
  Knowledge
PNDS. *See* Perioperative Nursing Data
  Set (PNDS)
POC. *See* Point-of-care (POC) data entry
Podcasts, 107
Point-of-care (POC)
  data entry, 27
  systems, 356–357
POMR. *See* Problem-oriented medical record
POP3 (Post Office Protocol), 109
Portable Document Format (PDF), 90
Portals
  health, 251
  patient, 251
Positive patient identifier (PPID), 350, 354
Post Office Protocol. *See* POP3 (Post
  Office Protocol)
POTS. *See* Plain old telephone service (POTS)
PowerPoint®, 133, 141
Practitioner instituted PHR, 241
President's information technology advisory
  committee (PITAC), 5
Printing, 69
  in word processing, 124–125

Print journal articles, 194
Privacy, 368
  email communication, 242
  PHR, 239, 240
Privacy Rights Clearinghouse, 438
Problem-Oriented Medical Information
  System (PROMIS), 12
Problem-oriented medical record
  (POMR), 12
Process interoperability, 267
Professional nursing organization,
  Websites, 195
Professional presentation
  computer-projected visuals, 134–135
  PowerPoint®, compatibility, 141
  presentation, 141–142
    handout creation, 141
    storyboarding, 141
    web transfer, 142
  slide creation, 135–141
Progressive disclosure, in professional
  presentation, 140
Project goal, 338–339
Project Kickstart™, 415
Project management, 336–337
  institute, 336
Project Management Body of Knowledge
  (PMBK), 336–337
Project scope, 339
PROMIS. *See* Problem-oriented medical
  information system
Protocols, 80
  IMAP, 109
  POP3, 109
  SMTP, 109
Provider-sponsored groups, 258–259
PsycINFO, 206
Public Health Information Network (PHIN),
  281, 366
PubMed, 205–206

Quality
  of care information, 250
  measurement issue, of HIT, 364
Quattro Pro®, 425
Queries, databases, 167–168, 173–175
  Boolean logic, 168–169
  mathematical operators, 173
  SQL for, 180
QuickBase®, 415
QWERTY keyboard, 219

Radianse Reveal™ Patient Flow, 355
Radio frequency identification (RFID),
  370–371
Radio frequency identifier (RFID)-tagged
  bracelets, 354
RAM. *See* Random access memory (RAM)
Random access memory (RAM), 30–31
  handheld computers, 218
Randomized controlled trials (RCT), 210
Readability, 190–191, 239
Read-only memory (ROM), 30
  handheld computers, 218
Real Player™, 399
Real Simple Syndication. *See* RSS
Real-time information, 333
Real-time telehealth, 377
Record requirements, databases,
  169–171
Redo (Ctrl + Y) keys, 64
Referenced cell, 147–148

Reference terminology, 270, 282, 292
Regional Coordinating Center for Hurricane
  Response (RCC), 367
Regional Health Information Organizations
  (RHIO), 277–278, 332
Rehabilitation Act of 1973, 402
Reimbursement, 362, 385
Relational databases, 162, 176–178
  queries in, 177–178
  terms, 177
Relative formula, 148
Reports, databases, 166–167
Request for information (RFI), 340
Request for proposal (RFP), 340
Research practice gap, 211
Restricted license, 439
Retinal scan, 370
Retrieving, word processing documents,
  122–123
Return on investment (ROI), 339, 362
RFI. *See* Request for information
RFP. *See* Request for proposal
RHIO. *See* Regional Health Information
  Organizations (RHIO)
RIA. *See* Rich Internet Application (RIA)
Rich Internet Application (RIA), 85
Rich text file (RTF), 111
Robotics, 382–383
Roger's diffusion of innovation theory,
  informatics, 314–315
  individual changes, 315
  societal changes, 315
ROI. *See* Return on investment
ROM. *See* Read-only memory (ROM);
  Read-only memory (ROM), handheld
  computers
Row, spreadsheets, 146
  freeze, 150
RP-7 robot, 382–383
RSS feeds, 105–106
RTF. *See* Rich text file (RTF)

Sakai Project, 392
Sans-serif fonts, 137
Satellite Internet connections, 84–85
Saving
  files
    in different formats, 70
    at specific location, 73
  object/document, 67–68
  word processing documents, 122–123
Scanners, 37–38
Scholarly article, 193. *See also* Online journals
  peer review of, 194
  search engine results, 194
  vs. ezine, 194–195
  vs. Web sites, 194–195
Scope and Standards of Nursing Informatic, 312
Scope creep, database, 176
Screen readers, 261–262
Scroll bars/box, 60
  horizontal and vertical, 61
Search engine results, for journal articles, 194
Search interface (engines), 203–204
  online help resources, 203
  stop words, 203, 204
Secondary data use, 179
Secondary memory, 32
Secure web pages, 90
Security pitfalls, 96–97
Selection, object, 66–67
Self-created PHR, 238–239

Semantic interoperability, 267
Semantic Web, 107
Seminal work, 208
Senteo™, 401
Sentinel event alert, 334
Serial port, 38
Serif fonts, 137
Servers, 26
SGML. *See* Standardized Generalized Markup
 Language (SGML)
Sharable content object reference model
 (SCORM®), 397–398
Sharable Content Object Repositories for
 Education (SCORE), 403
Shareware, 56
Sharing media, 104
Short message service (SMS), 102
Sigma Theta Tau International (STTI),
 Web site, 195
SimMan®, 401
Simple Mail Transfer Protocol (SMTP), 109
Simulation-based learning (SBL), 401
Simulations, 396
Single sign-on, 369
Sketchcast, 104
Skill enhancement, in word processing, 130
Sleep option, 75
Slide creation, for professional presentation
 background layers, 136
 charts, 139
 content layers, 136
 images, 138–139
 layout layers, 136
 nonlinear presentation, 140–141
 slide views, 135–136
 speaker notes, 140
 special effects. *See* Special effects, in
  professional presentation
 tables, 139
 texts, 137–138
Slideshare, 104
SLIECP. *See* State Level Health Information
 Exchange Consensus Project (SLIECP)
Smart cards, 239–240
Smartphones. *See also* Handheld computers
 defined, 216
 history, 216
SMS. *See* Short message service (SMS)
SMTP. *See* Simple Mail Transfer
 Protocol (SMTP)
SNOMED CT. *See* Systematized
 Nomenclature of Medicine Clinical
 Terms (SNOMED CT)
Social informatics, 313–314
Societal changes, Roger's theory, 215
Sociotechnical theory, informatics, 313–314
Software application programs, 51–53
Sony® Playstation Portable, 395
Sorting data, 171–172
 primary, 172
 secondary, 172
 tertiary, 172
 in word processors, 128
Sound, in professional presentation, 139–140
Spam, 114–115
Speaker notes, in professional
 presentation, 140
Spear phishing tactics, 372
Special effects, in professional presentation
 animations, 140
 color, 139–140
 sound, 139–140

transitions, 140
 video, 140
Spell check, in word processors, 126
Spreadsheets
 automatic data entry, 150–151
 cells, 145
  active, 146
  address, 146
  formatting with content type, 150
  linking from other source, 151
  range, 146
 column, 146
  freeze, 150
 database functions, 151
 data protection/security, 151
 designing, 151–152
 formulas. *See* Formulas, spreadsheets
  freeze, 150
 row, 146
  freeze, 150
 software, 145
 uses, 147–148
 workbook, 146
 worksheet, 146–147
Spyware, online security and, 93–94
SQL. *See* Structured Query Language (SQL)
Stacked chart, 154
Stakeholder, 338
Standardized Generalized Markup Language
 (SGML), 86
Standard Register that produces
 SmartWorks®, 415
Standards
 acronyms for, 268–269
 defined, 267
 developing, 273
 for healthcare. *See* Healthcare
  standardization
 international. *See* International standards
 overview, 267–268
Stand by, 75
Stark Law, 362
Star Model of Knowledge
 Transformation©, 195
State Level Health Information Exchange
 Consensus Project (SLIECP), 278
Statistical Analysis Software (SAS®), 425
Statistical Package for Social Sciences
 (SPSS®), 424–425
Status bar, 60–61
 insertion point, 60–61
 Overtype mode, 61
Stethoscope, 22
Stop words, 203, 204
Store and forward (S&F), 377
Storyboarding, 141
Streaming, 90
 video, 399, 403
Structured Query Language (SQL), 180
StudyMate Author®, 395, 397, 398
Subject headings, 201
 MeSH, 201, 203
Sudden Infant Death Syndrome
 (SIDS), 429
Supercomputers, 26
Superusers, system, 342
Support groups, Internet, 257–258
 message content analysis, 258
 online medical opinions, 260
 provider-sponsored groups, 258–259
Symbols, flow chart, 338, 341
Synchronization, handheld computers, 219

Syndromic surveillance, 366
Systematic review, defined, 206
Systematized Nomenclature of Medical
 Clinical Terms–Reference Terminology
 (SNOMED-RT), 299–300
Systematized Nomenclature of Medicine
 Clinical Terms (SNOMED CT), 273
Systems life cycle
 healthcare information system and,
  337–345
 implementation in, 343–345
  big-bang conversion, 344–345
  parallel conversion, 344
  phased conversion, 344
  pilot conversion, 344
 initiating phase, 338–340
  project goals identification in, 338–339
  project requirements, 339–340
  project scope identification in, 339
 maintenance/evaluation, 345
 overview of, 337–338
 planning, 340–343
  system design, 342–343
  system selection, 341–342
  system testing, 342–343
  training, 343
  workflow analyses, 340
System tray, 62

Tab key, 64
Tables
 in databases, 162–164
  antibiotics, 163, 164
  AutoNumber, 163, 164
  lookup, 164
  master, 163, 164
  relationship, 164
 in professional presentation, 139
 in word processors, 127–128
Tabs
 on dialog box, 63
 menu, 62
Tags, 72–73
Tangibles, 362
Tape drive, 32
Task bar, 62
Taxonomies, 291–292
Tax Relief and Health Care Act of 2006, 348
TCP. *See* Transmission Control Protocol (TCP)
Technical interoperability, 267
Technology, Education, and Copyright
 Harmonization (TEACH) Act, 443
Technology, informatics, guiding educational
 reform (TIGER), 10
Technology neutral, 368
Technorati, 105
TechSmith® Camptasia, 398
Teleconferencing, 103
Telehealth, 377
 clinic visits, 381
 disaster healthcare, 384
 in education, 384–385
 E-intensive care units, 381–383
 issues, 385–386
 real-time, 377
 store and forward technology, 377
 telehomecare, 378–381
 telenursing, 384
 teletrauma care, 383–384
Telehomecare
 biometric garment technology, 379
 for chronic disease management, 379–381

Telehomecare (*continued*)
  pill dispensers/reminders, 379
  portable monitoring devices, 378–379
Telemedicine, 377
Telemedicine Information Exchange, 377
Telemental health, 381
Telenursing, 384
Telenursing, 377
Telephony, 102–103
Telepresence, 377
Teletrauma, 383–384
Template, 147
Temporary memory, 30
Terminologies
  concepts, 290
    granularity, 292
    taxonomies, 291–292
  lists, 293
  standardization, 293
    ANA-recognized, 294–301
    ANA role, 293–294
    benefits of, 302–303
    issues in, 301–302
Testing
  integration, 342
  regression, 342
Text
  appearance, changing, 122
  characteristics, word processors
    copying, texts, 122
    cutting, texts, 122
    fonts, 122
    pasting, texts, 122
    text appearance, 122
    text-entering modes, 121–122
  editing, 62–64
    erasing text, 63
    moving insertion point, 63
    word wrap, 63–64
  erasing, 63
  in professional presentation, 137–138
Text-entering modes, in word processors,
    121–122
Thesaurus, in word processors, 126
Thin clients, 26
Threaded messages, 116
TIGER. *See* Technology, informatics, guiding
    educational reform
Toolbars, 61
Towers model, 27
Transitions, in professional
    presentation, 140
Translation, language. *See* Language
    translation, in word processing
Transmission Control Protocol
    (TCP), 80
Trojan horse, 93, 94
Tutorials, 201, 396
TXT. *See* Plain text (TXT)
Typefaces. *See* Fonts
Typeover, in word processing, 121

UHDDS. *See* Uniform Hospital Discharge
    Data Set (UHDDS)
UMLS. *See* Unified Medical Language
    System (UMLS)
Undo (Ctrl + Z) keys, 64
Unified Medical Language System (UMLS),
    281–282
Uniform Hospital Discharge Data Set
    (UHDDS), 296
Unique patient identifier, PHR, 237

United States standardization, for healthcare
  AHIC, 275–276
  CCHIT, 280
  CHI, 280–281
  FHA, 281
  HIE, 277–278
  HITSP, 279–280
  NCVHS, 281
  NHII, 276
  NHIN, 276, 277
    benefits, 277
  OASIS, 281
  PHIN, 281
  RHIO, 277–278
  SLIECP, 278
Universal key presses, 73
Universal Resource Locator (URL), 88–89
Universal resource locator (Web address), 253
Universal serial bus (USB) port, 34, 38,
    231, 235
  and self-created PHR, 239
Urban legends, hoax, 95
URL. *See* Universal Resource Locator (URL);
    Universal resource locator
    (Web address)
U.S. Department of Health and Human
    Services (HHS), 349
Usability, web, 318
USB. *See* Universal serial bus (USB) port
User Id, 109

VA. *See* Veteran's administration
VeriChip™ Corporation, 370
VeriMed™ implantable RFID microchip,
    440–441
Versus® Information System (VIS™), 355
Vertical bar, 60
Veteran's administration (VA), 332
Videos, in professional presentation, 140
Videotext terminals, 26
Virtual private network (VPN), 91
Virtual reality (VR), 399–401
Virus hoaxes, 95
Vocera™ Communications, 356
Vodcasts, 107
Voice communication systems, 356
Voice over Internet protocol (VoIP),
    103, 356
Voice recognition, 369
VoIP. *See* Voice over Internet protocol (VoIP)
VPN. *See* Virtual private network (VPN)

WAN. *See* Wide Area Network (WAN)
Warm boot, 41
Water's Edge game, 397
Web 2.0, 103
Web 3.0, 107
Web-based information, and clients,
    253–254
Webcast, 103
Web conferencing, 103
Web cookies, 90
Webinar, 103
Web navigation, 87–89
Web 2.0 office suites, 104
Web page design
  accessibility factors, 261
    color blindness, 262
    screen readers, 261–262
  principles of, 260–261
  usability, 262–263
Web pages, secure, 90

Web sites, 260. *See also* World Wide Web
    (WWW)
  design. *See* Web page design
  government sponsored organizations,
    192–193
  health information check list, 192
  health literacy, 189
  laws, rules, and regulations, 192
  non-for-profit organizations, 192–193
  of professional nursing organization, 195
  on readability, 190
Web transfer, 142
WEP. *See* Wired Equivalent Privacy (WEP)
White hat hacker, 41, 372
Wide Area Network (WAN), 78
Wi-Fi™, 102
WiFi networking, 221
Wi-Fi Protected Access (WPA), 80
Wikipedia, 104
Wikis, 104
Windows Mail®, 108, 114
Windows Media Player®, 107
Windows® Media Player, 399
WindowsXP®, 46, 50, 53
Wired Equivalent Privacy (WEP), 80
Wireless transmission, 80
Wizards, 65
Word processing
  document, 121
  features, 126–130
  language translation, 131
  page properties, 123–124
  paragraphs. *See* Paragraphs, in word
    processing
  printing, 124–125
  retrieving, files, 122–123
  saving, files, 122–123
  skill enhancement, 130
  text characteristics. *See* Text
    characteristics, word processors
Word processors, 120
Word wrap, 63–64, 124–125
Workbook, spreadsheets, 146
Workflow
  analyses, 340
  redesign, 335–336, 364
Worksheet, spreadsheets, 146–147
World Wide Web (WWW), 85–90, 102
  cookies, 90
  extranet, 91
  favorites (bookmarks), 89–90
  FTP program and, 80
  intranet, 91
  markup languages, 86–87
  navigation, 87–89
  secure web pages, 90
  streaming, 90
  virtual private network (VPN), 91
  Web browsers, 86
  web page tools, 89–90
Worm, online security and, 93
WPA. *See* Wi-Fi Protected Access (WPA)
WWW. *See* World Wide Web (WWW)

XML. *See* Extensible markup language;
    Extensible Markup Language (XML)

YouTube, 106

Zip disks, 33
Zipping, file, 113
Zoho®, 104
Zotero, 201